SAFETY AND EFFICACY OF RADIOPHARMACEUTICALS 1987

DEVELOPMENTS IN NUCLEAR MEDICINE

Series editor Peter H. Cox

Cox, P.H. (ed.): Cholescintigraphy. 1981. ISBN 90-247-2524-0

Cox, P.H. (ed.): Progress in radiopharmacology 3. Selected Topics. 1982. ISBN 90-247-2768-5

Jonckheer, M.H. and Deconinck, F. (eds.): X-ray fluorescent scanning of the thyroid. 1983. ISBN 0-89838-561-X

Kristensen, K. and Nørbygaard, E. (eds.): Safety and efficacy of radiopharmaceuticals. 1984. ISBN 0-89838-609-8

Bossuyt, A. and Deconinck, F.: Amplitude/phase patterns in dynamic scintigraphic imaging. 1984. ISBN 0-89838-641-1

Hardeman, M.R. and Najean, Y. (eds.): Blood cells in nuclear medicine I. Cell kinetics and bio-distribution. 1984. ISBN 0-89838-653-5

Fueger, G.F. (ed.): Blood cells in nuclear medicine II. Migratory blood cells. 1984. ISBN 0-89838-654-3

Biersack, H.J. and Cox, P.H. (eds.): Radioisotope studies in cardiology. 1985. ISBN 0-89838-733-7

Cox, P.H., Limouris, G. and Woldring, M.G. (eds.): Progress in radiopharmacology 1985. 1985. ISBN 0-89838-745-0

Cox, P.H., Mather, S.J., Sampson, C.B. and Lazarus, C.R. (eds.): Progress in radiopharmacy. 1986. ISBN 0-89838-823-6

Deckart, H. and Cox, P.H. (eds.): Principles of radiopharmacology. 1987. ISBN 0-89838-774-4

Heiss, W.-D., Pawlik, G., Herholz, K. and Wienhard, K. (eds.): Clinical efficacy of positron emission tomography. 1987. ISBN 0-89838-898-8

Gerber, G.B., Métivier, H. and Smith, H. (eds.): Age-related factors in radionuclide metabolism and dosimetry. 1987. ISBN 0-89838-953-4

Kristensen, K. and Nørbygaard, E. (eds.): Safety and efficacy of radiopharmaceuticals 1987. 1987. ISBN 0-89838-986-0

Safety and efficacy of radiopharmaceuticals 1987

edited by
KNUD KRISTENSEN
ELISABETH NØRBYGAARD

The Isothope Pharmacy
The National Board of Health
Copenhagen, Denmark

1987
MARTINUS NIJHOFF PUBLISHERS
A MEMBER OF THE KLUWER ACADEMIC PUBLISHERS GROUP
DORDRECHT / BOSTON / LANCASTER

Distributors

for the United States and Canada: Kluwer Academic Publishers, P.O. Box 358, Accord Station, Hingham, MA 02018-0358, USA
for the UK and Ireland: Kluwer Academic Publishers, MTP Press Limited, Falcon House, Queen Square, Lancaster LA1 1RN, UK
for all other countries: Kluwer Academic Publishers Group, Distribution Center, P.O. Box 322, 3300 AH Dordrecht, The Netherlands

Library of Congress Cataloging in Publication Data

Safety and efficacy of radiopharmaceuticals 1987 / edited by Knud
   Kristensen and Elisabeth Nørbygaard.
        p.   cm. -- (Developments in nuclear medicine ; 14)
   Papers presented at the Third European Symposium on Radiopharmacy
and Radiopharmaceuticals, held May 1-4, 1987 in Elsinore, Denmark.
   Includes index.
   ISBN-13: 978-94-010-8016-3
   1. Radiopharmaceuticals--Safety measures--Congresses.
2. Radiopharmaceuticals--Testing--Congresesss.   I. Kristensen, Knud.
II. Nørbygaard, Elisabeth.   III. European Symposium on Radiopharmacy
and Radiopharamaceuticals (3rd : 1987 · Helsingør, Denmark)
IV. Series.
RM852.S217 1987
615.8'424--dc19   87-27318
                                                                  CIP
ISBN-13: 978-94-010-8016-3   e-ISBN-13: 978-94-009-3375-0
DOI: 10.1007/978-94-009-3375-0

Copyright

© 1987 by Martinus Nijhoff Publishers, Dordrecht.

Preface

Safety and Efficacy of Radiopharmaceuticals was established as a very important and comprehensive subject at the First European Symposium on Radiopharmacy and Radiopharmaceuticals in Denmark in 1983.

The interest in this subject has grown considerably since then due to the growing interest among national authorities to deal with radiopharmaceuticals. The introduction in recent years of nuclear medicine techniques based on radioactive labelled cells and on monoclonal antibodies has stressed the importance of a well functioning approval system for the clinical trial and use of new radiopharmaceuticals. The process of transferring the experience from the non radioactive drug field into the area of radiopharmaceuticals is still ongoing. International organisations such as the World Health Organisation is also including this into their quality assurance programme from both the radiopharmaceutical and the radiation hygiene point of view. In order to give an up-to date survey of these areas, experts were invited to prepare review papers under the following headings: Safety and Efficacy of Radiopharmaceuticals with Emphasis on Biological Products, Radiopharmacy/Radiation Hygiene, Legal Aspects of the Introduction of New Radiopharmaceuticals and some selected aspects of Good Radiopharmacy Practice.

Summaries of these review papers were presented and discussed at the Third European Symposium on Radiopharmacy and Radiopharmaceuticals, Elsinore, Denmark 1.-4. May 1987. This Meeting was organized by the Danish Society of Clinical Physiology and Nuclear Medicine under the auspicies of the European Joint Committee on Radiopharmaceuticals of European Society of Nuclear Medicine and the the Society of Nuclear Medicine, Europe. The Isotope-Pharmacy, The National Board of Health, Copenhagen, provided the secretariate for the meeting.

This book contains the full text of these review papers and it is hoped that they will be useful as reference papers for future development in this field.

The editors should like to thank all the authors for their willingness to contribute and for the meticulous care with which they all prepared the reviews.

June 1987
Elisabeth Nørbygaard
Knud Kristensen

CONTENTS

X

CONTRIBUTORS

Ernst Bachmann
The DAK-laboratory
Copenhagen, Denmark

Karl Heinz Bremer
Radiochemische Laboratorium
Hoechst AG
Frankfurt (M), FRG

Trygve Bringhammer
National Board of Health and Welfare
Uppsala, Sweden

J.F. Chatal
Centre René Gauducheau
Nantes, France

H. Bjørn Christensen
Royal Danish School of Pharmacy
Copenhagen, Denmark

Peter H. Cox
Institute of Radiotherapy
Rotterdam, The Netherlands

H.J. Danpure
MRC Cyclotron Unit
Hammersmith Hospital
London, United Kingdom

Harriet Dige-Petersen
Glostrup Hospital
Glostrup, Denmark

Klaus R. Ennow
National Institute of Radiation Hygiene
Copenhagen, Denmark

F.A. Garritsen
Interuniversity Reactor Institute
Delft, The Netherlands

Hans Hvid Hansen
Århus University Hospital
Århus, Denmark

Stuart Hesslewood
Dudley Road Hospital
Birmingham, United Kingdom

G.A. Janoki
"Frederic Joliot Curie"
National Inst. for Radiobiology and Radiohygiene
Budapest, Hungary

B. Johannsen
Humboldt University
Berlin, DDR

Per Juul
Royal Danish School of Pharmacy
Copenhagen, Denmark

A. Kanclerz
University of Alberta
Edmonton, Canada

E.E. Knaus
University of Alberta
Edmonton, Canada

M. Kremer
INSERM, Faculte de Medicine
Nantes, France

Knud Kristensen
The Isotope-Pharmacy
Copenhagen, Denmark

Colin R. Lazarus
Guy's Hospital
London, England

K. Luu
University of Alberta
Edmonton, Canada

S.J. Mather
St. Bartholemews Hospital
London, United Kingdom

Søren Mattson
University of Gothenburg
Gothenburg, Sweden

R. Neirinckx
Amersham International
Amersham, United Kingdom

Elisabeth Nørbygaard
The Isotope-Pharmacy
Copenhagen, Denmark

S. Osman
MRC Cyclotron Unit
Hammersmith Hospital
London, United Kingdom

Roger Pickett
Amersham International
Amersham, United Kingdom

Jørgen Rygaard
Copenhagen City Hospital
Copenhagen, Denmark

Erling Sundrehagen
Norsk Radiopharmasi
Oslo, Norway

J.C. Saccavini
Oris-CEA Sacley
GIF/Yvette, France

Charles Sampson
Addenbrooks Hospital
Cambridge, United Kingdom

A. Schwarz
Radiochemisches Laboratorium
Hoechst AG
Frankfurt (M) FRG

Ove Svendsen
Scantox
Lille Skensved, Denmark

John Turner
Department of Health and Social Security
London, United Kingdom

Leonard Wiebe
University of Alberta
Edmonton, Canada

Jesper Zeuthen
Novo Research Institute
Copenhagen, Denmark

Asker Aarkrog
Research laboratory RISØ
Roskilde, Denmark

PART 1

SAFETY AND EFFICACY OF RADIOPHARMACEUTICALS WITH
EMPHASIS ON BIOLOGICAL PRODUCTS

Introduction

All the development phases of a new radiopharmaceutical from its design to its clinical trial and final approval for general clinical use was reviewed in 1983 (1). Products of biological origins presents special problems.

Therefore an up date with particular emphasis on this group of radiopharmaceuticals has been made.

The two main substances labelled are monoclonal antibodies and human cells. Each of them presenting particular problems with regard to efficacy and safety evaluation. Monoclonal antibodies are apart from their present use in neoplastic diseases foreseen to have potential use in localisaton of trombus, in the diagnosis of myocardial infarction and by cardiovacular diseases. The discussion here is particularly related to the use in cancer diagnostic procedures and possible use for cancer therapy.

General aspects of the design is dealt with in chapter one. Allthough at this stage not particularly related to biological products a review of new Tc-99m radiopharmaceuticals is also included. The selection of radionuclide and labelling method is much discussed. The development of chelating agents may change the emphasis from iodine radionuclides with its obvious problems of dehalogenation and may make the use of other radionuclides than the already used Indium-111 and Tc-99m, possible. It is essential that such radionuclides are carrierfree or have a very high specific activity. Different radionuclides may have different application. Testing of radiopharmaceuticals for safety and efficacy presents many problems as useful models at present are not readely available. Immunoreactive products are bound to interfere with a biological system. Safety testing using conventional methods may therefore not be useful or relevant. The restrictions on the use of animals for experimental work does also make the search for alternative methods required. In vitro methods should be used where ever possible.

Specifications and quality control methods are for products of biological origin much more difficult to establish than for other radiopharmaceuticals. Human cells is in particular a new area for establishment of pharmaceutical specifications that should be studied. Also here different radionuclides may be useful for different purposes. Quality control requires methods not so far used in radiopharmacy illustrating how complex a field this is and how it requires cooperation between specialists from many fields to obtain useful results. As an example quality control methods for labelled cells must at present be of two types. Those very time consuming and only for specialist to perform such as Phagocytosis, Chemotaxy, Migration studies. Others give incomplete information such as labelling efficiency, clumping of cells and behaviour in patients. But these must be used in daily work to follow the technique used. This illustrate very well the necessity of using principles of good radiopharmacy practice such as validation and methods control.

Reference
Safety and Efficacy of Radiopharmaceuticals. Kristensen K, Nørbygaard E (eds) Nijhof, Hague, 1984.

1. DESIGN AND DEVELOPMENT OF RADIOPHARMACEUTICALS BASED ON MONOCLONAL ANTIBODIES

J.C. SACCAVINI, J.F. CHATAL, M. KREMER

1. INTRODUCTION

The concept to use antibodies recognizing antigens associated with tumours for imaging and therapy, has gained great interest with the development of monoclonal antibodies. Originally one believed that hybridoma technology could give monoclonal antibodies reacting specifically with a particular tumour. Today the experience shows that most of monoclonal antibodies produced are tumour associated. This suggests that some cross reactions with normal tissues exist.

With polyclonal antisera heterogenesity of the antibody population specific for the same antigen is a limiting factor in the determination of the affinity of these antibodies for the antigen. Only an estimation of the mean value is obtained. The homogenous nature of monoclonal antibodies makes the determination of several parameters of the antigen-antibody reaction possible. Hereby the affinity and determination of the number of receptor determinants per single tumour cell can be determined.

Before human use, the in vivo performance of radiopharmaceuticals must be determined in an animal model. The models provided by human tumours grown as xenografts in immune-deprived mice gives some insight into this problem.

For the application in immunoscintigraphy, the antibodies must be radiolabelled. The progress in immunochemistry makes now the labelling of monoclonal antibodies with various isotopes possible.

As the antibodies are injected in man, strict quality control of the raw material and final product is necessary to ensure the innocuousness and efficiency of the product. All these different points will be discussed in details.

2. IMMUNOLOGICAL CONSIDERATIONS

2.1 Antibody class and species

Antibodies are generally produced through mouse ascites. The problem is to know if small amounts of mouse antibodies injected to humans will be well tolerated or not. At this time with two products developed and about five hundred patients examined in Europe no immunological side effects were observed. The problem may be the immunization of the patient after repetitive injections, even when antibody fragments are used.

Using the techniques of animal immunization for mouse monoclonal antibody production, antibodies of the IgG and IgM class are generally obtained, but the larger IgM molecules are unsuitable for in vivo imaging.

2.2 Antibody affinity and avidity

The affinity and avidity of the antibody for tumour cells are important factors to know, because they contribute largely to the success of tumour localization. The binding of antibody to the tumour cell is affected by the nature of the antigenic site, its expression (cytoplasmic or on the cell membrane), its turnover as well as the affinity of the antibody for it. The ideal case is a molecule of antigen expressed on the membrane with a low turnover and where many epitopes are expressed, favourable to the bivalent binding of antibodies. These two factors, the maximal number of antibody binding sites per cell and the afficity constant are determined by the method of Scatchard (1).

Powe (2) investigated whether difference in binding reactivities to tumour cells accounts in the performance of radioimaging using antimelanoma antibodies and nude mice grafted with human melanoma tumours. He found statistically significant correlation between the monoclonal antibody affinity, the receptor density on tumour cells and the ability of antibodies to localize tumours in vivo (Fig. 1).

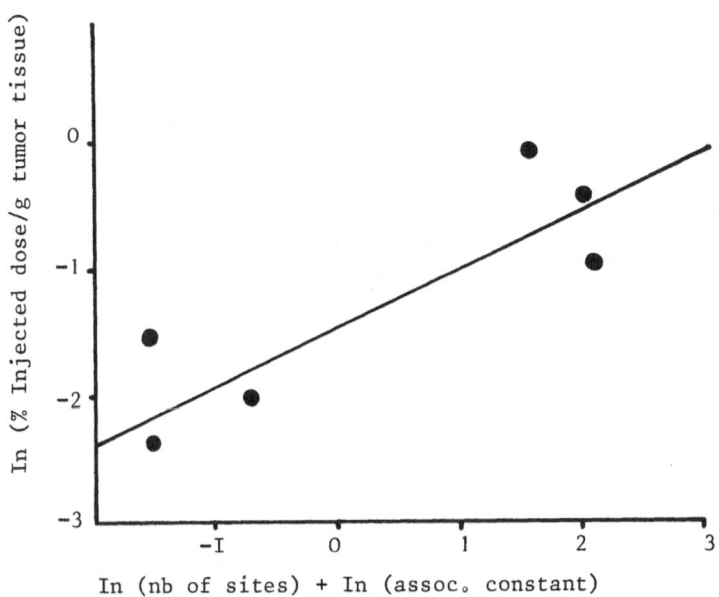

FIGURE 1. CORRELATION BETWEEN MONOCLONAL ANTIBODY AFFINITY AND RECEPTOR DENSITY ON TUMOR UPTAKE IN NUDE MICE GRAFTED WITH HU MAN MELANOMA

He found that the association constant alone appeared useful but the correlation was not significant, suggesting that both binding affinity and avidity to tumour receptors cells are together important factors in tumour localization.

3. ANTIBODY AFFINITY AND SPECIFICITY

3.1 Immunohistochemistry

In fact very few monoclonal antibodies are tumour specific. Most of the antibodies developed are tumour associated, which means they can also recognized a small number of normal tissues. It is important for each antibody to determine, by immunohistochemistry, its reactivity with a panel of normal tissues. With the two monoclonal antibodies: anti-CEA and 19.9 (directed against colorectal tumours) the immunohistochemistry performed

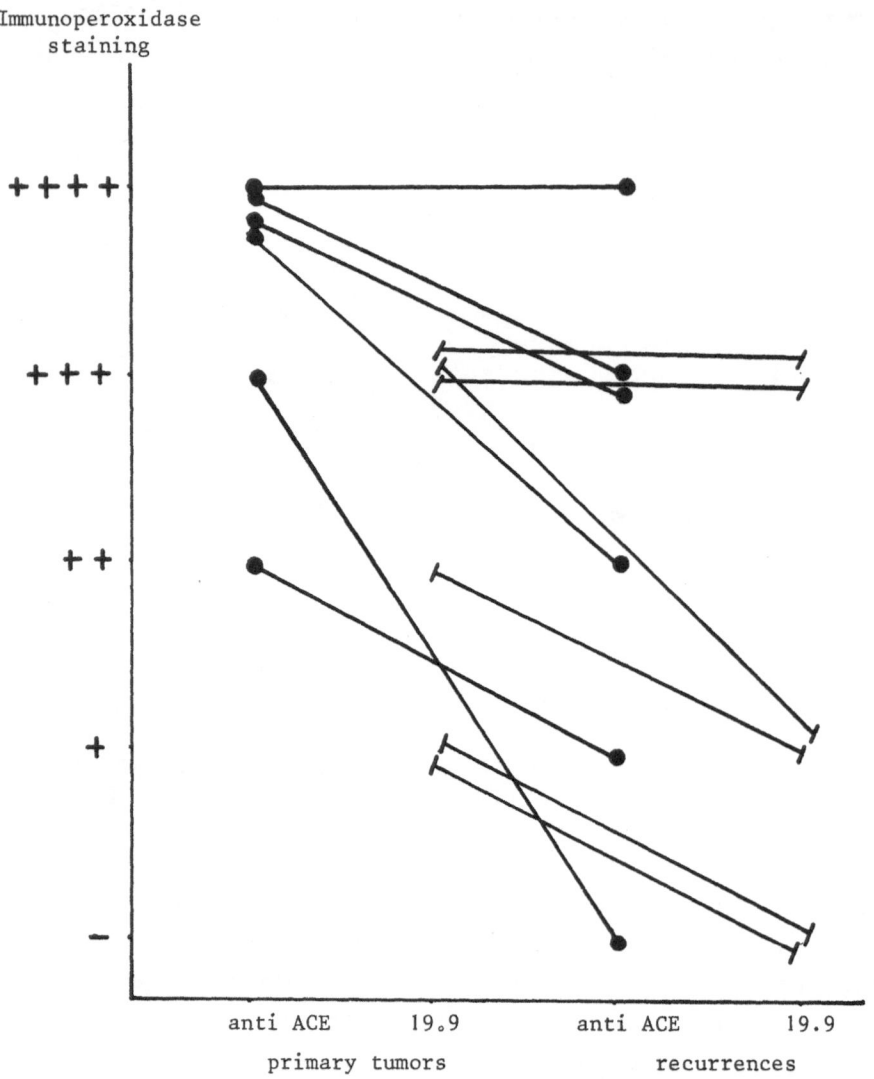

FIGURE 2. DIFFERENCES IN ANTIGENIC EXPRESSION ANTI-CEA AND 19.9 ANTIBODIES BETWEEN PRIMARY COLORECTAL TUMOURS AND METASTASES FROM THESE TUMOURS

on a large panel of normal tissues indicated a weak reactivity of the anti-CEA with normal colon epithelium and for the 19.9 a strong reactivity with normal pancreatic ducts. Despite this fact the immunoimaging of human colorectal and pancreatic tumours is possible. A reactivity of an antibody with a normal tissue does not constitute a limitation of the in vivo use of this antibody, it depends on the extent and on the intensity of the antibody reactivity.

In general antibodies recognize antigens expressed on the cells of tumours (adenocarcinomas, adenomas, etc). Antibodies are not specific for a tumoral organ, so it is of interest to test the antibody against a panel of organs presenting the same tumoral pattern. For example the B 72-3 antibody (3) was developed using a metastatic human breast tumour as the immunogen, and the antibody recognized 50% of breast tumours but also 80% of colon tumours. Today this radiolabelled antibody is mainly used for the localization of colorectal tumours. Another example is the case of the anti-HMFG$_2$(4). The antibody was developed using human milk fat globule (HMFG) as the immunogen and today it is used mainly for the detection of ovarian carcinomas.

3.2 Antibody mixtures

Tumours are very heterogeneous, they consist of a mixture of cells in various stage of the cell cycle and they may differ antigenically. We have found some differences in the antigenic expression between the primary tumour and the metastases of this tumour (see Fig. 2).

This difference may be due to quantitative variation in the expression of the antigen or may result from antigenic modulation.

Munz (5) demonstrated in an animal model that tumour localization was improved by using a mixture of monoclonal antibodies each directed against distinct colorectal tumour associated antigen. These results were confirmed clinically (6), using 19.9 and anti-CEA alone and a mixture of these two monoclonal antibodies. The sensitivity in the detection of colorectal carcinomas was increased by using the mixture. Furthermore Moyle (7) showed that a mixture of monoclonal antibodies recognizing separate epitopes results in an increase in the affinity of these antibodies for the antigen.

3.3 Animal models

Testing in experimental animal models precede any application of in vivo products in human subjects. The model of nude mice human tumours offers the possibility to test the capacity of antibodies to react and to bind selectively to the tumour using the paired labelling method described by Pressman (8). Hereby one can determine the optimal time interval between antibody infusion and external photoscanning in kinetic studies of radiolabelled antibodies. This experimental model however, has its limitations since in a mouse grafted with a human carcinoma, the only human tissue is the tumour. The necessity of the immunohistochemical study on a panel of human tissue was previously described.

The in vivo specificity of the antibody towards the tumour is determined on the animal model using the paired labelled antibody. This method consists in the injection on the same animal at the same time of the labelled tumour associated antibody and an antibody unreactive with the tumour (irrelevant antibody) labelled with a different isotope. The irrelevant antibody acts as a blood pool background. Theoretically, if both antibodies have the same element (I 131, I 125 for example) they will be handled identically, so a relative excess of the specific antibody in the tumour represents the specific interaction between the antibody and the tumour.

Using the specific 19.9 antibody and an irrelevant anti-hepatitis A_2 C_6 antibody we investigated the paired labelled antibody method on nude mice grafted with colorectal tumours. The results expressed as the localization index described by Moshakis (9) were calculated as the ratio of 19.9 uptake to anti-hepatitis uptake at the tumour or organ site divided by the ratio in the blood (see Fig. 3).

We found that the 19.9 antibody was 4 to 5 times more concentrated in the tumour compared to the anti-hepatitis antibody, but in normal tissue the distribution of the two antibodies was the same.

This approach can be also applied to some patients about to undergo surgery. After surgery the radioactivity in the biopsy specimen is measured for each radiolabelled antibody.

Larson (10), Chatal (6), reported simultaneous injection of paired labelled antibodies in patients. They found in both the melanoma and colorectal models a concentration of the specific antibody in the tumour 2 or 3 fold higher than the irrelevant antibody.

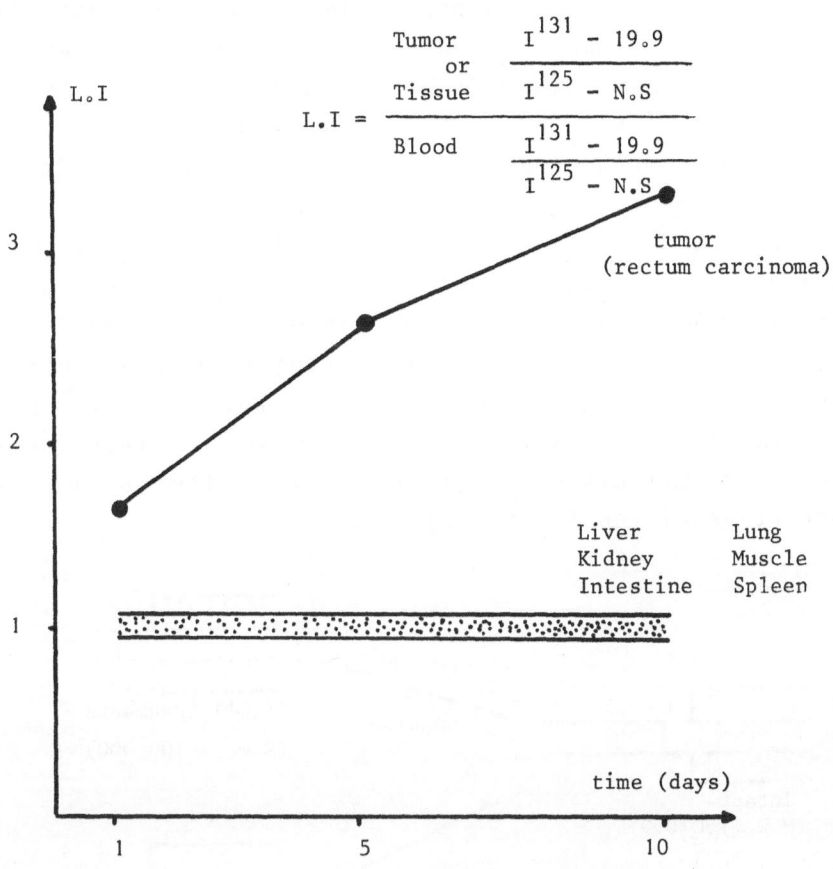

$$L.I = \frac{Tumor\ or\ Tissue}{Blood}\ \frac{\dfrac{I^{131} - 19.9}{I^{125} - N.S}}{\dfrac{I^{131} - 19.9}{I^{125} - N.S}}$$

FIGURE 3. LOCALIZATION INDICES (L.I.) OBTAINED WITH THE 19.9 ANTIBODY IN TUMOUR BEARING NUDE MICE ACCORDING TO THE PAIRED LABELLING METHOD

4. ANTIBODY SHAPE

Antibody fragments diffuse more easily into the tumour because of their smaller size, and their clearance from blood and normal tissues is faster. Thus the tumour to blood ratio may be increased as a result of these two concurrent events.

4.1 Production of antibody fragments

Antibodies may be cleaved in fragments of different size using proteolytic enzymes. Intact IgG1 and IgG2a are divided in 2 F(ab')$_2$ fragments using pepsin and 2 Fab fragments with papain (11). The IgG2b antibodies are cleaved in 2 Fab/c fragments using pepsin and the IgM in 5 F(ab')$_2$ fragments (12). Hereafter the F(ab')$_2$ fragments can be reduced in presence of a reducing agent such as beta-mercaptoethylamine in 2 F(ab') fragments (13) (see Fig. 4).

Generalley F(ab')$_2$ fragments generated after pepsin digestion retain their immunoreactivity, but with Fab or Fab' fragments it is not always the case. For example the 19.9 antibody recognizes an antigen CA 19.9 with repetitive epitopes; so bivalent binding of the antibody occurs. But with the Fab fragment a monovalent binding is only possible and this involves a decrease of the affinity constant and by the way of the immunoreactive of the short fragment.

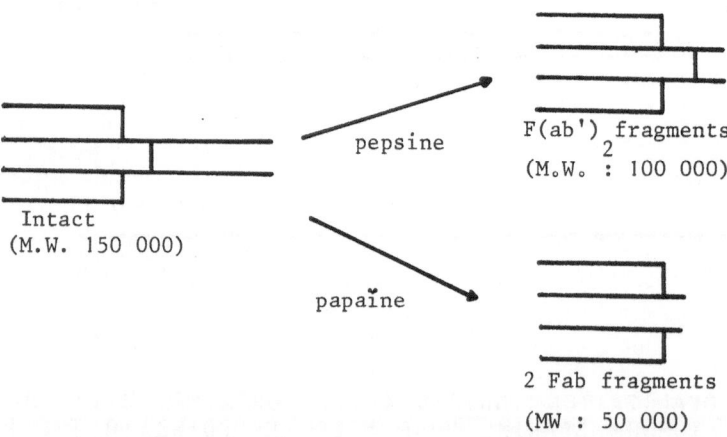

Intact
(M.W. 150 000)

pepsine

F(ab')$_2$ fragments
(M.W. : 100 000)

papaïne

2 Fab fragments
(MW : 50 000)

FIGURE 4. PRODUCTION OF ANTIBODY FRAGMENTS USING PEPSIN AND PAPAIN

4.2 Kinetics of the different fragments

Intact radiolabelled monoclonal antibodies and their fragments were injected into nude mice grafted with a colon carcinoma.

Biodistributions including tumour and normal tissues were performed and some mice were externally photoscanned. All the results obtained with $F(ab')_2$ fragments were superior to that obtained with intact immunoglobulins. But there is no concensus of opinion whether to use $F(ab')_2$ or Fab fragments.

Buchegger (14), Pimm (5) reported that Fab were superior to $F(ab')_2$ but Whal et al. (16) found that $F(ab')_2$ were superior to Fab. The difference in the results is probably due to the quality of Fab fragments produced. The results of biodistribution expressed as tumour to blood or organ ratios gave for $F(ab')_2$ and Fab fragments markedly higher values than those obtained with intact antibody and are achieved faster than with intact antibody. However this is not due to a absolute higher uptake of antibody into the tumour. In fact the percentage of injected dose in the tumour is lower with the fragments compared to the intact antibody. The conquence of this is that the earliest gamma camera tumour images are obtained with fragments. Today most of the clinical studies reported in the literature are performed with $F(ab')_2$ fragments and someones with Fab fragments. In the melanoma model with anti-P.97 Fab, Larson (10) reported a higher tumour to blood ratio compared to the intact antibody, but he noted that the absolute uptake of Fab into the tumour was lower by a factor four or five, confirming the results of biodistributions obtained in nude mice.

5. ANTIBODY LABELLING

The most commonly used isotope for labelling antibodies is iodine 131. Protein iodination is abundantly described in the literature (17,18,19) the labelling methods are simple, rapid and can be adapted to each antibody to keep its quite integral immunoreactivity. But the iodinated antibodies are unstable in vivo and the free iodine released from the antibody involves a decrease in tumour to blood ratio and this impairs the resolution of small tumours, and its high gamma-ray energy is not well adapted to gamma cameras.

In recent years the possibility to label antibodies through chelating agents has permitted the extension of studies to radiometallic nuclides such as indium and gallium and to some extent technetium. The best chelating agent is a molecule containing a chelating group that binds the nuclide tightly and a functional group for its conjugation to the proteins. The chelating agents most used are polyaminocarboxylic acids (DTPA or EDTA) which ar well known to form very strong complexes with most of the metallic ions. The DTPA can be activated in the anhydride form (20) and many EDTA derivatives were synthetized by Meares (21).

The in vivo stability of these compounds was studied with In-DTPA-antibody, the rate of indium exchange with other plasma proteins like transferrin is between 2.5-5% per day and for the In-EDTA benzyl-antibody the rate of exchange is lower (about 0.1% to 0.2% per day (22)).

For the labelling, the physical properties of indium (half-life 2.8 day, gamma ray 172 and 247 keV) make this isotope ideally suited for imaging purpose. Especially for Fab fragments, technetium can also be used despite its short half-life (6 hours).

The only problem with this kind of labelling is the presence of a high liver uptake. In patients the liver uptake with indium antibody is about 15-20% of the injected dose (23).

Some new approaches are proposed to avoid the problem of unspecific liver uptake such as the in vivo labelling using anti-chelate antibodies (24) or the use of the avidin-biotin system where the avidin-antibodies are first injected and then the biotin-DTPA-Indium-111 is injected for the in vivo labelling (25).

6. QUALITY CONTROL OF ANTIBODIES AND LABELLED ANTIBODIES

6.1 Antibody quality control

In accordance with good manufactoring practice all raw materials used must be analyzed to establish the identity, purity and in some instance the efficiency. For monoclonal antibodies the following biochemical and biological controls are to be performed:

- Purity of the protein:

The determination of the presence of proteins other than IgG is extremely important and also the presence of IgG other than those required. The protein purity can be estimated by a combination of analytical methods such as HPLC, gel filtration and ion exchange or polyacrylamide gel electrophoresis (SDS-PAGE) under reducing and non-reducing conditions with iso-electrofocusing.

- Immunoreactivity:

The immunoreactivity represents the specific activity of the antibody preparation. The immunoreactivity can be determined as the binding capacity of the antibody for a given antigen. The antibody titer defined as a total mass of antibody that binds a given mass of antigen can be determined by a radioimmunoassay. In our system we perform antibody competition with radiolabelled antibody of the precedent production to a given amount of antigen and we define for each batch of antibody the maximum binding ratio and the antibody concentration corresponding to the half maximum binding ratio (see Fig. 5).

- Biological controls

Since the antibody is intended for human injection it must be assured to be sterile, pyrogen free, presenting no abnormal toxicity and free of murine virus and DNA fragments. If the antibody is produced through mouse ascites many murine viruses must be tested (see chapter 9).

6.2 Radiolabelled antibody quality control

To assure the good performance of the radiolabelled antibody it is important to apply quality assurance tests, first to certify its radiopharmaceutical quality and also to predict its

in vivo performance. The control analysis of the final product
are: radiochemical purity, radioimmunoreactivity, sterility,
pyrogenicity and abnormal toxicity. The radiochemical purity
may be defined as the proportion of the total radioactivity
linked to the antibody. Electrophoresis for radioiodinated
antibodies and paper chromatography for radiometallic antibodies are recognized procedures to measure the radiochemical
purity. The radioimmunoreactivity represents the percent of
labelled antibody that is associated with a specific antigen.
When the antigen is known and isolated, the radioimmunoreactivity can be measured by affinity chromatography in which the
antigen is coupled to for instance cyanogen bromine activated
Sepharose. When the antigen is unknown, the radioimmunoreactivity can be measured by incubation of the labelled antibody
with a human tumour cell line (26). The pyrogenicity is measured using the L.A.L. test and toxicity testing performed only
on mice.

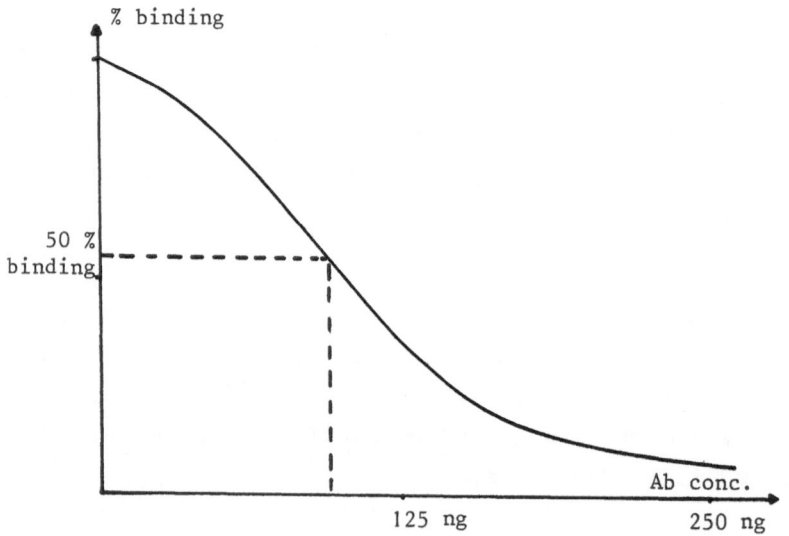

FIGURE 5. DETERMINATION OF UNLABELLED OC 125 ANTIBODY IMMUNOR
ACTIVITY

7. CONCLUSION

The perspectives of labelled antibodies in diagnostic imaging and therapy are large. In this paper we have outlined several criteria which are important to consider in the selection of monoclonal antibodies for in vivo use. The main problem is that today we generally only have available a number of tumour associated antibodies and no truly specific antibodies. Therefore the best compromise must be reached between the affinity of the antibody for tumours with the minimal antibody cross reactivity with normal tissues.

The choice of radionuclides: indium, iodine or technetium for labelling depends on the clinical application. Generally immunoscintigraphy of cancers requires late imaging times and this will exclude radionuclides with shorter half-lives.

An adequate quality control for the maintenance of antibody immunoreactivity, innocuousness and radiopharmaceutical efficiency is necessary. The quality control testing described in this paper is today recommended be different European countries.

REFERENCE
1.   Scatchard G. The attraction of proteins for small molecules and ions. Ann N Y Acad Sci 1949; 51: 660-672.
2.   Powe J, Herlyn D, Munz D et al. Radioimmunodetection of human tumour xenografts by monoclonal antibodies correlates with antibody density and affinity. Immunoscintigraphy, New York Gordon and Breach Science Publications, 1985; 139-156.
3.   Keenan A M, Colcher D, Larson D M, Schlom J. Radioimmunoscintigraphy of human colon cancer xenografts in mice with radioiodinated monoclonal antibody B 72-3. J Nucl Med 1984; 25: 1197-1203.
4.   Epenetos A, Shepherd J, Britton K, and al. Radioimmunodiagnosis of ovarian cancer using I-123 labelled tumour associated monoclonal antibodies. Cancer Detect and Prev 1984; 7: 45-49.
5.   Munz D L, Alavi A, Koprowski H, Herlyn D. Improved Radioimmunoimaging of human tumour xenografts by a mixture of monoclonal antibody $F(ab')_2$ fragments. J Nucl Med 1986; 27: 1739-1745.
6.   Chatal J F, Saccavini J C, Fumoleau P et al. Immunoscintigraphy of colon carcinoma J Nucl Med 1984; 25: 307-314.
7.   Moyle W R, Chenfang L, Corson R L et al. Quantitative explanation for increased affinity shown by mixtures of monoclonal antibodies. Mol Immunol 1983; 20: 439-452.
8.   Pressman D. Radiolabeled antibodies. Ann N Y Acad Sci 1957; 69: 644-650.

9.   Moshakis V Mc Lielhinney A J, Raghaven D et al. Monoclonal antibodies to detect human tumours: an experimental approach J Clin Pathos 1981; 34: 314-319.

10. Larson S, Brown J P, Wright P W et al. Imaging of melanoma with I 131 monoclonal antibodies. J Nucl Med 1983; 24: 123-129

11. Parham P, On the fragmentation of monoclonal IgG1, IgG2a and IgG2b from BALB/c mice. J of Immunol 1983; 2895-2902.

12. Ballou B, Reiland J, Levine G et al. Tumour localisation using $F(ab')_2$ from a monoclonal IgM antibody: Pharmacokinetics. J Nucl Med 1985; 26: 283-292.

13. Ishikawa E, Imagawa M, Hashida S et al. Enzyme labeling of antibodies and their fragments for enzyme immunoassay and immunohistochemical staining. J of Immunoass. 1983; 4 (3): 209-327.

14. Buchegger F, Hasekll Ch M, Schreger M et al. Radiolabeled fragment of monoclonal antibodies against carcinoembryonic antigen for localisation of human carcinoma grafted into nude mide. J Exp Med 1983; 158: 413-427.

15. Andrew S M, Pimm M, Perkins A C, Baldwin R W. Comparative imaging and biodistribution studies with an anti-CEA monoclonal antibody and its $F(ab')_2$ and Fab fragments in mice with colon carcinoma xenografts. Eur J Nucl Med 1986; 12: 168-175.

16. Whal R L, Parker C W, Philpott G W. Improved Radioimaging and tumour localisation with monoclonal $F(ab')_2$. J Nucl Med 1983; 24: 316-325.

17. Hunter W M, Greenwood F C. Preparation of I-131, labeled human growth hormones at high specific activity. Nature 1962; 194: 495-496.

18. Fraker P J, Speck J C. Protein and cell membrane iodinations with a sparingly soluble chloroamide 1,3,4,6 tetrachloro-3, 6 diphenyl glycoluril. Biochem. and Biophys Res Comm 1978; 80: 849-857.

19. Marchalonis J J. an ezymic method for the tracer iodination of immunoglobulins and other proteins. Biochem J 1969; 113: 299-305.

20. Hnatowich D S, Layne W W, Chilos R L et al. The preparation and labeling of DTPA-coupled albumin Int J Appl Rad Isot 1982; 33: 327-332.

21. Meares C F, Mc Call M J, Reardan D T et al. Conjugation of antibodies with bifunctional chelating agents isothiocyanate and Bromoacetamide Reagents. Methods of analysis an subsequent addition of metal ions. Analyt Biochem 1984; 142 (I): 68-78.

22. Goodwin D A, Meares C F, Mc Tigue M et al Metal decomposition rates of In 111 DTPA and EDTA conjugates of monoclonal antibodies in vivo. Nucl Med Comm 1986; 7: 831-838.

23. Hnatowich D J, Griffin T W, Koscinczyk C et al. Pharmacokinetics of an In 111 labeled monoclonal antibody in cancer patients. J Nucl Med 1985; 26: 849-858.

24. Reardan D T, Meares C F, Goodwin D A et al. Antibodies against metal chelates. Nature 1985; 316: 265-267.

25. Hnatowich D J, Altering the in-vivo behaviour of radio-
     labeled antibodies through the use of avidin-biotin. World
     federation Congress of Nuclear Medecine and Biology. 2-7
     Novembre 1986 Buenos-Aires.
26. Lindmo T, Boven E, Cuttitta F et al. Determination of the
     immunoreactive fraction of radiolabeled monoclonal anti-
     bodies by linear extrapolation to binding at infinite
     antigen excess. J of Immunol Meth 1984; 72: 77-88.

2. NEWER TECHNETIUM-99m RADIOPHARMACEUTICALS

B. JOHANNSEN

1. INTRODUCTION

Just now, we are having the semicentenary of the discovery of the element 43, later on named "technetium" (1,2). In 1937, Perrier and Segrè showed that radioactive isotopes of element 43 could be formed by neutron or deuteron bombardment of molybdenum. They investigated the activity in order to collect some information on the chemistry of 43. By the introduction of technetium-99m into nuclear medicine in the early sixties the chemistry of technetium, especially its coordination chemistry, has been promoted into new spotlight.

Since a decade or so it has generally been accepted that much more profound knowledge of basic chemistry is imperative for further progress in Tc-99m-radiotracer design. Consequently, reactions at various oxidation states of Tc have been studied and new classes of Tc complexes have been synthesized and characterized.

Referring to the previous review given in 1985 (3) this paper attempts to illustrate to what extent such a research activity has actually brought about a new generation of Tc-99m-radiotracers during the last two or three years.

2. FOCUS ON AGENTS FOR SPECT

As stated by Henry N. Wagner Jr. at the SNM meeting last year (4), advances in positron emission tomography (PET) are being translated into single-photon emission computed tomography (SPECT) - initially with iodine-123 compounds, and now with technetium-99m agents.

One consideration in this context is the relatively long acquisition time necessary to produce images of sufficient quality with conventional instrumentation. Since the biodistribution patterns of Tc-99m must not alter significantly during this interval of approximately 25 min, Tc-99m tracers designed for SPECT need not only display the desired organ uptake but remain with a fixed distribution within the target organ for a sufficiently long time. The fixation is either only a help to image initial perfusion or is itself focus of clinical study. Recent research has been dominated by the former approach that appears to be quite easier than the development of Tc-99m agents which have to be capable of binding specifically to receptors, enzymes etc., and providing information on such interactions.

Radiochemical meetings (5,6) have been evidence of the recent increase in chemical knowledge concerning technetium complexes. Significant progress in developing SPECT agents has been attained by modifying and optimizing compounds already under study since a while rather than exploiting new types of complexes. Such "optimized" agents have been moved into the realm of routine use for rCBF and myocardial perfusion imaging. The most promising candidates today are Tc-99m HM-PAO, Tc-99m N-piperidinylethyl-DADT, a new Tc-99m isonitrile called RP-30, and a mixed-ligand Tc-99m DMPE complex.

3. Tc-99m HM-PAO

There are several requirements for a radiopharmaceutical that can be used for rCBF imaging. A prerequisite is to make Tc complexes capable of crossing the intact blood-brain barrier (BBB). This can be accomplished by neutral and lipophilic complexes which have been shown to penetrate the BBB by passive diffusion. Today's Tc-99m brain perfusion imaging agents belong to the class of five-coordinate Tc(V) oxo compounds with the general structure shown in Fig. 1.

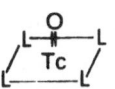

FIGURE 1. Square-pyramidal Tc(V) oxo complex: Source of rCBF agents (L=donor atoms of ligand)

The coordination environment around the Tc(V) centre is that of an approximate square pyramid with the oxo oxygen atom at the apex and four donor atoms of the ligand forming the basal plane. Thorough "carrier" studies with long-lived Tc-99 have revealed the chemistry of this type of complexes. The oxo group dominates the chemistry by its large steric requirement and inducing a large structural trans effect.

Anionic, neutral and cationic Tc(V) oxo complexes can easily be synthesized with bidentate or tetradentate O, N, S, As or P donor ligands.

In 1983, propylene amine oxime (PnAO) was shown by Volkert et al. (7,8) to form a neutral, lipophilic technetium complex that can cross the blood-brain barrier. The complex resembles Xe-133: it freely diffuses across the BBB in both directions and thus washed out quickly from the human brain after initial high brain uptake. This implies that the agent has not been suitable yet for conventionel SPECT studies. What was required next was modification of the promising backbone ligand structure (Fig. 2) with the aim of attaining a Tc complex which displays both high uptake in brain, and is retained sufficiently long to allow SPECT imaging.

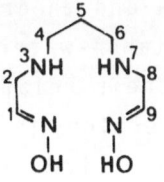

PAO

FIGURE 2. General structure of the tetradentate-N_4 bis (oxime) ligands

We can paraphrase the desired agent as "chemical micros-
phere" (9) that is trapped in its first passage through the
brain like labelled microspheres in the capillary network next
to their site of injection, and shows good gray to white matter
differentiation and little or no redistribution.

Amersham International has synthesized a series of over 100
PAO compounds in order to meet the great challenge. It was discovered that hexamethylpropyleneamine oxime (HM-PAO) (Fig. 3)
displays the most promising features.

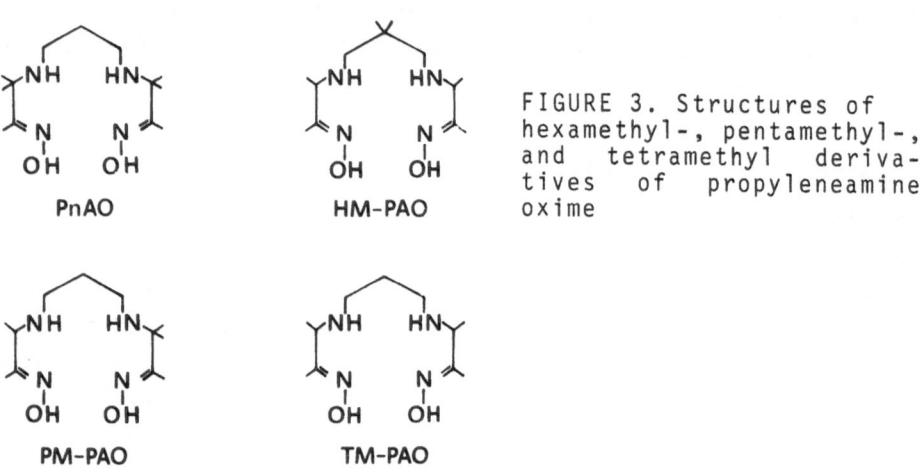

FIGURE 3. Structures of
hexamethyl-, pentamethyl-,
and tetramethyl deriva-
tives of propyleneamine
oxime

The studies also brought about some information on substitution effects on lipophilicity, permeability through BBB, and
stability of the complexes. Derivatization at the 1 and 9 position yielding alkyl-derivatives of PnAO increases the lipophilicity linearly with the length of the substituting alkyl
chains as proved by HPLC data and theoretically calculated (9).
The relationship between octanol-water partition coefficient,
log P, of the complexes and their relative brain-uptake in rats
2 min after intravenous injection is in accordance with the
concept that the ideal lipophilicity ranges between log P = 0.9
and 2.5.

Since increasing molecular weight (M.W.) and plasma protein binding both hindering or preventing transmembrane diffusion beyond threshold values parallel increasing lipophilicity or alkyl chain length, respectively, a M.W. cut-off of approximately 500 Daltons and a dramatical increase in protein binding between log P = 0.5 and 3.5 with a sharp BBB permeability deterioration occur.

In order to combine high brain uptake with prolonged retention of activity in brain, in vivo reactivity is required. As for such reactivity, with technetium complexes we encounter the problem of kinetic inertness according to Taube's definition. Ligand exchange that has been observed with technetium (V) oxo complexes of O-donor and some other ligands is unlikely to play a role in short-term biodistribution of the complexes in question. It appears reasonable to consider two solutions to the problem - reactivity of suitable pendant moiety and instability of the complexes in vivo. The latter is the case with Tc(V) oxo HM-PAO (Fig. 4) and some other derivatives as discovered by Neirinckx et al. (9,10)

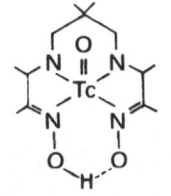

FIGURE 4. Neutral, lipophilic Tc (V) oxo complex of HM-PAO

Tc-HM-PAO

As proved by X-ray crystal structure analysis, Tc(V) in the Tc HM-PAO complex is coordinated to a single oxygen atom and four nitrogen atoms. By ring closure through hydrogen bonding of the oxime functionalities, an additional ring is formed. The trapping mechanism within the brain is thought to be caused by a conversion of this complex to a hydrophilic one, possibly by opening this hydrogen bond and subsequent rearrangement leading to stable 6-membered rings (Fig. 5).

The conversion is still subject to speculation and needs more investigation. With respect to complex stability, there is a major difference of very stable Tc-PnAO and Tc-HM-PAO.

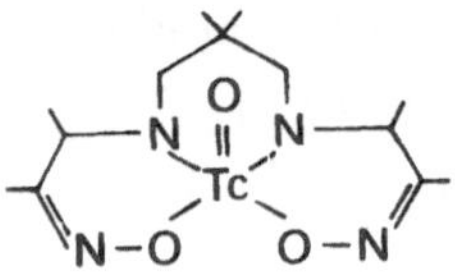

FIGURE 5. Hydrophilic, "secondary" Tc HM-PAO complex possibly formed by intracellular conversion

Demethylated derivatives such as TM-PAO and PM-PAO also form "reactive" complexes (11). Great difference has been observed between the conversation rate in vitro and in vivo. The intra-cellular conversion is much faster. Proteins are assumed to ca-talyze the re-arrangement reaction.

Following the discovery and preliminary clinical trial of Tc-99m HM-PAO as a rCBF agent, stereoisomerism of the ligand has been taken into account (12). As shown in Fig. 6, the two chiral centres at C-2 and C-8 of the ligand can give rise to meso and d,l diastereoisomers. According to animal and human studies the d,l form is superior in terms of brain retention and minimal redistribution. It is consequently now preferred in radiopharmaceutical preparation.

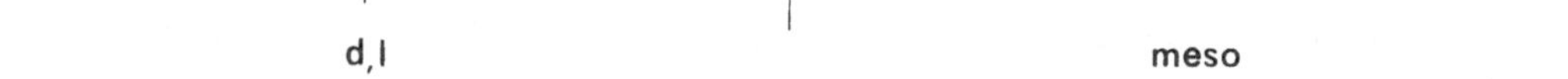

FIGURE 6. Diastereoisomers of HM PAO

Another point is the preparation of the tracer. There are problems due to the vulnerability of "no-carrier-added" Tc-99m at oxidation state +5 and the need to simplify labelling proce-dures for routine use.

Labelling of HM-PAO is performed in alkaline solution. With Sn^{2+} being the reducing agent some obstacles have to be tackled in preparing ready-to-use kits: Stannous chloride has the drawback of hydrolysis, Sn(II) tartrate is of low solubility and ligand exchange as an alternative approach starting from Tc gluconate would be too slow (13). Conversion of the lipophilic Tc-HM-PAO to a hydrophilic product also occurs in vitro. All these factors require careful optimizing of the ingredients and reaction conditions and restrict the useful life of the reconstituted agent to half an hour or so.

A multi-centre trial and clinical experience gathered up until now have highlighted Tc-99m-HM-PAO as a SPECT agent that significantly reflects the distribution of human cerebral blood flow and could have an important impact on the diagnostic efficacy and treatment of patients suffering from various cerebrovascular and neurological disorders (14 - 19). Iodine-123 iodoamphetamine can be largely replaced.

Technetium-99m HM-PAO or other neutral, lipophilic Tc-99m complexes are not brain-specific. It appears reasonable to expand their application. Because of the agent's membrane permeability, blood cells can easily be labelled with Tc-99m-HM-PAO. There are first reports on labelling of leucocytes for imaging inflammation (20,21).

The data obtained with Tc-99m rCBF agents also sustain our hope to image receptors with Tc-99m tracers provided receptor-binding complexes will be possible to develop (4).

4. N-PIPERIDINYLETHYL-DADT

Among the neutral lipophilic Tc(V) oxo complexes a different class containing a N_2S_2 backbone (Fig. 7) has been chosen by the research group at The Johns Hopkins Medical Institutions in Baltimore to develop a SPECT agent to assess cerebral blood flow (22-25).

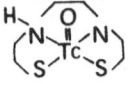

Tc(V)oxo-N_2S_2

FIGURE 7. Structure of lipophilic Tc(V) oxo complexes with tetradentate diaminodithiol (DADT) ligands

Tetradentate diaminodithiol ligands form very stable complexes which cross the blood-brain barrier. In order to combine brain uptake with retention, modified derivatives of DADT and their Tc complexes have been synthesized and tested.

The approach other than that for in vivo labile Tc-HM-PAO was based on the fact that some alkylamines accumulate in and are retained by the brain. By functionalizing hexamethyl-DADT with a pendant piperidinylethyl side chain (Fig. 8) a promising candidate was developed. When labelled with Tc-99m or Tc-99 two isomers are formed in a ratio of 4:1 with the major product showing the higher uptake in and slower clearance from brain

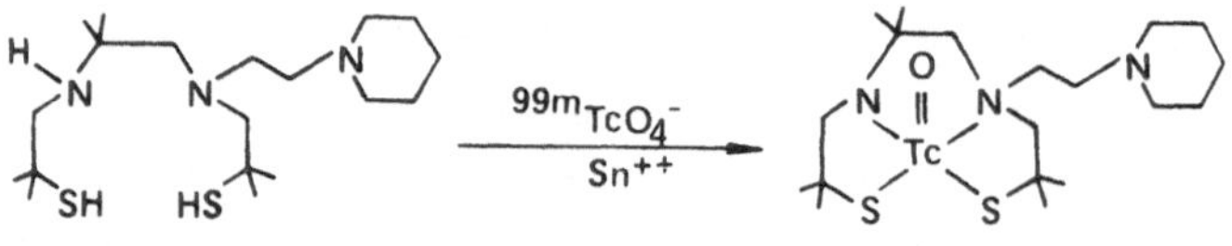

N-piperidinylethyl-DADT

FIGURE 8. Preparation of Tc(V) oxo complex (isomers) of N-piper idinylethyl-DADT

Comparison of the superior isomer with isomers of 10 other new N-aminoethyl derivatives showed that the N-piperidinyl-DADT complex had the highest uptake in mouse brain whereas retention up to two hours can be increased significantly by alteration of the amino ethyl moiety (24).

One can hypothesize that the progress achieved in designing relatively small, neutral complexes with an appropriate side-group attached to promote binding to cellular counterparts will pave the way for specific receptor-binding Tc-99m radiotracers.

Labelling of the DADT ligands has been easily performed with Tc-99m pertechnetate in the presence of reducing agents such as stannous or dithionite ions followed by HPLC or other purification. As S-protected compounds are used as precursors or storage form of the free dithiol ligands successful efforts have been made to develop a versatile synthetic route and a convenient deprotection procedure (26,27).

Both Tc-99m brain perfusion agents discussed above belong to the same type of compounds, namely neutral Tc(V) oxo complexes. Neither the Tc(V) oxidation state nor the Tc=O bond is, however, essential for passive diffusion across the BBB (28). Various neutral, lipophilic technetium compounds are being under investigation.

5. CATIONIC MIXED-LIGAND TC(III) COMPLEXES

Recent progress in the search for a Tc-99m agent to replace Tl-201 for myocardial perfusion imaging can be noticed within both the class of cationic Tc(III) complexes and Tc(I) complexes as well as in some understanding of the underlying mechanism. All the types of compounds indicated in Fig. 9 except the Tc(V) oxo complexes have been shown to exhibit myocardial uptake with both characteristic differences between the Tc(III) and Tc(I) groups and quite different suitability of their individuals for myocardial imaging in humans (29-32)

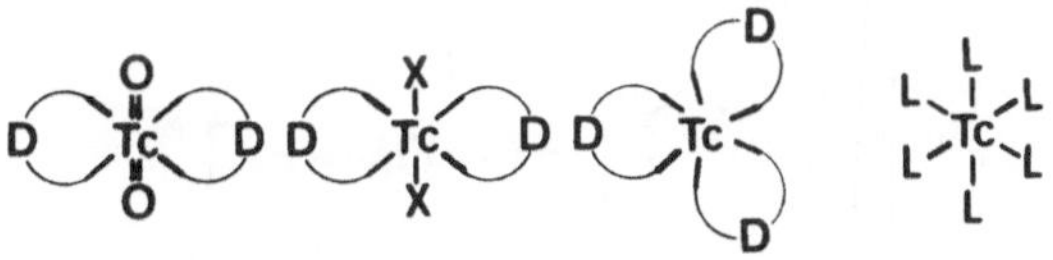

$(Tc^V O_2 D_2)^+$ $(Tc^{III} X_2 D_2)^+$ $(Tc^I D_3)^+$ $(Tc^I L_6)^+$

FIGURE 9. Types of cationic technetium complexes (D = bidentate ligand, L = monodentate ligand, X = Cl, Br or OH)

In addition, diarene complexes of technetium(I) provide a class with interesting structure-myocardial uptake relationships (33).

A disappointing feature that has emerged with Deutsch's Tc(III) DMPE agent is a high liver uptake which interfers with imaging of the cardial apex, and a very marked species dependence implying poor quality myocardial imaging in humans. Another drawback of Tc (DMPE) $_2$Cl$_2$$^+$ is the fast washout from the myocardium that is likely to occur because the cationic complex is reduced _in vivo_ to a neutral Tc(II) form (29). In order to overcome this problem two solutions appear to be at hand: An apparently minor but in fact important alteration (OH for Cl) in the DMPE complex as described by Münze et al. (34) and non-reducible Tc(III) cations based on tetradentate Schiff base ligands and monodentate phosphines as suggested by Deutsch et al. (29, 35).

As for the former approach, in studies directed to minimize the quantity of toxic DMPE and accelerate the labelling reaction by oxalic acid and mannitol, a new, in vivo stable complex has been obtained. Oxalic acid can also be replaced by aminopolycarboxylic or polyaminopolycarboxylic acids such as NTA, IDA, EDTA or DTPA. Analytical data obtained with carrier reaction scheme given in Fig. 10 where one chlorine atom and one hydroxyl group being the monodentate ligands in the Tc(III) DMPE complex.

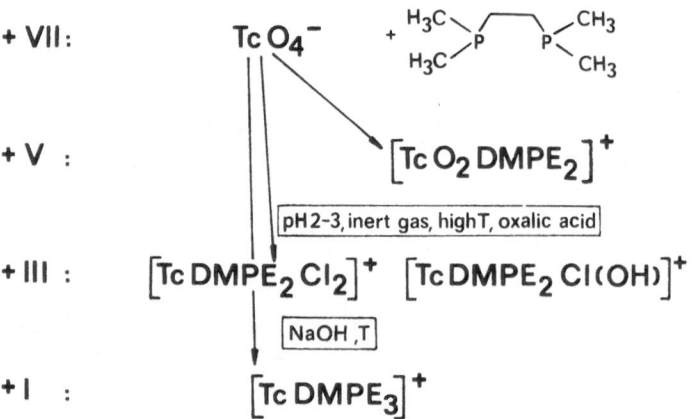

FIGURE 10. Reaction routes for the system TcO_4/DMPE

The new Tc-99m myocardial imaging agent prepared from a lyophilized kit has been evaluated in patients (36, 37).

Deutsch's search for non-reducible Tc(III) agents arose from comparative biodistribution studies of Tc(III) and the Re(III) analog DMPE complex. The data established that in-vivo-accessibility of the redox potential of the Tc(III) centre is crucial for undesired myocardial washout. In a series of Tc(III) complexes of the type $Tc^{III}LY_2^+$, where L represents a tetradentate Schiff base ligand and Y represents monodentate tertiary phosphine ligands, the effect of substituents in the ligands on the redox potential has been evaluated (38). Among the non-reducible complexes are those of the Schiff base ligand shown in Fig. 11 and trialkylphosphines.

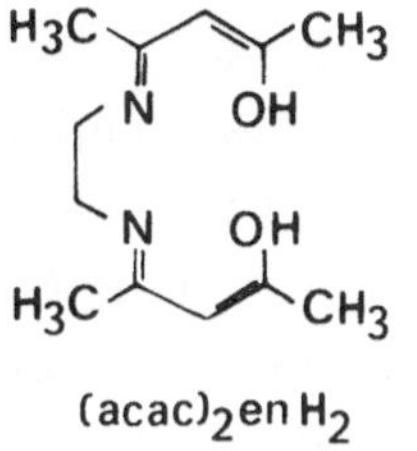

FIGURE 11. The Schiff base ligand N,N' -ethylenebis (acetyl-acetone iminato)

(acac)$_2$en H$_2$

The octahedral complex (Fig. 12) does not wash out of the myocardium.

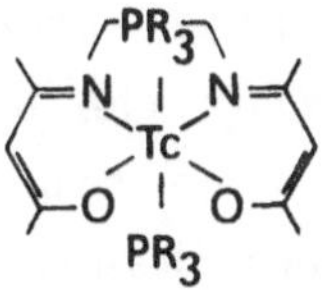

FIGURE 12. Structure of non-reducible mixed-ligand Tc(III) complexes with the tetradentate ligand (acac)$_2$en

According to animal studies variation of the phosphine ligand allows to adjust the lipophilicity "window" for good myocardial image (29). Slow clearance of lung activity and very high initial liver activity remain an obstacle.

6. NEUTRAL, SEVEN COORDINATE Tc(III) COMPLEXES: The BATO type

Nunn, Treher et al. at The Squibb Institute for Medical Research have taken an alternative route that is based no longer upon cationic but neutral Tc(III) complexes (39-43). The new complexes showing myocardial uptake are Boronic Acid Adducts of Technetium Oximes (BATOs). The coordination sphere of the technetium atom consists of three (N-bonded) dioxime molecules and one chlorine atom. At one end the dioximes are held together by two proton bridges, analogous to Tc-HMPAO, and at the other end they are capped by a derivatized boron atom. One member of BATOs is currently undergoing clinical investigation as myocardial perfusion imaging agent. The compound is TcCl $((cdo)_3mb)$ where cdo represents cyclohexyldioxime and mb represents methyboronic acid. The agent called SQ 30217 or Tc-99m-CARDIOTEC[R], respectively, has been fully characterized (41-43). Conductivity measurements show that the complex is neutral. There is no significant presence of a dipole condition within the molecule. Increased electron density on the halogen is indicative in weakening of the metal-chlorine bond.

The radiopharmaceutical is easily prepared by reconstituting a lyophilized Sn^{2+} containing kit with generator eluate and heating at $100°C$ for 15 minutes. The new agent shows no interspecies differences in myocardial uptake. Because of myocardial washout with half-lives of approximately 3 min and 80 min the agent does not represent a pronounced SPECT agent of the kind discussed above. SPECT imaging can be initiated when washout from the myocardium is dominated by the slow component.

The tracer is not significantly taken up or retained by the lungs, it is cleared rapidly from the blood, and is mainly excreted via the liver. There is no significant redistribution. These features allow good planar images of the myocardium to be obtained in less than 5 min after injection. An exercise study can already be followed about $1-\frac{1}{2}$ hours later by second injection at rest.

7. CATIONIC Tc(I) ISONITRILES

Cationic Tc(I) complexes of different types often behave similarly in that they are trapped within the heart. Most of them are disappointing because of slow blood clearance in humans resulting in poor images even several hours after injection, and interference from lung and liver activity.

Although also suffering from some limitations, Tc(I) isonitriles which were introduced by Jones (Boston), Davison (Cambridge, MA) and co-workers in 1981, brought about a breakthrough. The alkyl group R of the CNR ligand in complexes of the type Tc^IL_6+ (Fig. 9) has been systematically altered. When R = t-butyl, a candidate is formed that has been promising in clinical studies, though not ideal for myocardial perfusion imaging. Its biokinetics is unique thanks to rapid clearance from the blood into the lung with subsequent move of the activity to the liver where the background remains relatively high. Its high lung and liver uptake and rapid myocardial redistribution preclude, however, its use during stress.

By screening a series of 40 isonitrile derivatives Du Pont radiopharmaceutical company succeeded in developing a most promising compound: Tc-99m hexakis-2-methoxy-2-methylpropyl-1-isonitrile, referred to as RP-30 or N-30 (44-46). In animal and human studies the new agent (Fig. 13) has shown the favourable myocardial uptake and blood clearance characteristics of the t-butyl isonitrile complex, but with much lower background activity in lung and liver. In correlative studies in humans (normal, ischemia, scar) excellent agreement between Tl-201 and the Tc-99m agent has been observed (47).

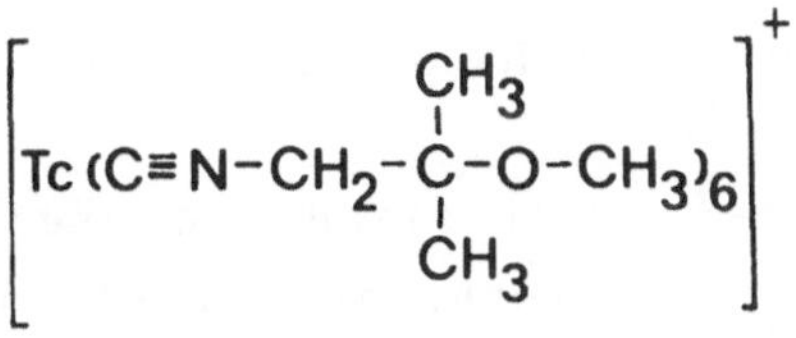

$$\left[Tc\,(C\equiv N-CH_2-\underset{\underset{CH_3}{|}}{\overset{\overset{CH_3}{|}}{C}}-O-CH_3)_6 \right]^+$$

FIGURE 13. Tc-hexakis-2-methoxy-2-methylpropyl isonitrile (RP-30)

Based on initial experience in the human (48), hexakis (carbomethoxyisopropyl isonitrile) technetium(I) - Tc-99m-CPI - is another promising member of the Tc-isonitrile family. It demonstrates high myocardial uptake and differs from Tc-99m-TBI in that it does not redistribute into zones of ischemia for at least several hours after injection and clears rapidly through the lung and liver. The activity is rapidly cleared from the myocardium thus permitting reinjection of the tracer 3 or 4 hrs after the first injection. The advance having achieved up to now will encourage ongoing research on these and other types of compounds to find the best attainable myocardial perfusion Tc-99m tracer.

34

8. A NEW RENAL FUNCTION AGENT: Tc-99m MAG$_3$

Starting from anionic Tc-99m-DADS (Fig. 14, R = H) a more potential carboxyl derivative with R = COOH was subsequently suggested as a replacement for I-131 hippurate. The occurance of complex isomers wiht different renal excretion patterns due to the carboxyl sustituent disqualifies the agent, however, for wide clinical use. Continuing efforts resulted in a Tc-99m complex of the N$_3$S ligand mercaptoacetyltriglycine (MAG$_3$) thus avoiding the problem of stereoisomerism (49 - 53).

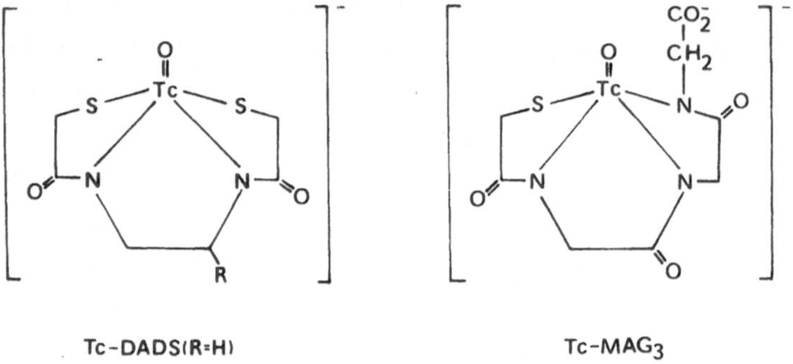

FIGURE 14. Structures of Tc-DADS and Tc-MAG$_3$

The ligand has been synthesized and used for labelling as the S-benzoyl protected precursor. Labelling occurs at 95°C either by direct reduction of pertechnetate in alkaline solution of the precursor or by ligand exchange (49). Experience with a kit preparation as well as updated clinical results which sustain the suggestion that Tc-99m MAG$_3$ may become a replacement for I-131 or I-123 iodohippurate are to be published by Taylor and co-workers (54).

To study the structural requirements for optimal renal tubular transport related compounds such as isomeric derivatives of Tc-99m MAG$_3$ have also been synthesized and studied (55).

9. BIFUNCTIONAL CHELATE APPROACH

The bifunctional chelate approach is concerned with covalent attachment of chelating groups to interesting molecules in order to enable or improve labelling of these molecules.

Already established in labelling proteins with indium- and gallium isotopes the approach also became of great interest in preparing either proteins with stable bonded Tc-99m and intact biological activity or Tc-99m labelled small biomolecules such as fatty acids, steroids and various amino acids (43-49).

One problem with DTPA-coupled proteins is competing non-specific binding of Tc-99m to the protein (46). The peculiarity of the coordination chemistry of technetium and advances in the field of neutral and compact Tc complexes has led to preference of such chelating agents as dithiosemicarbazones (45, 50 - 53), diaminodithiols (DADT) and diaminodisulfides (48).

10. THE Tc-NITRIDO-CORE - AN ENRICHMENT IN TRACER DESIGN?

The nitrido ligand (N^{3-}) is isoelectronic with the oxo ligand that dominates the chemistry of Tc(V) radiopharmaceuticals. N^{3-} is a powerful pi-electron donor which tends to stabilize metals in high oxidation states. Baldas and Bonnyman at the Australian Radiation Laboratory have reported the preparation and characterization of a number of Tc-nitrido compounds (66-68). They also studied the effect of the Tc-N bond on the behaviour of Tc-99m radiopharmaceuticals. Other groups (69, 70) have contributed further information on this new class of Tc compounds.

Whether the use of the nitrido ligand and its observed influence on some in-vivo-properties is actually going to fulfill the expectations for a new approach in design of Tc-99m radiopharmaceuticals is somewhat difficult to predict.

11. CONCLUSION

To sum up, the most significant development that has emerged recently in the field of Tc-99m radiopharmaceuticals relates to brain and myocardium perfusion imaging agents. Research efforts have also been devoted to other scopes and objectives such as renal function, improvements in labelling, new types of complexes as well as those not outlined here such as tumor localization (e.g. 71-73), receptor binding (74, 75) or basic synthetic and analytical chemistry.

Acknowledgement

I would like to express my gratitude to all authors who sent me their latest papers or other helpful information.

REFERENCES
1. Perrier C, Segrě E, Radioactive isotopes of element 43. Nature 1937; 140: 193.
2. Perrier C, Segrě E, Technetium: the element of atomic number 43. Nature 1947; 159: 24.
3. Johannsen B, Advances in radiochemistry of Tc-99m. in: Cox PH, Mather SJ, Sampson CB, Lazarus CR (eds), Progress in radiopharmacy, 1986. Martinus Nijhoff Publishers 1986; 135-154.
4. Wagner Jr HN, SPECT and PET advances herald new era in human biochemistry; The Society of Nuclear Medicine scientific meeting highlights. J Nucl Med 1986; 27: 1227.
5. 2nd Intern. symposium on technetium in chemistry and nuclear medicine. Padova, Italy, Sept 9-11, 1985.
6. 6th Intern. symposium on radiopharmaceutical chemistry. Boston, June 29-July 3, 1986.
7. Volkert WA, Troutner DE Hoffman TJ, Seger RM, Holmes RA, Tc-99m-propyleneamine oxime Tc-99m-PnAO): A potential brain radiopharmaceutical. J Nucl Med 1983; 24: 128.
8. Volkert WA, Hoffman TJ, Seger RM, Troutner DE, Holmes RA, Tc-99m-propyleneamine oxime Tc-99m-PnAO): A potential brain radiopharmaceutical. Eur J Nucl Med 1984; 9: 511.
9. Neirinckx RD, Nowotnik DP, Pickett RD, Harrison RC, Ell PJ, Development of a lipophilic Tc-99m-complex useful for brain perfusion evaluation with conventional SPECT imaging equipment. in: Proc. workshop of the Rheinisch-Westf. Ges. f.Nuklearmedizin, Oct 12-13, 1984. Walter de Gruyter, Bonn 1984.
10. Nowotnik DP, Canning IR, Cumming SA, Harrison RC, Higley B, Nechvatal G, Pickett RD, Piper IM, Bayne VJ, Forster AM, Weisner PS, Neirincks RD, Volkert WA, Troutner DE, Holmes RA, Development of a Tc-99m-labelled radiopharmaceutical for cerebral blood flow imaging. Nucl Med Commun 1985; 6: 499.
11. Chaplin SB, Oberle PA, McKenzie EH, Hoffman TJ, Volkert WA, Holmes RA, Canning LR, Pickett RD, Nowotnik DP, Neirinckx RD, Regional cerebral uptake and retention of Tc-99m-tetramethyl - and pentamethyl-propylene amine oxime chelates. Nucl Med Biol 1986; 13: 261.
12. Sharp PF, Smith FW, Gemmell HG, Lyall D, Evans NTS, Gvozdanovic D, Davison J, Tyrrell DA, Pickett RD, Neirinckx RD, technetium-99m HM PAO stereoisomers as potential agents for imaging regional blood flow: Human volunteer studies. J Nucl Med 1986; 27: 171.
13. Gruner KR, Die Entwicklung heutiger Radiopharmaka aus der Sicht des Herstellers. Der Nuklearmediziner 1986; 9: 297.
14. Ell PJ, Hocknell JML, Jarritt PH, Cullum I, Lui D, Campos-Costra D, Nowotnik DP, Pickett RD, Canning LR, Neirinckx RD, A Tc-labelled radiotracer for the investigation of cerebral vascular disease. Nucl Med Commun 1985; 6: 437.

15. Ell PJ, Costa DC, Kinetics of Tc compound favor its use in SPECT. Diagnostic Imaging, June 1986: 112-117.

16. Neirinckx RD, Clinical experience with Ceretec^{TM}, the first widely available Tc-99m agent for rCBF measurement. RAD, April 1986; 18-20.

17. Reichmann K, Biersack HJ, Basso L, Hartmann A, Matthews ITW, Neirinckx RD, Pickett RD, Winkler C, A comparative study of brain uptake and early kinetics of Tc-99m-dl HM-PAO and other PnAO derivatives in baboons. Nucl Med 1986; 25: 134.

18. Podreka I, Suess E, Goldenberg G, Steiner M, Brücke Th, Müller Ch, Deecke L, Initial experience with Tc-99m-hexamethyl-propyleneamine oxime (Tc-99m-HMPAO) brain SPECT, (abstract) J Nucl Med 1986; 27: 887.

19. deRoo M, Verbruggen A, van Pamel G, Mortelmans L, deSaedeler J, Dom R, Malfroid M, Lammens M, Multidetector SPECT gray matter imaging with Tc-99m-HM-PAO in dementia, (abstract) Nucl Med 1986; 25: A 34.

20. Peters AM, et al., Clinical experience with Tc-99m-hexamethyl-propylene-amineoxime for labelling leucocytes and imaging inflammation. in press.

21. Schümichen C, el al., Tc-99m HM-PAO labelling of leucocytes for detection of imflammatory bowel disease. in press.

22. Epps LA, Burns HD, Lever SZ, Goldfarb HW, Kervitsky TM, Wong DJ, Kramer AV, Wagner Jr HN, The chemistry and biology of technetium(V) oxo complexes of N-piperidinylethyl diaminodithiolate for brain imaging. in: Nicolini M, Bandoli G, Mazzi U (eds.), Technetium in chemistry and nuclear medicine. 2. Raven press, New York, 1986: 171.

23. Lever SZ, Burns HD, Kervitsky TM, Goldfarb HW, Woo DV, Wong DF, Design, preparation, and biodistribution of a technetium-99m triaminedithiol complex to assess regional cerebral blood flow. J Nucl Med 1985; 26: 1287.

24. Goldfarb HW, Scheffel U, Lever SZ, Burns HD, Wagner Jr HN, Comparison of Tc-99m aminoethyl diaminodithiol analogues for blood flow imaging, (abstract). J Nucl Med 1986; 27: 1050.

25. Bok BD, Scheffel U, Goldfarb HW, Burns HD, Lever SZ, Wong DF, Wagner Jr HN, Comparative pharmacokinetics of Tc-99m-aminoethyl-diaminodithiol (DADT) derivatives and I-123-iodoamphetamine for regional brain blood flow imaging, (abstract). Nucl Med 1986; 25: A 77.

26. Baidoo KE, Lever SZ, Kramer AV, Epps, LA, Burns HD, Wagner Jr HN, Synthesis of Tc-99m-N_2S_2 complexes via the p-methoxybenzyl protected thiol ligand, (abstracht). J Nucl Med 1986; 27: 1050.

27. Lever SZ, Baidoo KE, Kramer AV, Burns HD, Epps LA, Scheffel U, Wagner Jr HN, Synthesis and evaluation of new technetium-99m complexes. 3. Eur Symp Radiopharmacy and Radiopharmaceuticals. Elsimore 1987.

28. Neves M, Libson K, Deutsch E, Technetium-99m radiopharmaceuticals for brain perfusion imaging. in: Nicolini M, Bandoli G, Mazzi U (eds.), Technetium in chemistry and nuclear medicine. 2. Raven press, New York, 1986; 122.

29. Deutsch E, Libson K, Vanderheyden JL, Technetium-99m myocardial imaging agents. Personal communication.

30. Münze R, Syhre R, Seifert S, Klötzer S, Mohnike W, Schmidt H, Myocardial imaging agents labelled with technetium-99m. Proc. Conf. Radiopharm. and Labelled Compounds 1984, Tokyo. IAEA Vienna 1985; 249.

31. Münze R, Kretzschmar M, Syhre R, Kampf G, Klötzer D, Güthert I, Bergmann R, Biokinetic data of various radioactive cationic molecules. An attempt at evaluation of significant chemical properties of myotropic agents. in: Nicolini M, Bandoli G, Mazzi U (eds.), Technetium in chemistry and nuclear medicine. 2. Raven press, New York, 1986; 197.

32. Gerundini P, Deutsch E, Savi A, Tyrrel DA, Fazio F, Evaluation of new Tc-99m-radiopharmaceuticals for heart and brain studies. in: Nicolini M, Bandoli G, Mazzi U (eds.), Technetium in chemistry and nuclear medicine. 2. Raven press, New York, 1986; 333.

33. Dean RT, Wester DW, Nosco DL, Adams MD, Coveney JR, Robbins MS, McElvany KD, De Jong R, Progress in the design, evaluation and development of Tc-99m radiopharmaceuticals. in: Nicolini M, Bandoli G, Mazzi U (eds.), Technetium in chemistry and nuclear medicine. 2. Raven press, New York, 1986; 147.

34. Seifert S, Schneider F, Syhre R, Muenze R, The development of a new myocardial imaging agent based on DMPE. Annual report, Centrel Instute of Nuclear Research, Rossendorf, G.D.R, 1986.

35. Deutsch E, Vanderheyden JL, Gerundini P, Libson K, Hirth W, Savi A, Zecca L, Fazio F, Development of nonreducible 99m-technetium(III) cations as myocardial perfusion imaging agents, (abstract). J Nucl Med 1986; 27: 894.

36. Münze R, Mohnike W, Syhre R, Schmidt J, Seifert S, Successful imaging of the human heart by using an improved technetium phosphine radiopharmaceutical, (abstract). Nucl Med 1986; 25: A 46.

37. Syhre R, Seifert S, Schneider F, Münze R, Mohnike W, Schmidt J, Gisske H, Bach H, Ein Tc-99m-Radiopharmakon auf DMPE-Basis - geeignet zur planaren Szintigraphie und zu SPECT-Untersuchungen des Herzens. NucCompact 1986; 17: 199.

38. Jurisson SS, Dancey K, McPartlin M, Tasker PA, Deutsch E, Synthesis, charaterization, and electrochemical properties of technetium complexes containing both tetradentate Schiff base and monodentate tertiary phosphine ligands: Single-crystal structure of trans- (N,N' -ethylene bis (acetylacetone iminato)) bis (triphenylphosphine) technetium (III) hexafluorophosphate. Inorg Chem 1984; 23: 4743.

39. Nunn AD, Treher EN, Feld T, Boronic acid adducts of technetium oxime imaging capabilities, (abstract). J Nucl Med 1986; 27: 893.

40. Narra RK, Feld T, Wedeking P, Matyas J, Nunn AD, SQ 30,217, a technetium 99m labelled myocardial imaging agent which shows no interspecies differences in uptake, (abstract). J Nucl Med 1986; 27: 1051.

41. Thompson M, X-ray photoelectron spectroscopy of potential technetium-based organ imaging agents. Anal Chem 1986; 58: 3100.

42. Unger SE, McCormick TJ, Treher EN, Nunn AD, A comparison of desorption ionization methods for the analysis of neutral seven-coordinate technetium radiopharmaceuticals. Anal Chem (In press).

43. Nunn AD, personal communication.

44. Williams SJ. Mousa SA, Morgan RA, Caroll TR, Maheu LJ, Pharmacology of Tc-99m-isonitriles: Agents with favorable characteristics for heart imaging, (abstract) 1986; 27: 877.

45. Mousa SA, Williams SJ, Myocardial uptake and retention of Tc-99m-hexakisaliphatic isonotriles: Evidence for specificity, (abstract). J Nucl Med 1986; 27: 995.

46. Williams SJ, Mousa SA, Mahent J, Carroll TR, Morgan RA, Identification of a Tc-99m hexakis-isonitrile with favorable pharmacokinetics for myocardial perfusion scintigraphy, (abstract). Nucl Med 1986; 25: A 45.

47. McKusick K, Holman BL, Jones AG, Davison A, Rigo P, Sporn V, Vosberg H, Moretti J, Comparison of 3 Tc-99m isonitriles for detection ischemic heart disease in humans, (abstract). J Nucl Med 1986; 27: 878.

48. Holman BL, Sporn V, Jones AG, Sia STB, Perez-Balino N, Davison A, Lister-James J, Kronauge JF, Mitta AEA, Camin LL, Campbell S, Williams SJ, Carpenter AT, Myocardial imaging with technetium-99m CPI: initial experience in the human. J Nucl Med 1987; 28: 13.

49. Fritzberg AR, Kasina S, Eshima D, Johnson DL, Synthesis and biological evaluation of technetium-99m MAG_3, as a hippuran replacement. J Nucl Med 1986; 27: 111.

50. Taylor Jr A, Eshima D, Fritzberg AR, Christian PE, Kasina S, Comparison of iodine-131 OIH and technetium-99m MAG_3 renal imaging in volunteers. J Nucl Med 1986; 27: 795.

51. Taylor Jr A, Eshima D, Christian PE, Fritzberg AR, Kasina S, Comparison of Tc-99m mercaptoacetyltriglycerine (MAG_3) and OIH in normal subjects and patients, (abstract). J Nucl Med 1986; 27: 1986.

52. Fritzberg AR, Rao TN, Adhikesavalu D, Camerman A, Vanderheyden JL, Synthesis and characterization of Re And Tc complexes of N2S2 and N3S ligands. 6th Intern. Symp. Radiopharm. Chem. Boston 1986, paper 45 (abstract).

53. Nosco DL, Manning RG, Fritzberg A, Characterization of the new Tc-99m dynamic renal imaging agent: Tc-99m MAG_3, (abstract). J Nucl Med 1986; 27: 939.

54. Taylor Jr A, personal communication

55. Verbruggen A, Dekempeneer P, Cleynhens B, Hoogmartens M, De Roo M, Synthesis and renal excretion characteristics of isomeric methyl derivatives of Tc-99m-mercaptoacetyl triglycerine. 6th Intern. Symp. Radiopharm. Chem. Boston 1986, paper 45 (abstract).

56. Yokoyama A, Recent progress in the development of bifunctional radiopharmaceuticals. Proc. Conf. Radiopharm. and labelled Compounds 1984, Tokyo. IAEA Vienna 1985; 251-265.

57. Arano Y, Magata Y, Furukawa T, Horiuchi K, Yokoyama A, Endo K, Torizuka K, Bifunctional chelating agents for Tc-99m-labelled monoclonal antibodies. Proc. Conf. Radiopharm. and Labelled Compounds 1984, Tokyo. IAEA Vienna 1985; 143-151.

58. Yokoyama A, Hosotani T, Arano Y, Horiuchi K, Technetium DTS-bifunctional radiopharmaceuticals: Role of amino containing side chain on biodistribution. 6th Intern. Symp. Radiopharm. Chem Boston 1986, paper 47 (abstract).

59. Childs RL, Hnatowich DJ, Optimum conditions for labelling of DTPA-coupled antibodies with technetium-99m. J Nucl Med 1985; 26: 293.

60. Liang FH, Virzi F, Hnatowich DJ, The use of diaminodithiol for labelling small molecules with technetium-99m. $Nucl_2$ Med Biol 1986, in press.

61. Zollinger K, Huber G, Iftimia M, Bläuenstein P, Beer HF, Schubiger PA, Protein labelling with technetium-99m using different reducing agents and coupled bridging ligands, (abstract) Nucl Med 1986; 25: A 76.

62. Hosotani T, Yokoyama A, Arano Y, Horiuchi K, Saji H, Torizuka K, Search for Tc-99m labelled DTS bifunctional radiopharmaceutical: Role of functional groups in myocardial accumulation. Int J Appl Radiat Isot 1986; 37: 505.

63. Arano Y, Yokoyama A, Magata Y, Horiuchi K, Saji H, Torizuka K, In the procurement of stable Tc-99m-labelled protein using bifunctional chelating agent Int J Appl Radiat Isot 1986; 37: 587.

64. Hosotani T, Yokoyama A, Arano Y, Horiuchi K, Wasaki H, Saji H, Torizuka K, In the procurement of a neutral and compact monomeric complex of dithiosemicarbazone (DTS) derivative: Tc-99m-KTS. Int J Nucl Med Biol 1986; 12: 431.

65. Arano Y, Yokoyama A, Magata Y, Saji H, Horiuchi K, Torizuka K, Synthesis and evaluation of a new bifunctional chelating agent for Tc-99m labelling proteins: p-Carboxyethylphenyl glyoxal-di (N-methylthiosemicarbazone). Int J Med Biol 1986; 12: 425.

66. Baldas J, Bonnyman J, Substitution reactions of Tc-99m-NCL_4 - A route to a new class of Tc-99m-radiopharmaceuticals. Int J Appl Radiat Isot 1985; 36: 133.

67. Baldas J, Bonnyman J, Effect of the Tc-nitrido group on the behaviour of Tc-99m-radiopharmaceuticals. Int J Appl Radiat Isot 1985; 36: 919.

68. Baldas J, Bonnyman J, Williams GA, Studies of technetium complexes. 9. Use of the tetrachloronitrido technetate(VI) anion for the preparation of nitrido complexes of technetium. Crystal structure of bis (8-quinolinethiolato) nitridotechnetium(V). Inorg Chem 1986; 25: 150.

69. Abram U, Spies H, Münze R, Kaden L, Lorenz B, Wahren M, Nitrido complexes of technetium. in: Nicolini M, Bandoli G, Mazzi U (eds.), Technetium in chemistry and nuclear medicine. 2. Raven press, New York, 1986: 81.

70. Abram U, Spies H, Görner W, Kirmse R, Stach J, Lipophilic technetium complexes. III. Chelate complexes of technetium(V) containing the Tc-nitrido core. Inorg Chim Acta 1985; 109:L 9.

71. Schümichen C, Weiss H, Tumor localization and biodistribution of Tc-99m muramylpolypeptide (MPP) in the rat. Nucl Med 1986; 25: 28.
72. Jeghers O, Puttemans N, Urbain D, Ham HR, Letter to the editor: Technetium-99m DMSA uptake by metastatic carcinoma of the prostata. J Nucl Med 1986; 27: 1223.
73. Clarke SEM, Fogelman I, Lazarus CR, Edwards S, Maisey MN, A Comparison of I-131 MIBG and Tc-99m-pentavalent-DMSA for imaging patients with medullary cell carcinoma of the thyroid, (abstract). Nucl Med 1986; 25:A 22.
74. Stadalnik RC, Trudeau WL, Vera DR, Pauly MP, TcNGA functional imaging of the liver: A model for testing the clinical role of receptor-binding radiotracers, (abstract). J Nucl Med 1986; 27:67.
75. Galli G, Valle G, Maini CL, Orlando P, Giordano, Tc-99m-asialo-alpha-1-acid-glycoprotein: A   receptor-specific radiopharmaceutical for liver scintigraphy Nucl Med 1986; 25: A55.

3. LABELLING METHODS WITH RADIOACTIVE IODINE

K.H. BREMER AND A. SCHWARZ

1. IODINE RADIONUCLIDES

Iodine radionuclides have been used for many years for the simple and rapid labelling of biological substances, particularly antibodies. Amongst the thirty-two known isotopes of iodine, iodine-123 and iodine-131 are the most routinely used because of their physical properties (Figure 1).

		I-131	**I-123**
half–life	⇒	8.02 days	13.3 hours
gamma energy	⇒	364 keV	159 keV
beta energy	⇒	606 keV	
manufactured in	⇒	reactor	cyclotron
price	⇒	low	very high

FIGURE 1. Comparison of I-131 and I-123.

Iodine-123, which is a pure gamma-emitter and possesses a favourable gamma energy level of 159 keV has a low radiation load.

The use of iodine-123 to label antibodies is, however, considerably limited by the fact that it has a relatively short half-life of 13 hours, and cyclotrons are required for its production.

Iodine-131 with its high-energy gamma radiation of 364 and 637 keV together with its high-energy beta radiation and a relatively long half-life of 8 days is in more than one respect not an ideal radionuclide for in vivo diagnostics. Despite this, it will continue to retain a certain diagnostic importance and it is used for labelling antibodies, because it is available with adequately high specific radioactivity. The labelling procedure itself is relatively simple and cheap.

2. LABELLING PROCEDURES

There are many different methods available for labelling biological substances with radioactive iodine. Some of the most widely used are shown in Figure 2.

| 1.1 Chloramine T–reagent | Oxidation of the radioiodide with N–chloro–p–toluenesulfonamide–sodium in the presence of the protein to be labelled. |
| 1.2 Iodo–Gen–method | 1.3.4.6–tetrachloro–3o, 6o–diphenyl–glycoluril, is used as "solid phase" oxidizing agent or dissolved in a small volume of acetone. |

| 2.1 "Bolton–Hunter"–technique | The N-hydroxysuccinimidylester of 3–(4–hydroxy–phenyl)–propionic acid is radioiodinated and purified. Then the coupling reaction is carried out and the labelled protein is separated by gel filtration. |
| 2.2 Substitution of an organometallic group for iodine | Variant of the "Bolton–Hunter" method with exchange of an organometallic group, e.g. $(Bu)_3$–Sn for radio iodine. |

FIGURE 2. Methods of protein iodination.
        1. Oxidizing techniques based on chloro-compounds
        2. Labelling by conjugation with activated esters

Proteins are mainly labelled by means of electrophilic substitution, i.e. by substituting iodine for hydrogen in the presence of mild oxidation agents. This procedure is usually performed in the amino acids tyrosine and histidine. The most common methods employed are the Iodo-Gen and chloramine T methods in which the substances to be labelled react directly with the iodine.

The Iodo-Gen method shows the advantages that the labelling procedure is very simple and that a mild oxidation medium causes only slight damage to the biological material. The yield is almost 100% and easily reproducible even with large amounts of activity.

The Bolton-Hunter method is based on a different principle. Firstly, an activated ester is labelled, which then reacts with a functional group of the protein in a second step. Although this method allows the proteins to be labelled with very little damage, it is a very elaborate procedure, since complex purification steps are always necessary. A variation on the Bolton-Hunter method is to introduce the iodine nuclide into the activated ester by means of halogen exchange via an organometallic compound. This does not, however, make the above mentioned purification procedures any simpler.

3. EXPERIMENTAL PART

Only small amounts of Iodo-Gen - dissolved in acetone and added to the aqueous reaction solution - are required for the iodination reaction, which involves little waste, even when using 15 mg or more IgG per batch (Figure 3). The reaction takes place in the homogeneous phase and results in reproducible yields of 90 to 95%. A reaction time of 10 minutes is adequate. The mixture is then purified using polyacryl amide gel. The protein is eluted by means of PBS buffer as a uniform fraction in the column. The inactive Iodo-Gen is specifically eluted in a second run, and is identified by UV absorption. Radioactive iodide and iodate are hardly detectable in the remaining eluate.

The solution is diluted with PBS buffer, human albumin is added and it is sterile-filtered. Purity testing is performed using a Bio-Gel P-2-column (230 x 26 mm) for gel filtration.

Elution is with PBS buffer with a pH of 7.9 at a rate of 1 ml/min. HPLC is performed on TSK 250 columns, the eluent in this case being citrate buffer with a pH of 6.8.

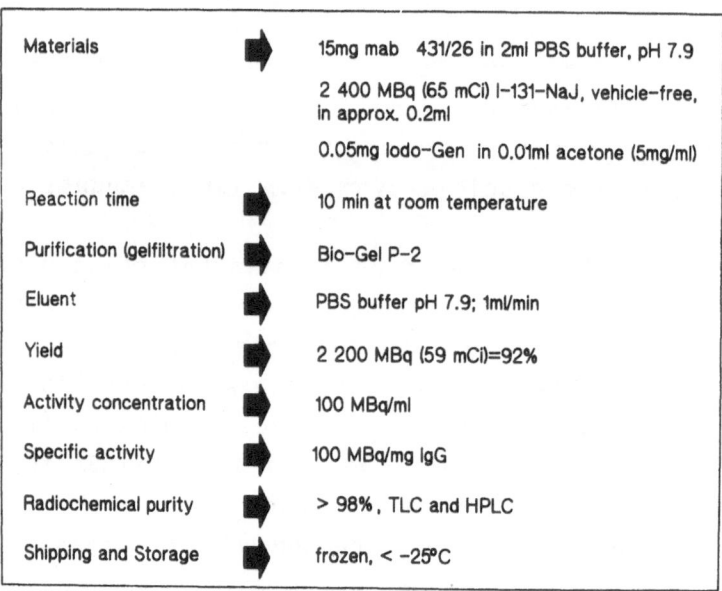

Materials	➡	15mg mab 431/26 in 2ml PBS buffer, pH 7.9
		2 400 MBq (65 mCi) I–131–NaJ, vehicle–free, in approx. 0.2ml
		0.05mg Iodo–Gen in 0.01ml acetone (5mg/ml)
Reaction time	➡	10 min at room temperature
Purification (gelfiltration)	➡	Bio–Gel P–2
Eluent	➡	PBS buffer pH 7.9; 1ml/min
Yield	➡	2 200 MBq (59 mCi)=92%
Activity concentration	➡	100 MBq/ml
Specific activity	➡	100 MBq/mg IgG
Radiochemical purity	➡	> 98%, TLC and HPLC
Shipping and Storage	➡	frozen, < –25°C

FIGURE 3. Labelling of antibodies with I-131 by a modified Iodo-Gen-procedure.

4. QUALITY CONTROL

Such iodine-labelled substances are intended for use in humans and are therefore subject to stringent quality control (Figure 4). The biological and chemical purity criteria in European and other national pharmacopoeias apply to all pharmaceuticals. They must be sterile and pyrogen-free, and the content of active substance, and nature and amount of impurities must be determined in suitable assays.

In addition, purity of the radio nuclide and radiochemical purity must be assured for radiopharmaceuticals. Whilst the purity of the radionuclide can be determined directly on the basic material, a series of modern analytical techniques must be used to establish the radiochemical purity of the end product.

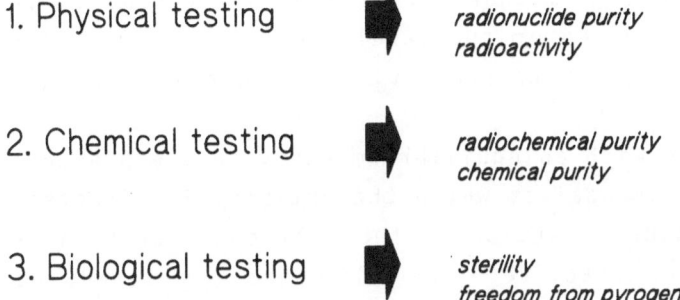

1. Physical testing ➡ *radionuclide purity*
radioactivity

2. Chemical testing ➡ *radiochemical purity*
chemical purity

3. Biological testing ➡ *sterility*
freedom from pyrogens

FIGURE 4. Quality control

The gel filtration used for purification is also suitable as a quality control assay, and is particularly useful for detecting low molecular impurities (Figure 5). Rapid determination of the free iodine content is possible with thin-layer chromatography. This method can be used for stability testing. HPLC, however, provides the most comprehensive information on the quality of the product. Not only secondary products and free iodine, but also polymer fractions can be detected and quantified with this method.

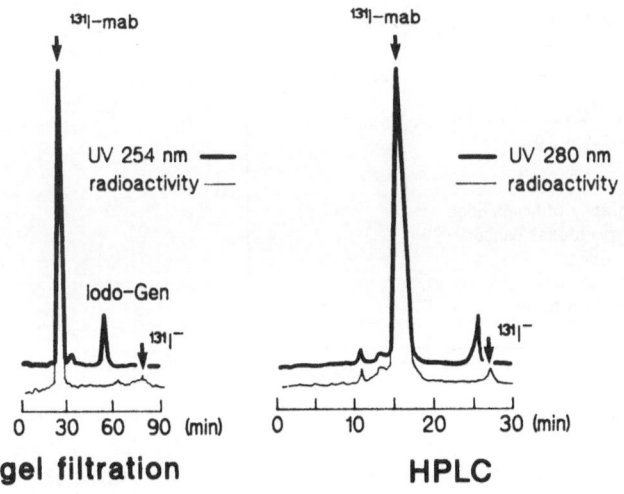

FIGURE 5. Purification of a I-131-labelled monoclonal antibody

5. BIOLOGICAL BEHAVIOUR

In the case of labelled monoclonal antibodies it is very important that the inherent immunoreactivity of monoclonal antibodies must not be impaired by the labelling process, in other words, as much of their immunoreactivity as possible must be retained.

This is determined with an equilibrium assay in the presence of surplus tumour cells against which the antibody is directed. Using a constant amount of antibody, the cell concentration is increased until every reactive - or undamaged - antibody is able to bind to a cell. After centrifuging, the cell bound fraction and the antibody in the supernatant which is not reactive, are separated, and the activity is determined. Immuno reactive levels of 80-90% are usually measured. If the levels are lower, this usually means that the antibody has been damaged in the labelling process or has been contaminated with nonspecific proteins.

Monoclonal antibodies	Applications	Radionuclides
BW 431/31 IgG₁ ✱	anti–CEA; detection of colorectal carcinomas	I, In
BW 431/26 IgG₁ ✱	anti–CEA, detection of colorectal carcinomas	I, In, Tc
BW 494/32 IgG₁ ✱	detection of pancreas carcinoma associated mucus antigen	I, In, Tc
BW 495/36 IgG₃	immunoscintigraphy of lymph node metastases from breast cancer	I
BW 575/100 IgG₁	radioimaging of lung tumors	I, In, Tc

✱ = F(ab')₂

FIGURE 6. Labelled monoclonal antibodies and their immunoreactivities

For the testing and differentiation of new monoclonal anti-bodies basic screening procedures have to be applied and the iodination procedure used must be more comprehensive than the above mentioned routine tests. Basic information on the beha-viour of the iodinated preparation is obtained by determining organ distribution in healthy animals. Usually rats are used for this purpose. The xenograft model of the nude mouse has proved particularly useful for substances intended for tumour imaging. With this model, it is possible to map the time course of the activity in the implanted tumour in the living animal with a gamma camera.

6. CRITICAL EVALUATION

A series of intact monoclonal antibodies and their fragments were labelled with iodine-131 by using the Iodo-Gen method (Figure 6). For comparison reasons the same monoclonal anti-bodies and their fragments were also labelled with Indium-111 and Technetium-99m. These labelled preparations were tested preclinically and in the case of BW 431/31, 431/26 and 494/32 also clinically. The results of the clinical tests show that iodine-131 has clear disadvantages in comparison with the other two nuclides used for labelling. It therefore seems appropriate to list the advantages and disadvantages of monoclonal antibo-dies labelled with iodine-131 (Figure 7).

Advantages:

1. Simple and rapid labelling procedure
2. Possible use in immune therapy

Disadvantages:

1. Physical properties of the radionuclide
2. Poor in vivo stability
3. Expensive batch-production process

FIGURE 7. Advantages and disadvantages of I-131-labelled monoclonal antibodies

An advantage is the simplicity of the labelling procedure. This means that the method of iodine labelling is the first choice for the testing of a new antibody. A preliminary overview of the accumulation in the target organ, the kinetic behaviour of the preparation and the distribution pattern in other organs is achieved rapidly. It must also be borne in mind at this point that monoclonal antibodies labelled with iodine-131 may have a future role in tumour therapy.

The physical properties of iodine-131 are the most serious disadvantages. In addition to the undesirable beta radiation, it posesses high gamma energy. The poor in vivo stability of these preparations is also a very negative aspect. A further negative factor is that every preparation has to be prepared and shipped individually which involves considerable expense.

REFERENCES
1. Fraker P J, Speck J C, Protein and cell membrane iodinations with a sparingly soluble chloroamide Biochem Biophys Res Commun 1978; 80: 849.
2. Bolter A E, Hunter W M, The labelling of proteins to high specific radioactivities by conjugation to a I-125-containing acylating agent Biochem J 1973; 133: 529.
3. Richardson A P, Mountford P J, Baird A C, Heyderman E, Richardson T C, Coakley A J, An improved Iodogen method of labelling antibodies with I-123 Nucl Med Commun 1986; 7: 355.
4. Mather S J, Radioiodinated Monoclonal Antibodies: a Critical Review Appl Radiat Isot 1986; 37: 727.
5. Andrew S M, Pimm M V, Perkins A C, Baldwin R W, Comparative imaging and biodistribution studies with an anti-CEA monoclonal antibody and its $F(ab')_2$ and Fab fragments in mice with colon carcinoma xenografts Eur J Nucl Med 1986; 12: 168.
6. Steinsträsser A, Schwarz A, Kuhlmann L. Monoclonal Antibodies: Optimizing of Labelling Procedures by Quality-control Methods (Poster) 3. Eur Symp Radiopharmacy and Radiopharmaceuticals, Elsmore 1987.

4. LABELLING WITH INDIUM-111.

S.J.Mather

1. INTRODUCTION

Indium-111 can be considered to be the second most important isotope in Nuclear Medicine. It has two gamma photons at energies suitable for scintigraphy, an acceptable patient radiation dose and a half-life of 67 hours which permits imaging at time points later than is possible with shorter lived isotopes such as Tc-99m and I-123.

Methods developed for labelling with Indium-111 have the advantage that they will also be directly useable for other potentially useful nuclides of indium such as Indium-113m and -114m and may also be applicable for other metallic radioisotopes with similar chemistry such as, for example, Gallium-67 and Yttrium-90.

Indium-111 is used as a label for simpe ligands such as DTPA where its principal advantage is that its relatively long shelflife permits prospective pyrogenicity testing prior to its use as an intrathecal tracer(1). It has also found some application as a label for the tumour seeking reagent Bleomycin (2).

The isotope has found more general application for labelling materials of biological origin such as blood-cells or proteins, either where alternative labelling methods damage the reagents or are unstable, or do not suit the extended pharmacokinetics of the tracer.

Established methods for labelling cells with indium involve chelation of the isotope by hydrophobic ligands to produce a neutral lipophilic complex which diffuses through the wall of the cell, but then following metabolism, becomes imprisoned

within to produce a stable tracer (3). Recently reported methods for labelling cells such as platelets (4) and leucocytes
(5) seem likely to replace existing techniques in the near future.

The main area of expansion in indium-labelling technology at
the present time is that used for labelling monoclonal antibodies. While antibodies themselves are undoubtedly of interest
as radiopharmaceuticals in their own right, they also serve as
useful models for other labelled proteins since antibodies are
large glycoproteins possessing the full range of chemically
functional groups suitable for label attatchment, they possess
a well defined receptor-binding domain, and they are multifunc-
tional proteins interacting with a range of biological systems.
Any method developed for labelling antibodies with indium, therefore, is likely to be applicable to other proteins of interest in Nuclear Medicine.

Current methods of antibody labelling follow the general
schema:

1) DERIVATISATION: Attachment of a suitable chelating group
to the protein.

2) PURIFICATION: Removal of unbound chelate.

3) RADIOLABELLING: Attachment of radioindium to the protein-
bound chelate groups.

2. DERIVATISATION

In describing a system of derivatisation, consideration must
be given to A) the chelating species itself, and B) the means
of its attachment to the protein. These two aspects can be considered independently.

Chelating agents can be considered in three groups:
(i) Established polycarboxyclic acid ligands - EDTA, DTPA.
(ii) Novel open chain ligands.
(iii) Macrocyclic ligands.

2.1 Established polycarboxyclic ligands

The structures of Ethylenediaminetetracetic acid (EDTA) and
diethylenetriaminepentaacetic acid (DTPA) are shown in Figure
1. Bifunctional chelating agents (BCA's) based on these ligands
have found the most widespread application. EDTA analogues in-

clude the series described by Meares and Co-workers, namely p-
diazobenzyl EDTA (6) p-(bromoacetamido) benzyl EDTA (7), p-
(isothiocyanato) benzyl EDTA(7) and p-(carboxymethoxy) benzyl
EDTA (8), (Figure 2).

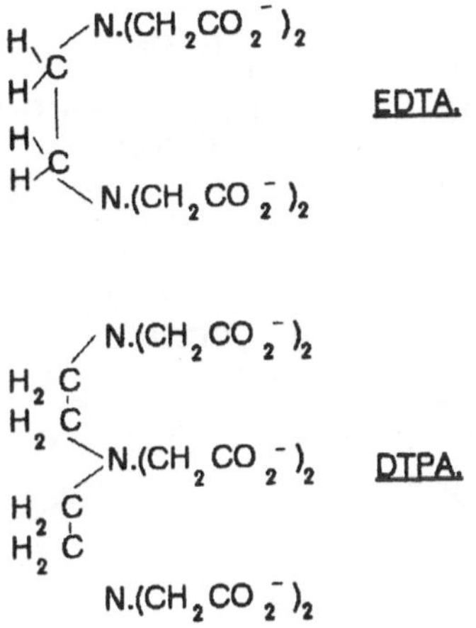

$$H_2C \begin{array}{c} N.(CH_2CO_2^-)_2 \\ | \\ N.(CH_2CO_2^-)_2 \end{array} \quad \text{EDTA.}$$

$$\begin{array}{c} N.(CH_2CO_2^-)_2 \\ H_2C \\ H_2C \\ N.(CH_2CO_2^-)_2 \quad \text{DTPA.} \\ H_2C \\ H_2C \\ N.(CH_2CO_2^-)_2 \end{array}$$

FIGURE 1. Chemical structures of Ethylenediaminetetraacetic a-
cid (EDTA) and diethylenetriaminepentaacetic acid (DTPA).

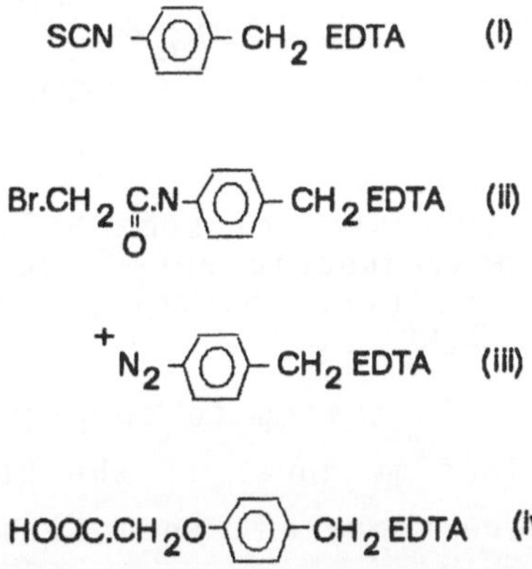

SCN ─⟨O⟩─ CH$_2$ EDTA   (i)

Br.CH$_2$ C.N─⟨O⟩─ CH$_2$ EDTA   (ii)
        ‖
        O

$^+$N$_2$─⟨O⟩─ CH$_2$ EDTA   (iii)

HOOC.CH$_2$O─⟨O⟩─CH$_2$ EDTA   (iv)

FIGURE 2. Chemical structures of some bifunctional chelates of
EDTA. (i) p-Isothiocynatobenzyl-EDTA, (ii) p-bromacetamidoben-
zyl-EDTA, (iii) p-diazobenzyl-EDTA (iv) p-carboxymethoxybenzyl-
EDTA.

DTPA derivatives include the bicyclic (9) and mixed acid
(10) anhydrides, the N-hydroxysuccinimide ester (11) and p-
(isothiocynato)benzyl DTPA (12), (Figure 3).

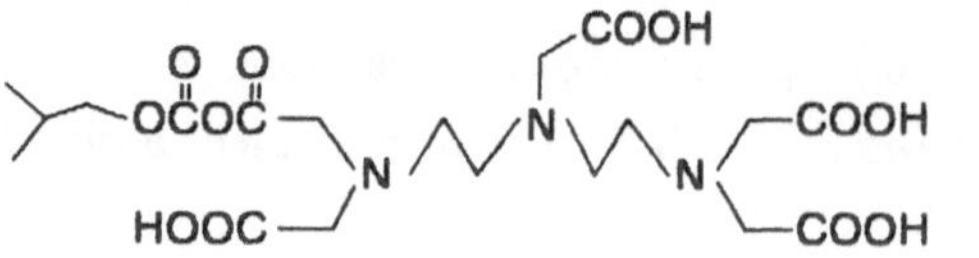

FIGURE 3. Chemical structures of some bifunctional chelates of DTPA. (v) Mixed carboxycarbonic anhydride of DTPA, (vi) N-hydroxysuccinimide ester, (vii) bicyclic dianhydride, (viii) p-isothiocyanatobenzyl DTPA.

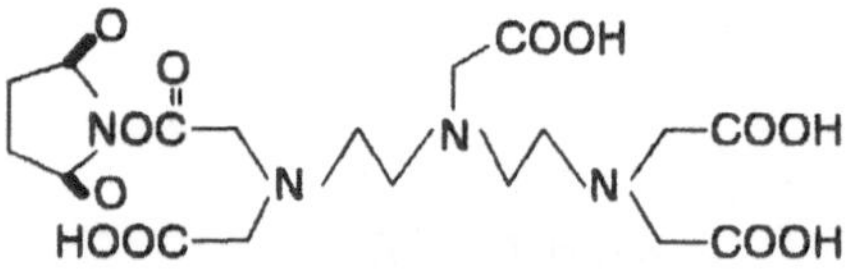

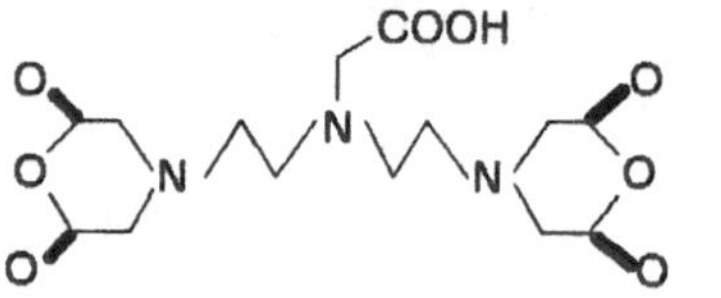

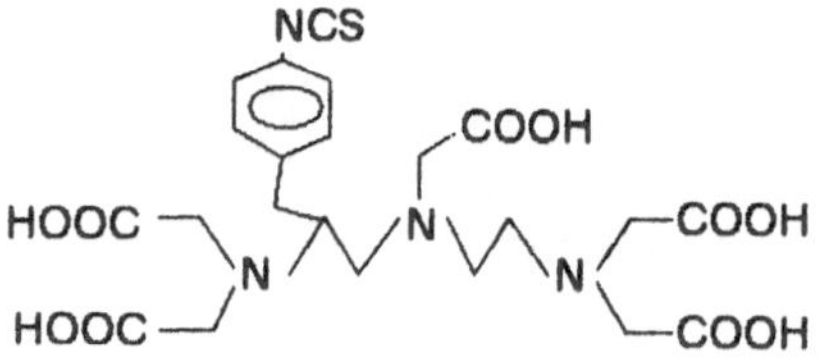

Difficulties arise in trying to compare the theoretical advantages of the various methods. If the stability constants of the native ligands are compared, then although the actual quoted figures vary, the equilibrium constant of DTPA and indium is generally 2-3 orders of magnitude greater than that of EDTA. While the stability constants of the bifunctional chelating agents themselves have not, in general, been determined, it must be expected that they will differ from the unsubstituted chelates.

An important difference between the various BCA's is that while some (such as the DTPA anhydrides and NHS ester) utilise one of the indium-binding carboxyl groups in order to form an amide bond with the protein, others have a linking group inserted into the backbone of the chelate in order to leave all the co-ordination sites available for binding indium (Figure 4). The removal of one of the chelating carboxylate groups from DTPA still leaves sufficient coordination sites for indium binding (10), however, it would be expected that the stability constant of the resultant ligand would be somewhat reduced by this and by other stereochemical considerations.

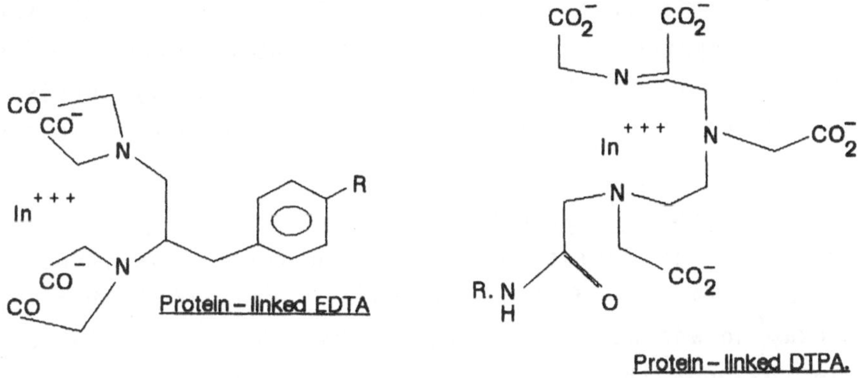

FIGURE 4. Chelation of indium after linkage of protein to backbone substituted EDTA and carboxyl substituted DTPA.

On the other hand, it has been suggested that the insertion of a linking group onto the backbone of a chelate may actually increase the thermodynamic stability of metal complexes (13) presumeably due to an increase in their structural rigidity.

The stability of antibodies labelled with indium using the cyclic DTPA anhydride and isothiocyanatobenzyl EDTA have been compared by incubating the conjugates in serum. Indium-benzyl-EDTA-antibody was found to be more stable than In-DTPA-antibody (13,14). A comparison of antibody labelled with the two DTPA anhydrides, p-isothiocyanatobenzyl EDTA and p-isothiocyanato-benzyl DTPA has been performed in tumour-bearing nude mice. The p-SCN-Bz-DTPA conjugate produced the best results in terms of image quality and tumour:tissue ratios (12).

It must be noted that all of the bifunctional chelating agents described possess stability constants lower than that of transferrin (15) and are therefore at a thermodynamic disadvantage with respect to this protein. That loss of indium to transferrin is not found to be greater must be due to the slow kinetics of the exchange reaction.

In practice, the labelling method that has received most widespread application is that which uses the bicyclic anhydride of DTPA (16), this being the only one of the bifunctional chelating agents to be commercially available (Sigma Chemical Co.). A protocol describing a detailed method for labelling antibodies with this reagent is appended below. All the other BCA's require synthesis and while those which utilise one of the carboxyl groups of DTPA are relatively simple, synthesis of the others requires the services of an experienced organic chemist.

2.2 Novel open-chain chelates

Other open-chain chelating agents used for indium labelling include a number of off-the-shelf reagents such as desferrioxamine and penicillamine(17) which have been linked to antibodies using either glutaraldehyde or carbodiimide(18). Of these, the most interesting candidate is desferrioxamine. This chelate forms highly stable complexes with iron (Log K = 31) and, presumeably, with indium also. It contains a single primary amino group through which a link can be made to the antibody without weakening the stability of the metal complex.

Triethylenetetraminehexaacetic acid (TTHA) continues the series EDTA-DTPA-TTHA. Since this reagent has a spare carboxyl group relative to DTPA, it might be expected that a carboxyl-linked TTHA would have advantages over a carboxyl-linked DTPA in terms of metal-binding stability. In a comparison of antibodies labelled with the N-hydroxysuccinimide esters of the two chelates in tumour-bearing nude-mice, however, DTPA gave higher tumour uptake and lower bone-marrow accumulation (19). In a comparison of the stability of indium labelled DTPA and DTTA, the DTPA complex was found to be the more stable, however indium labelled Human Serum Albumin using an azoimidate DTTA link was more stable (20).

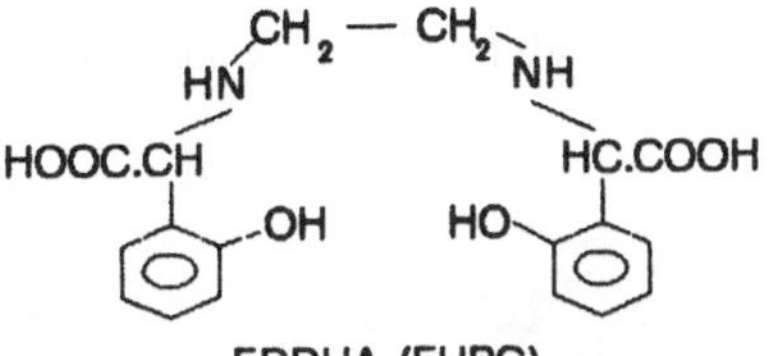

HN CH₂ — CH₂ NH

HOOC.CH   HC.COOH

OH   HO

EDDHA (EHPG).

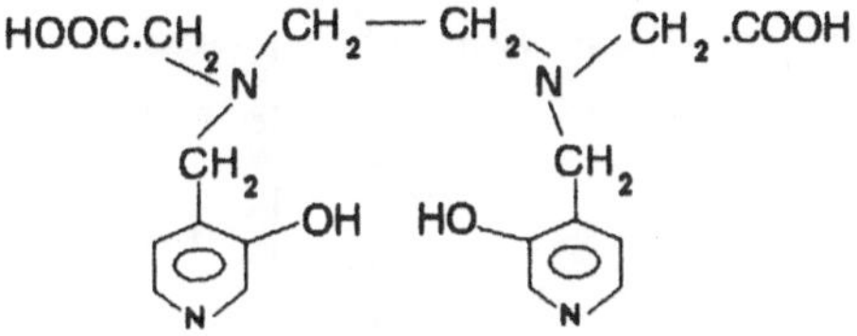

HOOC.CH₂ CH₂ — CH₂ CH₂.COOH

N   N

CH₂   CH₂

OH   HO

PLED.

FIGURE 5. Chemical structures of ethylenediamine N,N' di((o-hy-droxyphenyl) acetic acid), EDDHA and N,N' dipyridoxylethylene-diamine N,N' diacetic acid, PLED.

A number of chelating agents with stability constants for indium much higher than those of DTPA and EDTA have been de-scribed. These include the phenolic and pyridoxalic ligands shown in Figure 5. EDDHA (also called EHFG), ethylenediamine N,N' di((o-hydroxyphenyl) acetic acid) has a log K for indium of 33 and PLED, N,N' dipyridoxylethylenediamine- N,N' diacetic acid, log K=37 (21). Antibodies labelled with gallium-67 via EDDHA using carbodiimide compared well with iodinated antibody in tumour bearing mice (22). Antibody labelled with indium-111 via EDDHA attached to oligosaccharide gave better tumour loca-lisation than antibody labelled via DTPA attatched to lysine residues (23) but whether the improvement in localisation should be ascribed to the ligand or the means of its attachment is not described.

2.3 Macrocycles

A likely future development will be the preparation of func-tionalised macrocyclic ligands for the attachment of metal ions to proteins (24). The closed ring structure of macrocycles re-

sults in very high thermodynamic stabilities of metal complexes
which would effectively prevent catabolism of the metal ion and
may radically alter the biodistribution of radioactive antibody
metabolites.

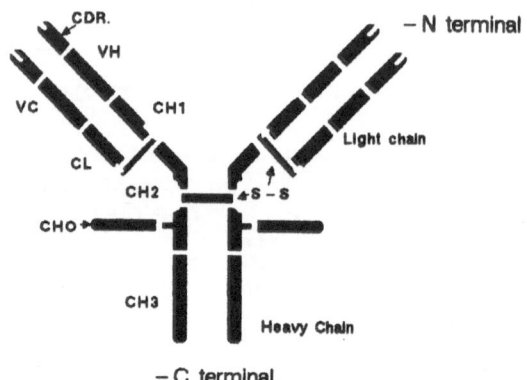

FIGURE 6. Diagrammatic representation of an antibody molecule.

Antibodies possess a number of functional groups which can
be used as a point for attachment of the chelate of choice. Numerous techniques exist for modification of many of the amino-
acid side-chains that make up the antibody molecule, but relatively few of these have been applied for radiolabelling purposes. The principal requirement of a derivatisation procedure is
that it should employ mild chemical conditions in order to limit damage to the antibody itself. It should also be selective
in terms of the functional chemical group it modifies and side
reactions such as those that produce intra or inter-protein
links should be minimal. Finally the reaction should be efficient in order to make the most of expensive chemical intermediates and to simplify purification procedures.

The terminal amino group of lysine residues has received
most interest as a site for chelate attatchment. Several types
of reaction have been described (Figure 7), the most popular
involving the bicyclic anhydride of DTPA (Fig 3(vii)). This reaction meets many of the requirements of an ideal derivatisation procedure with the exception that, owing to the bifunctional nature of the agent, extensive cross linking can occur at
higher anhydride:protein ratios.

LYSINE.

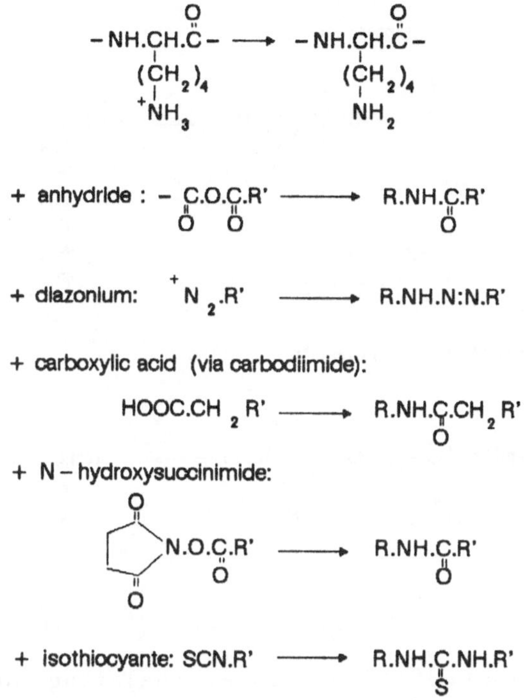

$$-NH.CH.\overset{O}{\overset{\|}{C}}- \longrightarrow -NH.CH.\overset{O}{\overset{\|}{C}}-$$
$$\overset{|}{(CH_2)_4} \qquad \overset{|}{(CH_2)_4}$$
$$\overset{|}{{}^+NH_3} \qquad \overset{|}{NH_2}$$

+ anhydride : $-\overset{}{\underset{O}{C}}.\overset{}{\underset{O}{O.C}}.R' \longrightarrow R.NH.\overset{}{\underset{O}{C}}.R'$

+ diazonium: $\overset{+}{N}_2.R' \longrightarrow R.NH.N:N.R'$

+ carboxylic acid (via carbodiimide):

$$HOOC.CH_2 R' \longrightarrow R.NH.\overset{}{\underset{O}{C}}.CH_2 R'$$

+ N – hydroxysuccinimide:

N.O.$\overset{}{\underset{O}{C}}$.R' $\longrightarrow$ R.NH.$\overset{}{\underset{O}{C}}$.R'

+ isothiocyante: SCN.R' $\longrightarrow$ R.NH.$\overset{}{\underset{S}{C}}$.NH.R'

FIGURE 7. Reactions of bifunctional chelating agents with lysine amino-acid redidues.

In all the reactions shown, the reactive species of the lysine amino group is unprotonated. The reactions are therefore performed at slightly basic pH with the reaction being directed by the pKa of individual lysine residues.

After lysine, the thiol group of cysteine residues has received most attention (Figure 8). Cysteines exist in native antibodies primarily in the oxidised, disulphide form. These must undergo a mild reduction before the derivatisation reaction can take place.

The carboxylic amino-acids aspartic and glutamic acid can be linked to amino groups via an O-acyclisourea intermediate produced by reaction with carbodiimide (18) (Figure 9). Unfortunately, this reaction is not very efficient and requires, in general, the use of high carbodiimide:antibody ratios which result in undesirable cross-linking of the protein.

CYSTEINE.

(I) Bromoacetamido derivative.

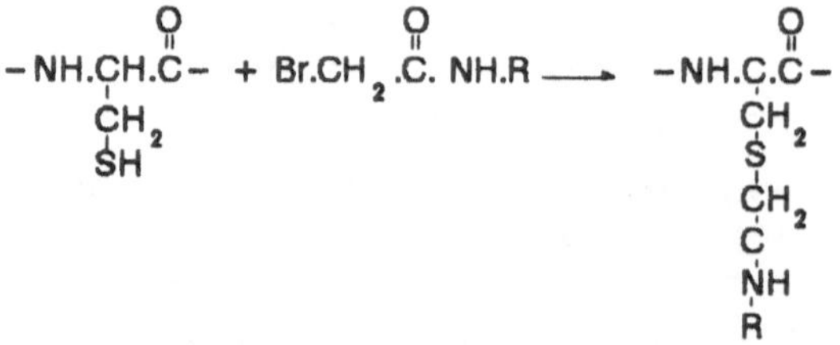

(II) Maleimide derivative.

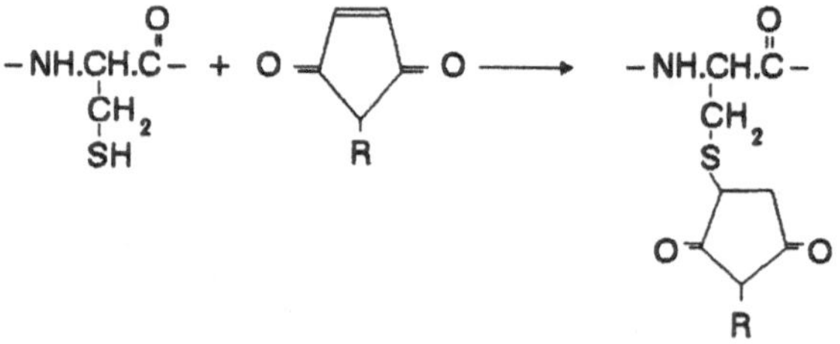

FIGURE 8. Reactions of bifunctional chelating agents with cysteine amino-acid residues.

A number of the reactions described are not 100% specific for particular amino-acids. Thus while the bromoacetamido reaction is highly specific for cysteine in reduced antibody preparations and the isothiocynate reaction normally specific for lysine, other secondary reactions can occur via nucleophilic attack on competing amino-acids such as tyrosine, histidine and methionine.

In general, amino-acids situated throughout the protein molecule will be modified by these reactions resulting in a homogeneous preparation of labelled antibody. While most of these amino-acids will be situated in the constant regions of the immunoglobulin, a proportion will be located in the Complementarity Defining Region (CDR) or antigen combining site (Figure 6). Derivatisation at this point may disrupt the immunoreactivity of the antibody. The development of site-specific labelling techniques which direct the radiolabel to areas distant

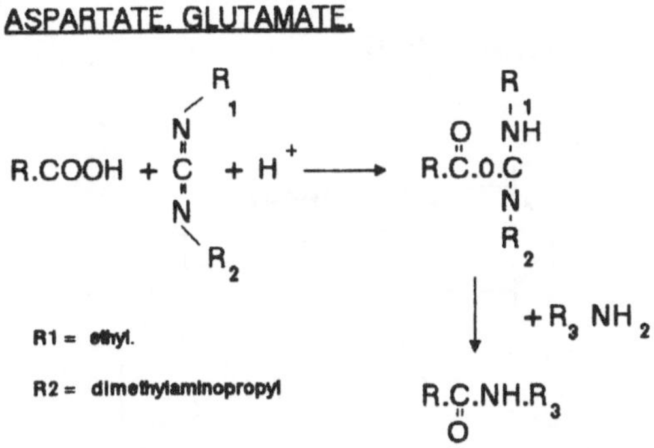

ASPARTATE, GLUTAMATE.

R1 = ethyl.

R2 = dimethylaminopropyl

FIGURE 9. Reactions of aminic bifunctional chelating agent with aspartate or glutamate using carbodiimide as intermediate.

from the CDR has potential advantages particularly in the production of radiolabelled antibodies of high-specific activity for use in radioimmunotherapy.

Bromoacetamido derivatisation of cysteine can be considered to be in-part site-specific because the intra-chain disulphide bonds are located in the centre of the antibody molecule away from the antigen combining site. An alternative method involves the attachment of the chelate to modified oligosaccharide side-chains in the CH2 region of the antibody. After oxidation of the carbohydrate to the aldehyde form a specific reaction with a suitable bifunctional chelating agents can be performed (Figure 10). Antibodies labelled in this manner have been shown to retain their ability to bind antigen to a higher degree than those using non-site-specific techniques (23).

3. PURIFICATION

Since none of the techniques described are 100% efficient in terms of the attachment of the chelate to the antibody, a purification step is normally used to remove free chelate prior to addition of the radiolabel. To this end, a number of publications describe extensive purification steps including column chromatography and dialysis. A complicating factor is that a number of the chelates described appear to bind non-covalently to the protein. Such weakly bound chelates dissociate in vivo resulting in increased non-target uptake of the radiolabel.

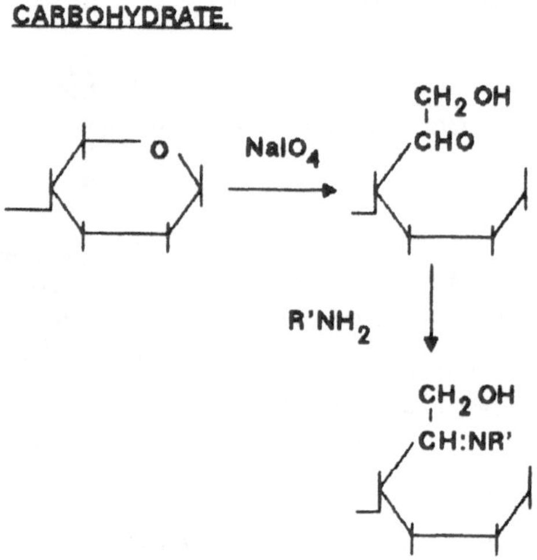

CARBOHYDRATE.

FIGURE 10. Reaction of aminic bifunctional chelating agent with oxidised carbohydrate moiety.

The ideal means of purification in this situation is the use of gel-filtration High Pressure Liquid Chromatography. This technique is highly efficient and in addition to removing the large majority of non-covalently bound chelate can also remove any antibody polymers formed during the derivatisation procedure. Unfortunately most HPLC systems are of steel construction. These may shed ferric ions into the samples resulting in occupation of the chelating groups by contaminating metals. HPLC systems of non-ferrous construction can be designed. One such system that is commercially available is the pharmacia FPLC system which is composed entirely of plastic. Apparatus such as this, although rather expensive, is highly recommended for purification of derivatised antibody preparations.

During the purification procedure, it is advantageous to change the buffer from that in which the derivatisation is performed to one suitable for the radiolabelling procedure such as a citrate or acetate buffer.

4. RADIOLABELLING

Radiolabelling is performed by the simple addition of the indium to the derivatised antibody solution. It is important, however, to avoid the formation of indium hydroxide precipitates that can occur at pH's around neutrality. This is normally achieved by the formation of an intermediate indium complex with a weak acid such as acetate or citrate prior to the antibody addition (8). If the pH of the antibody solution is sufficiently low, however, and providing a sufficient concentration of chelating ions is present, then this intermediate step can be omitted.

5. APPENDIX: LABELLING METHOD

In addition to the theoretical aspects of indium labelling of proteins, the main considerations of the radiopharmacist are frequently practical. The formulation of a reliable, reproduceable and pharmaceutically acceptable system of derivatisation, purification and labelling is essential. The following appendix describes such a system based upon the widely used DTPA anhydride method and highlights those aspects considered to be of particular importance.

NOTE: All reagents and materials should be as free of metal-ion contamination as is practically possible. The highest analytical grade of chemicals, and in particular water, should be used. Disposable plastic containers are preferable to glassware which, if unavoidable, should be of borosilicate glass, washed with 1M hydrochloric acid and rinsed with de-ionised water until neutral to litmus.

5.1 Derivatisation

a) The antibody should be obtained in a suitable buffer (eg Hepes, phosphate, bicarbonate) at a pH compatible with the biological properties of the antibody, but designed to optimise the reaction (pH 8-8.5). Protein concentration (measurable by optical density at 280nm) should be high - > 5 mgs per ml.

b) Cyclic DTPA anhydride (CDTPAA, Sigma chemicals) is dissolved in dry DMSO to a concentration of 2-10 mgs per ml. (DMSO is hygroscopic, anhydrous material should be purchased and stored over a molecular seive).

c) Sufficient CDTPAA solution to give an anhydride:antibody molar ratio of 2-4:1 is added dropwise to the stirred antibody solution. The mixture is then stirred for a further five minutes.

d) At this stage an estimation of the success of the derivatisation procedure is useful. This can be performed as follows: Adjust the pH of a small sample of the reaction mixture to pH 5-6 by the addition of 1M acetate buffer pH 5. Add a trace amount (approx 1MBq) of 111-In-acetate or 113m-In-acetate (See point 3 below) and incubate for 5 minutes. Separate the protein bound and unbound forms of indium either on a short gel-filtration column (eg Sephadex) or by an appropriate TLC method (eg ITLC paper developed with 0.1M citrate buffer). The proportion of activity associated with the protein should be at least 35%

5.2 Purification

The unbound DTPA is now separated from protein-bound DTPA by passage down a suitable chromatographic column. Ideally this should be a plastic-based HPLC column such as the FPLC Superose columns (Pharmacia). Alternatively a 30-60 cm Sephacryl or Sephadex column may be used. (The FPLC or Sephacryl columns will remove antibody aggregates formed during the derivatisation reaction, Sephadex columns will not).

The column should be first equilibrated and the sample then eluted with 0.1M acetate (or citrate) buffer pH 5-6. Fractions containing the monomeric antibody peak should be collected and pooled. After measurement of the protein concentration, the derivatised antibody can be aliquotted into suitable sized patient doses and frozen for future use. At this time samples can be sent for sterility and apyrogenicity testing if required.

5.3 Radiolabelling

To a vial of 111-In-chloride is added sufficient 5M acetate buffer pH 5.5 to produce a final concentration of 0.5M acetate. A vial of antibody is thawed and added dropwise to the indium acetate solution. The mixture is incubated for 10-30 minutes. The radiochemical purity of the preparation can be measured by a suitable TLC method (eg ITLC paper developed in 0.5M acetate buffer pH 6 containing 1 mg per ml EDTA or DTPA). If further purification is required, this can be performed on a Sephadex or HPLC column.

REFERENCES
1.   Hasain, F., Phil., D and Som., P. Chelated In-111. An i-deal radiopharmaceutical for cisternography. Brit J Radiol 1972;, 45: 677-679.
2.   Merrick, M.V., Lavender, J.P., Poole, G.W. et al In-111 labelled bleomycin; clinical experience as a diagnostic agent in tumours of the thorax and abdomen. Brit J Radiol 1975; 48: 279-285.
3   Danpure, H.J. in Radiopharmacy and Radiopharmaceuticals. Ed. Theobald A.E., Taylor and Francis, London 1985:51.
4.   Peters, A.M., Lavender, J.P. et al: Imaging thrombus with radiolabelled monoclonal antibody to platelets. Brit Med J 1986; 293: 1525-1527.
5.   Peters, A.M., Danpure, H.J., Osman., S et al. Clinical experience with Tc-99m-hexamethylpropyleneamineoxime for labelling leucocytes and imaging inflammation. Lancet 1986; ii: 946-949.
6.   Leung, C., Meares, C.F., and Goodwin, D.A. The attachment of metal-chelating groups to proteins: Tagging of albumin by diazonium coupling and use of the products as radiopharmaceuticals. Int J Appl Radiat Isot 1978; 29: 687-692.
7.   Meares, C.F., McCall, M.J., Reardan, D.T., et al: Conjugation of antibodies with bifunctional chelating agents: Isothiocynate and bromoacetamide reagents, methods of analysis and subsequent addition of metal ions. Anal Biochem 1984; 142: 68-78.
8.   Yeh, S.M., Sherman, D.G. and Meares, C.F. A new route to 'bifunctional' chelating agents: Conversion of aminoacids to analogues of ethylenedinitroltetraacetic acid. Anal Biochem 1979; 100: 152-159.
9.   Hnatowich, D.J., Layne, W.W., Childs, R.L. The preparation and labelling of DTPA-coupled albumin. Int Appl Radiat Isot 1982; 33: 327-332.
10. Krejcarek, G.E., Tucker, K.L. Covalent attachment of chelating groups to macromomolecules. Biochem Biophys Res Comm 1977; 77: 581-585.
11. Buckley, R.G., Searle, F. An efficient method for labelling antibodies with In-111. FEBS letters 1984; 166: 202-204.
12. Brechbiel, M.W., Gansow, O.A., Atcher, R.W. et al. Synthesis of 1-(p-isothiocynatobenzyl) DTPA - antibody labelling and tumour-imaging studies. Inorg Chem 1986; 25: 2772-2781.
13. Cole, W.C., DeNardo, S.J., Meares, C.F. et al. Comparative Serum stability of radiochelates for antibody radiopharmaceuticals. J Nucl Med 1987; 28: 83-90.
14. Yeh, S.M., Meares, C.F., Godwin, D.A. Decomposition rates of radiopharmaceutical indium chelates in serum. J Radioanal Chem 1979; 53: 327-336.

15. Welch, M.J., Welch, T.J. Solution chemistry of carrier-free indium. in Radiopharmaceuticals. Eds: Subramanian, Rhodes, Cooper, Sodd. Soc Nucl Med, New York, 1975.

16. Hnatowich, D.J., Childs, R.J., Lanteigne, D. and Najafi, A. The preparation of DTPA-coupled antibodies radiolabelled with Metallic radionuclides: an improved method. J Immunol Meth 1983; 65: 147-157.

17. Pritchard, J.H., Ackerman, M., Tubis, M. and Blahd, W.H. Indium-111-labelled antibody heavy metal chelate conjugates: A potential alternative to radioiodination. Proc Soc Exp Biol Med 1976; 151: 297-302.

18. Janoki, Gy.A., Harwig, J.F., Chanachai, W. and Wolf, W. Ga-67-desferrioxamine-HSA: Synthesis of chelon protein conjugates using carbodiimide as a coupling agent. Int J Appl Radiat Isot 1983; 34: 871-877.

19. Buckley, R.G., Barnett, P., Searle, F, et al: A comparative distribution study of In-111 labelled DTPA and TTHA monoclonal antibody conjugates in a choriocarcinoma xenograft model. Eur J Nucl Med 1986; 12: 394-396.

20. Paik, C.H., Herman, D.E., Eckelman, W.C., Reba, R.C. Synthesis, plasma clearance and in-vitro stability of protein containing a conjugated indium-111 chelate. J Radioanal Chem 1980; 57: 553-564.

21. Taliaferro, C.H., Motekaitis, R.J., Martell, A.E. New multidentate ligands. 22. N.N.'-dipyridoxylethylenediamine-N,N'-diacetic acid: a new chelating agent for trivalent metal ions. Inorg Chem 1984; 23: 1188-1192.

22, Matzku, S., Schumacher, J., Kirchgessner, H., Bruggen, J. Labelling of monoclonal antibodies with a Ga-67-phenolic aminocarboxylic acid chelate. Eur J Nucl Med 1986; 12: 397-412.

23. Rodwell, J.D., Alvarez, V.L., Lee, C. et al: Site specific covalent modification of monoclonal antibodies: In-vitro and in-vivo evaluations. Proc Natl Acad Sci 1986; 83: 2632-2636.

24. Moi, M.K., Meares, C.F., McCall, M.J. et al. Copper chelates as probes of biological systems: stable copper complexes with a macrocyclic bifunctional chelating agent. Anal Biochem 1985; 148: 249-253.

5. LABELLING METHODS WITH TECHNETIUM-99m.

ERLING SUNDREHAGEN

1. INTRODUCTION

Technetium-99m has favourable physical radiation characteristics (halflife = 6.02 h, nearly pure gamma radiation of 140 keV energy) and is distributed as Mo-99/Tc-99m generators to most nuclear medicine departments or radiopharmacy units. Though its radiation is simple, its chemistry is complicated and induces numerous pharmaceutical problems.

Technetium is a transitional element with an electron structure consisting of a krypton-like core with an additional 4d6 5s1 electron structure. This illustrates well the chemical stability of the pertechnetate ion (oxydation state VII), and also how interactions between the d-electrons in Tc's oxidation state III-V with the electrons from electron donating ligands give rise to rather stable electron structures around the nucleus of the technetium complexes.

2. LIGAND EFFECTS

Most methods for Tc-99m-labelling of biological or biochemical substances are based on reactions with the cationic technetyl group

$$O= Tc^{m+}(OH^-)_n$$

where m and n are integers between 0 and 4.

The values of m and n depend on the acidity of the solution, the reducing potential in the chemical surroundings, the ionic strength and the chemical characteristics of the other ions in the solution.

The cationic technetyl groups react with electron donating ligand material, either in the unmodified biological material itself, or with chelating agents linked to the substances to be labelled. The reaction rates and the stability of the end products are strongly dependent on the coordinative characteristics of the ligands.

Most coordinative compounds contain nitrogen, oxygen, sulfur or a halogen as bonding atoms. Different metallic ions prefer different bondings atoms (table 1). A closer consideration of the metal ion charge within the complex formed may explain the differences between the different metals.

Table 1. Preferences for different electron donors of some metallic cations.

Oxygen		Nitrogen	Sulfur	Phosphorous
Mg(II)	Cr(III)	Cu(II)	Cu(I)	Pd(II)
Ca(II)	Fe(II)	Cd(II)	Ag(I)	Pt(II)
Si(IV	Pt(IV)	V(II)	Au(I)	Au(I)
Sn(II)	Zn(II)	Co(III)	HG(I)	Ag(I)
U(V)	Re(V)	Ni(II)		Hg(II)
·Fe(III)				
Be(II)				

The column interposed between oxygen and nitrogen indicates that these cations do not have general preferences between oxygen and nitrogen as electron donors.

The technetyl group is characterized by a rather large ionic radius with low charge to radius ratio. The coordination binding to a ligand involves donation of electron pairs from the ligand to the charged nucleus of the complex, thus a considerable negative charge is transferred on to the metal atom.
In this way electronic structures resembeling those of nobel gases may be formed, resulting in considerable chemical stability, in contradiction to the more pure metallic cations to

which electron donation gives a more unstable chemical condition.

As a first consideration, it could seem favourable to have as high charge to radius ratic and as high ligand polarizability (ability to donate electrons) as possible.

However, if both these quantities rise, the electronegative charge transferred to the metal opppose further electron donation resulting in lower stability. For a given metallic cation, a favourable chemical combination is reached somewhere in the series

F, O, N, S, P.

First transition metals of low oxidation state prefer Nitrogen. Ions of high charge to radius ratio may prefer Oxygen. Ions of low charge to radius ratio (like technetyl groups) have their highest reactivity with sulfur-containing ligands and ions with more than 7 d electrons even with phosphourous ligands.

Alkyl substitution of the hydrogen in the electron donor generally results in lower stability of the complexes. However, free thiols are unstable and may introduce problems to pharmaceutical formulations.

3. DIRECT LABELLING METHODS.

3.1 General

Since nearly all proteins and most polypeptides have chains containing ligand structures as mentioned above, direct complex formation between reduced Tc-99m and the substance to be labelled may take place. Technetium-labelling with high radiochemical quality may be obtained if the protein to be labelled contains free sulfhydryl moities and can be used in a rather high concentration (1). However, most biochemicals to be labelled for radiopharmaceutical purposes should be labelled in low concentrations, since a limited number of receptors or antigens are to be depicted.

Direct labelling may be performed succesfully if the proteins are chemically stable in rather acidic conditions (2). Most such complex formation are, however, disturbed by side reaction, i.e. radiocolloid formations.

Reduced technetium hydrolyzes (3) and forms radiocolloids, especially with reducing stannous ions (4) at the pH corresponding to the stability pH - range of most proteins and cells.

Two radiopharmaceutical approaches have been made to overcome these problems in direct labelling.

3.2 Pre-tinning

Buck A Rhodes describes a pre-tinning ligand exchange technique (5): Stannous ions are reacted with the protenaceous material, and loosely bounded stannous ions are removed, i.e. by gel chromatography. Thus the amount of free stannous ions (and colloids) present in the solution are decreased. However, since rather high stannous concentrations must be applied, reductive cleavage of disulfide bridges within the molecules usually takes place.

3.3 Intermediate complexing

Weakly binding intermediate complexing agents may keep the reduced Tc-99m and stannous ions in solution, preventing radiocolloid formation, and if such intermediates comprise antioxidants, reducing agents with tendency to cause side reactions may be kept at low concentration (6). Thus reduced technetium in non-colloid form may be transferred to the protenaceous material to be labelled.

3.4 Results

The direct labelling methods utilize the ligand effects of the native molecules and cells, which may be sufficient or not, varying between different materials. Erythrocytes are special in this respect, being permeable for several stannous salts, and the stannous ions are bonded to · structures inside the cells. When pertechnetate is added, either in vivo or in vitro, reduction and binding of Tc takes place inside the erythrocytes.

These techniques have been optimalized by different authors (7,8), but are still suspectible to variations if the radiopharmaceutical quality assurance is neglected.

The same pretinning strategy has been applied to white blood cells (9,10) with limited success, mainly because of the low penetrance of stannous ions through the white blood cell membranes.

The introduction of lipophilic Tc-99m-chelates for brain imaging (11) rendered new perspectives for white cell labelling. Such chelates may present the reduced Tc-99m to ligand structures within the cells, thus increasing the labelling efficiency and the stability of the labelled cell. Initial studies are promising (12), but the results vary with variations in the pharmaceutical practice, once again indicating the importance of the quality assurance.

Direct labelling methods are usually lenient to structures to be labelled. The main problems concern radiochemical purity and stability. With regard to labelling of white cells, it must also be taken into consideration that the Auger and convertional electrons of the Tc-99m-radiation contribute to a substantial radiation dose to the labelled cells, in contrast to the low radiation dose to other organs of the patient (13).

4. BIFUNCTIONAL CHELATING AGENTS.

Chelating agents linked to the protenaceous material will regularily increase the stability of the Tc-99m-label of biological material. However, the chemistry of bifunctional chelating agents are presently too rough and time-consuming to be applied on living cells.

Proteins, however, have extensively been modified by such methods. Traditionally, anhydrid coupling of DTPA to proteins has been used and is thoroughly described (14,15). DTPA is a highly stable chelator for metallic ions of high charge to radius ratio, like In-111.

As an example, Myoscint - the pharmaceutical product made from monoclonal antibodies probably most extensively tested in vivo - is made from DTPA coupled monoclonal antimyocin antibody fragments. No reduction in immonoreactivity was reported with In-111-labelled conjugate (16).

These conjugates have also been used with Tc-99m as label (17). Acceptable results were obtained after preparative chromatography. However, in clinical trials inferior results were obtained compared to the results from In-111-label conjugate, and the biokinetics were different (18). This example illustrates how the pharmaceutical industry face new problems when In-111 is replaced by Tc-99m in labelling of monoclonal antibodies.

Other authors report drastic reduction of immunoreactivity by DTPA-coupling, even with In-111-labelling. Fawwaz & al (19) report a loss of titre by a factor 10. In general the results from DTPA-coupling may hardly be predicted and the judgements may also be influenced by the test methods applied (se below). Childs & Hnatowich have optimized the condition for Tc-99m-DTPA-protein formation (20). Unfortunately these conditions are not optimal for most biochemicals to be labelled.

As mentioned, oxygen is not a good electron donor to reduced technetium, hence bifunctional linkers containing sulfur or phosphorous have been investigated. Initiated by his success with compounds for functional kidney studies, Allan Fritzberg has explored the field of thiolated bifunctional linkers, and advocates especially NN-bis-mercapto-acetyl w, w-1-diaminoaliphatic carboxylic acids or amines (21). These ligands may be linked to proteins by water soluble carbodiimides. All thiolated linkers must, however, be handled under reducing conditions in acid solutions to inhibit disulfide bridge formation between protein molecules. Such acidic reducing conditions may, however induce reductive cleavage of the native disulfide bridges within the protein molecules (22). Monoclonal antibodies are usually stable at slightly acidic pH. Several other proteins must be kept at neutral pH, where the disulfide formation may be extensive.

Phosphorous-containing ligands are even easier to polarize. Benedict & al (23) have made diphosphonate-derivatized macromolecules (proteins, polysaccharides, plastic polymers and polypeptides) which can be radiolabelled with Tc-99m without denaturing or loss of biological activity. However, the inventors favourably add amines, thiols or carboxylic acid groups to the diphosphonate-derivatized ligands prior to conjugation. This indicates that phosphorous containing moities may have an inferior Tc-complexing ability compared to these mixed complexing moities.

All bifunctional linkers applied are by nature good metal binders, thus all chemical handeling of these substances should be in small volumes of thoroughly rinsed water, and of course with highest purity available of all chemicals added.

5. REDUCING AGENTS

Most Tc-99m labelling methods involve reduction of pertechnetate to lower oxydation states. The choice of reducing agents should be guided by the following considerations:

a) The electrochemical potential must be sufficient for nearly complete reduction, also when relatively large amount of Tc-99m, Tc-99 and radiation products, hyperoxides and oxygen contamination are present.

b) The electrochemical reducing potential should, on the other hand, not be so strong that disulfide linkages within the biochemical molecules are split.

c) The reducing agent should not form side reaction products with Tc-99m or with the biomolecules to be labelled. If so, chemicals preventing such side reaction should be added.

d) The reduction must take place under pharmaceutical acceptable conditions and should not involve preparative chromatography.

Since its introduction stannous chloride has gained widespread application as a reducing agent (24).

Colloid formation, however, remains a substantial problem, unless large amounts of strongly chelating ligands are linked to the biomolecules. Tartrate in the solution reduces colloid formation (25) and stabilizers may be added to minimize the amount of stannous ions necessary. Dithionite has been chosen in a monoclonal antibody preparation for imaging of necroses (17). Electrolyttical reduction, sodium borohydrid, reduction

by concentrated hydrochlorid acid and metallic cations apart
from stannous ions, have not yet been developed to pharmaceutical acceptable standards for clinical routine use.

6. NITRIDO LABELLING METHODS

Most reductive labelling methods are performed in - or aim
at - a single closed vial with lyophilized content to be combined with Tc-99m-solution. One of the most interesting new labelling techniques does presently not comply with such claims.
On the contrary, this method is performed with a rather complicated set-up for treatment of Tc-99m prior to the labelling of
biochemicals:
Bonnyman and Baldas has demonstrated that $(Tc-99mNX_4)$ - where X
is a halo group, is very useful for Tc-99m-labelling of biochemicals (26). The Tc=N moiety is extremely stable to hydrolysis,
and the nitrido group remains firmly attached to the Tc atom
throughout a number of substitution reactions.

The Tc=N compounds are formed by evaporation until dryness
of the pertechnetate eluate, followed by azide treatment in
presence of hydrochloric or hydrobromic acid. To complete the
reduction and to destroy excess azide the solution is refluxed
for several minutes.
Tc in $Tc-99mNX_4$ is in oxydation state VI. If the ligand has an
ability to act as a reducing agent, further reduction to oxydation state V takes place, followed by a ligand substitution
around the TcN core. Thus, ligands having weakly reducing
moities, i.e. thiols, are especially suited for this labelling
method. A greater impact on radiopharmaceutical practice will
be achieved when a simpler single vial system for Tc=N - formation is obtained.

7. QUALITY ASSURANCE

Quality assurance of Tc-99m-labelling of biological substances
should:
a)   Assure that the labelling method chosen results in a pro-
     duct of high chemical purity and stability with well

preserved biological and/or biochemical activities, and that the labelling process is performed in accordance to the guidelines of good radiopharmaceutical practice.

b) Include quality controls of the performance of the methods, both in the kit-producing industry and at the users site.

As an example the immunological activity of labelled monoclonal antibodies may be controlled by antigen affinity studies. The fraction of the antibodies remaining immunoreactive after the labelling process may be determined by linear extrapolation to conditions representing infinite antigen excess. Such methods are modifications of the Lineweaver-Burk plot, i.e. a double inverse plot of binding fraction versus antigen concentration. Correctly used, such methods will give results independent on the antigen concentration in the actual experiment, and are especially valuable for testing the reactivity of labelled antibodies to diseased cells and tissues (27).
Rapid tests for immunological quality control at the users site are still lacking.

8. RADIONUCLIDE TRANSIT TIME IN DISEASED CELLS

Protenaceous material that binds to cell membranes are usually rapidly internalized by endocytosis. It is well known that radioiodinated materials are deiodinated inside the cells followed by rapid excretion of the radionuclide from the cells, thus limiting the accumulation of radioactivity in the diseased tissue. This excretion may be limited by the design of an appropriate iodination chemistry.

Information on the influence from the technetium labelling chemistry on the cellular transit time of Tc-99m is limited. A biological evaluation of Tc-99m-labelling methods should take this aspect into consideration.

9. CONCLUSION

Several Tc-99m labelling methods are available for pharmaceutical application. The methods chosen must be thoroughly controlled, both chemically biochemically and biologically. We need a better understanding of the general chemistry of Technetium, and improvements in the linking technologies and pharmaceutical performances of the methods.

REFERENCES
1. Eckelman WC. Semin Nucl Med 1975; 5: 5.
2. Persson RBR, Darte L.: Int J Appl Radiat Isot 1977; 28: 97-104.
3. Gorski B, Kock H. J Inorg Nucl Chem 1989; 31: 3565.
4. Sundrehagen E. Int J Appl Radiat Isot 1979; 30: 739-743.
5. Rhodes BA. US Patent 1981; 4.305.922.
6. Sundrehagen E. J Nucl Med 1986; 27: 555-559.
7. Fischer J., Wolf R, Leon A. J Nucl Med 1967; 8: 229-232.
8. Srivastava SC, Chervu LR. Semin Nucl Med 1984; 14: 68-82.
9, Uchida T, Nemoto T & al. J Nucl Med 1979; 20: 1197-1200.
10. Farid NA, White SM, Heck LL & al. Nucl Med Comm 1985; 6: 443-447.
11. Nowothnik DF, Canning LR. & al. Nucl Med Comm 1985; 6: 443-447.
12. Schumichen C, Scholmerich J. Nuc Compact 1986; 17: 274-276.
13. Skretting A, Benestad HB, Sundrehagen E. Radiation doses to cells and body organs from Tc-99m-labelled granulocytes. In print.
14. Hnatowich DJ, Layne WW, Childs RL. Int J Appl Radiat Isot 1983; 33: 327-332.
15. Hnatowich DJ, Layne WW, & al Science 1983; 220: 613-615.
16. Khaw BA, Mattis JA & al. Hybrodoma 1984; 3: 11-22.
17. Khaw BA, Stauss HW & al. J Nucl Med 1982; 23: 1011-1019.
18. Strauss HW. Personal communication.
19. Fawwaz & al. J Nucl Med 1985; 26: 488-492.
20. Childs RL, Hnatowich DJ. J Nucl Med 1985; 26: 293-299.
21. Fritzberg E. European Patent Application 0 118256 A2, 1986.
22. Rhodes BA & al. J Nucl Med 1986; 27: 685-693.
23. Benedict JJ, Poser JW, Degenhandt.CT. European Patent Appl. 207557, 1987.
24. Eckelman W, Richards P. J Nucl Med 1970; 11: 761.
25. Pettit WA, Deland FH, Bennet SJ. Int Appl Radiat Isot 29: 344-345.
26. Bonnyman J, Baldas J. PCT/AU 84/00268.
27. Lindmo T, Boven E. & al. J Immunol Methods 1984; 72: 79-89.

6. ANIMAL MODELS FOR THE EVALUATION OF RADIOPHARMACEUTICALS

ROGER D PICKETT

1. INTRODUCTION

On the 24th November 1986 the Council of the European Communities adopted the directive(1) on the approximation of laws, regulations and administrative provisions of the Member States regarding the protection of animals used for experimental and other scientific purposes, with a view, amongst other things, to reducing to a minimum the number of animals so used. Paragraph 2 of Article 7 of the directive states, "An experiment shall not be performed if another scientifically satisfactory method of obtaining the result sought, not entailing the use of animals, is reasonably and practically available". In the United Kingdom, the Animals (Scientific Procedures) Act 1986(2) came into force on January 1st 1987 and the provisions for licensing particular types of work require that the applicant demonstrates that he has "adequately considered the feasibility of using alternative methods not involving live animals". These moves have been stimulated by the growing public opinion against the widespread use of laboratory animals. In some cases, the level of protest has achieved extreme proportions. The scientific community has also questioned the need for the numbers of animals used in experiments. One particular example in the U.K. has been the report of an Advisory Committee(3) on the use of the LD_{50} test. The Committee urged restraint suggesting that it was not necessary to produce an accurate and precise determination of an LD_{50} requiring the use of large numbers of animals but that a "limit test" to determine an approximate margin of safety would, in most cases, suffice.

On the other hand, there is a need to demonstrate adequately both the safety and efficacy of new products before they can be allowed to be used routinely in patients and indeed to provide those new products as a result of continuing research. Most people in the scientific community recognise the dilemma and indeed the responsibility placed on those working in the field of animal experimentation. There is a moral, and now legal, obligation to critically evaluate proposed animal studies in the light of in vitro alternatives and, if having decided to proceed, we must ensure that the data derived is relevant and useful.

2. RADIOPHARMACEUTICALS AND BIODISTRIBUTION

The efficacy of a diagnostic (or therapeutic) radiopharmaceutioal is dependant upon the physical characteristics of the radionuclide (type of emission, energy, half-life) but more importantly in the context of this discussion, the biological characteristics. These include preferential uptake into, passage through, retention in or exclusion from the biological system to be investigated. Diagnostic information is derived from the observed rate or extent of one or more of these processes. The major use of animals in connection with the evaluation of radiopharmaceuticals is therefore in the study of biodistribution or pharmacokinetics. Ideally the radiopharmaceutical should have no effect on the systems being studied and so, by design, they tend to be pharmacologically inert at the dose levels encountered in normal use. There is however a need to demonstrate the safety of radiopharmaceuticals by the performance of appropriate toxicity testing as well as an analysis of possible pharmacological effects. In vitro techniques can provide much valuable information during all phases of new radiopharmaceuticals research and development but there is also the need for the use of in vivo methods.

2.1. Biodistribution Studies; General Methods

It is important to recognise from the outset that no animal

'model' can be a true replica of the human situation. The results obtained from animal studies must therefore be treated with extreme caution if one endeavours to make predictions of performance in humans. The advantage of using animal models is that, under defined, controlled and usually reproducible conditions, comparisons can be made between the performance of different materials and it is this comparison of performance, rather than the absolute performance that can frequently be extrapolated to humans. For example, Tc-99m-labelled Human Serum Albumin from two different sources may clear from the blood of rats with biological half-lives of 132 minutes and 61 minutes respectively(4). These clearance half-lives will probably not extrapolate directly to humans. But the fact that the first clears more slowly probably will make extrapolation possible and this has been confirmed clinically for those two Tc- 99m-HSA products(5).

It has been stated(6) that "an animal model of a disease is only as useful as the questions we ask of it". We can also say that the choice of biodistribution method will depend on the type of question being asked. Thus the different phases in the development of a radiopharmaceutical require different answers and so different techniques will be used. The three most commonly used methods are shown in table 1. For each there tends to be a 'trade-off' between resolution and quantification:

Table 1. TISSUE DISTRIBUTION METHODS

	RESOLUTION	QUANTIFICATION
Dissection	Low	High
Gamma Scintigraphy	Medium	Medium
Autoradiography	High	Low

2.1.1. Dissection. This is the most widely used laboratory bio-distribution method. For gamma emitting nuclides it is reasonably straightforward requiring simply the administration of the test material by the chosen route followed, after an appropriate interval by sacrifice and dissection. Assaying the dissected and weighed organs or tissues for radioactivity provides a precise quantitative measure of the biodistribution. The advantages of the method, as applied to routine rat or mouse studies are that it is accurate, precise and reasonably quick. Capital outlay, apart from the gamma counter, is minimal. The main disadvantages stem from the fact that the animals need to be sacrificed. It is, therefore, only possible to obtain information from an animal at a single time point and a number of animals may be required, there being no possibility of using each animal as its own control unless simultaneous dual-isotope studies are performed. The resolution of the method is only as good as the dissection technique and some a priori knowledge of biodistribution is required.

2.1.2. Gamma Scintigraphy. Using a gamma camera, tissue distribution can be obtained qualitatively in the live animal. Our standard technique is to anaesthetise two male rats with urethane (ethyl carbamate, 1.0-1.5 g/kg i.p.).
This anaesthetic, although treated as a suspected carcinogen, conveniently produces complete anaesthesia and immobilisation without significantly affecting cardiovascular or respiratory function. It does however have some adverse effects on liver function and this should be borne in mind when studying compounds metabolised and/or cleared via this route. The anaesthetised rats are placed side-by-side in the prone position on the surface of a gamma camera fitted with a high resolution parallel hole collimator. The intravenous injection of approximately 30 MBq of technetium 99m to each animal provides sufficient counts for good images. Polaroid pictures are taken throughout a study lasting typically one hour and during this time data are also recorded on magnetic tape or computer disk. The resolution achieved is in many cases better than that achieved

during dissection studies, since when looking at the whole animal one does not have to decide in advance which organs to look at and distribution within an organ can often be detected. The particular advantages of the use of the gamma camera include the fact that it is not necessary to sacrifice the animals to obtain the data. One may, therefore, study the time course of distribution by continuous observation of the same animal or the use of the same animal on more than one occasion thereby reducing interanimal variations, or costs if one is using expensive animals. A further advantage is the immediate availability of qualitative information on the principal route, rate and extent of excretion and an indication of any possible organ specificity of uptake. Disadvantages include the need for anaesthesia or physical restraint, stresses which may perturb the distribution of the cardiac output and hence the distribution of the test article. Quantification may not be precise but of course the main disadvantage is the capital cost of the equipment.

Other external detecting devices such as the small animal whole body rectilinear scanner are available. The resolution achievable is probably inadequate for most research and development applications.

When interest is not so much in the qualitative biodistribution of activity throughout the body but rather in the rate of passage into or through a defined organ, for example the kidney, then a correctly positioned well collimated stationary probe can provide valuable information. The same information would also be available from regions of interest studies using a gamma camera but the sensitivity of a probe can be much greater.

2.1.3. Whole Body Autoradiography. At an appropriate time after the administration of the radioactive substance, the test animal (usually rat, mouse or guinea pig because of their size) is sacrificed, quick-frozen in a cardice/hexane freezing mixture and then embedded in a resin. This block of resin with the whole body inside it is then placed in a refrigerated microtome. Whole body sections are out and, after freeze-drying, the sections are apposed to X-ray film (we use Agfa Osray M3 or Kodak AX3 or CX1). Development of the film reveals the biodistribution of activity within the section. The principal advantage of this technique is the high resolution achievable and the quality of the results, which at a glance allow an overall appreciation of general biodistribution. Quantification is possible by use of pre-calibrated ladder sections and microdensitometry applied directly to the film. More recently, sophisticated systems have become available for the digitization of autoradiographic images to allow computer processing. As for dissection techniques, whole body auto- radiography suffers from the disadvantage of necessitating the sacrifice of the animal. Additionally it may take days or even weeks before the results are available.

The above basic methods may be applied in all phases of radiopharmaceuticals research and development. For a typical commercial diagnostic radiopharmaceutical there are four phases which may overlap. These are research, development, regulatory and production. The requirements for animal testing in each phase are different.

3. APPLICATION OF ANIMAL MODELS TO RADIOPHARMACEUTICALS
3.1 Research

From an industrial point of view the research phase of a project will probably involve the evaluation of a range of compounds or labelled entities for defined properties. Additionally all new compounds will be subjected to a rapid qualitative assessment of biologioal behaviour following intravenous administration to laboratory rodents - typically rats or mice. The gamma camera is ideal for this initial screen enabling the investigator to form an immediate opinion of biodistribution characteristics and approximate rate and mode of excretion. The qualitative data may be supplemented by dissection of the animals to provide quantitative data or by analysis of the computer stored data for particular regions of interest. More specific models may be used to screen compounds for more specific properties. For example, a Tc-99m-labelled complex for the imaging of cerebral bloodflow must cross the blood-brain-barrier and be retained within brain tissue. At Amersham the gamma camera was used to great effect in the initial screening of over 100 compounds for this property. Supplementary dissection studies provided quantitative data which could be related to the physico-chemical characteristics of the complexes to enable the generation of structure distribution relationships whereby the synthesis of further compounds could be rationalised.

Radiopharmaceuticals for other applications can be screened in a similar manner. In many cases normal, healthy animals can be, and have been successfully used. For example see the excellent reviews of Fritzberg and Bloedow(7) on hepatobiliary radiotracers and McAfee and Subramanian(8) on renal radiodiagnostic agents. For some other targets the situation is not quite so simple. For example the species variability in the heart uptake of compounds intended for use as myocardial perfusion agents is well known(9) The now famous "Noah's Ark" experiments have clearly demonstrated the need for caution in the interpretation of initial screening data.

In this respect the rat appears to be particularly non-selective, many labelled complexes showing acceptable accumulation in the myocardium only to be shown to be unpromising in subsequent screening in other species. The possibility of using human tissue must be considered as part of the screening protocol. In vitro studies using cultured myocytes or even the use of perfused human myocardium from transplant subjects must represent the most promising avenues in this area.

As we have said, animal models are used not as replicas of humans but as laboratory tools to provide information prior to an evaluation in humans. This is because one cannot perform speculative research in human subjects. However, there is one area where human tissue, in vivo can be used and this is in screening potential radiopharmaceuticals for the detection or localisation of tumours. In recent years there has been enormous interest in the potential of radiolabelled monoclonal antibodies for this application. As discussed by Moldofsky et al(10), the long tedious path that leads to the eventual selection of those few antibodies that may have uses in diagnostic imaging begins in the initial laboratory screening of secreting hybridomas both to select fairly specific antibodies and to eliminate many of those with lower affinities. Cross reactivity with normal human tissue should also be assessed in vitro with a view to excluding those antibodies showing unwanted reactivity, for example with circulating blood cells or bone marrow. Once purified antibody can be produced, then subsequent testing of the radiolabelled antibody must demonstrate preserved immunoreactivity and specificity. Most of these studies are more appropriately performed using in vitro techniques such as immunocytochemistry.

Although it can be argued that there are many differences between animal models and patients, it seems prudent to evaluate potential antibodies in an animal model to demonstrate both in vivo stability of the labelled antibody and significant localisation within tumour. Some researchers however feel that studies in animal models are not a necessary prelude to clinical evaluation in patients. A Joint Committee of the Cancer Research Campaign and the U.K. National Institute for Biological Standards and Control, in discussing the inadequacy of animal models, has suggested that "the only valid information obtainable from animals is .... an indication of antibody localisation in xenografts of human tissues(11). Similarly, Lentle (12) has suggested that "it may be that in the particular context of radioimmunodiagnosis, animal studies will be used for quality control of the radiopharmaceutical but will be ineffectual in predicting clinical effectiveness since human cancers transplanted into animals do not adequately model disease in human beings".

For fundamental research into mechanisms of uptake and retention animal tumours have undeniable application. For a detailed review see Wiebe(13). This includes a listing of more

than 200 animal tumours that have been used in radiotracer uptake studies. Such models may be of great beneficial use in the
evaluation of radiopharmaceuticals where localisation may be
nonspecific, relying on such factors as increased permeability
of capillary beds to macromoleoules; increased macrophage activity and necrosis; increased cell membrane permeability; hypoxia or anoxia; blood flow and blood vessel formation and increased metabolic activity. Where the localisation mechanism is
more specific, such animal models may sometimes be misleading.
For example, Spencer et al(14) reported on the lack of accumulation of I-131 MIBG in the transplanted NCI mouse neuroblastoma C1300 whereas adequate localisation was demonstrated in the
adrenal glands of the same mice. Since human neuroblastomas
accumulate I-131 MIBG the authors call into doubt the biochemical similarity of the mouse neuroblastomas and the human tumour although other possible explanations of the data were also
put forward. It is for this type of reason that we have found
it more convenient and useful to use human tumour tissue, xenografted into laboratory animals.

To overcome the problems of rejection, thymectomised or immunologically, chemically or radiologically immune compromised
animals may be used. We, however, have routinely used the gene-
tically immune compromised nude mouse as the xenograft host.
This mutant was first found in 1962 and lacks the thymus gland
which results in the inability of the nude mouse to recognise
the xenograft, in that mediated immune functions are severely
impaired. The first transplantation of a human malignant tumour was successfully demonstrated in 1969(15). Gallagher(16)
has listed a number of requirements of a model which are met by
the human tumour-nude mouse system.

1. Human solid tumours are readily accepted.
2. Many tumours can be transplanted serially.
3. Tumours have a constant and predictable growth rate that
   can be followed by simple measurement.
4. Human characteristics are preserved in mouse-grown tu-

mours as judged from microscopic examination, chromosome analysis, isozyme studies, and immunological investigations.

5. Extensive and long range investigations are possible.
6. There is no need for difficult, time consuming or continuous immunosuppressive treatment that might influence results.

It has also been suggested that, for certain tumours, there is a higher viability in nude mice compared to immunosuppressed animals.

The literature contains many examples of the successful use of xenografted human tumours from a variety of origins.

Tumour Origin	Reference(s)
Osteogenic Sarcoma	17, 18
Colon Carcinoma	19, 20, 24, 29, 30, 33, 34
Soft Tissue Sarcoma	21
Choriocarcinoma	22, 23
Lung adenocarcinoma	25
Urinary Bladder Carcinoma	26
Pancreatic Carcinoma	27, 28
Breast Tumour	31
Melanoma	32, 34
Lymphoma	34
Glioma	35

I do not propose to analyse each of these models with respect to their applicability to radiopharmaceuticals research but rather to highlight some of the more general problems that may be encountered in their use.

If the researcher decides to proceed with a xenograft model, the choice of tumour cell line must of course be based on factors such as suitability with respect to antigenic determinants, growth rate and availability. Consideration should be given to the possibility of antigen secretion or "shedding". Interaction of a labelled antibody with circulating antigen could lead to diminished availability of the injected antibody and to a marked change in distribution and/or excretion characteristics(33).

Special handling facilities are required to maintain the animals, firstly because of the susceptibility of immune compromised animals to infection, particularly murine hepatitis and secondly to protect staff from the potential hazards of handling human tissue, particularly from viral infection or the transmission of oncogenic material to the operator. We have found plastic film isolators, maintained under negative pressure and HEPA filtration at both inlet and outlet, to be a practical approach not only for the maintenance of the animals but all our experimental work is also carried out using such a system. On a practical note, some of the problems encountered in the literature appear to centre on the size of tumour and the expression of results of quantitative studies. For example, recent correspondence in the Journal of Nuclear Medicine(36,37) has emphasized the problem of comparing the uptake of radioisotope in tumours of differing weight. In very small tumours the percentage uptake expressed per gram of tumour can lead to some surprisingly high values, whereas in large tumours this value may be disappointingly low. When expressed as absolute percentage uptake in the tumour, it must be remembered that a mouse tumour of 1g corresponds, on a weight for weight basis, to a 2-3 kg tumour in a human and thus high percentage uptake figures must be treated with caution in extrapolations to man. The effect of tumour weight on the uptake of a monoclonal antibody to CEA has been studied by, amongst many others, Duewell et al(24) and as tumour size increased absolute percentage uptake increased but relative uptake (per g) decreased. These authors have remarked that the higher relative uptake in small tumours is obvious because in small tumours practically all the tissue will be viable and active thus allowing the circulating specific antibody to reach the corresponding epitopes. In bigger tumours only the surface and well vascularised parts of the tumour are reached. Moreover, central necrotic parts of larger tumours may have lost much of their antigenic properties. A high concentration of circulating antigen produced by the larger tumours will also result in the formation of immune complexes which are mainly deposited in the liver thus making less antibody available for uptake by the tumour.

To overcome these problems it is imperative that studies are performed on tumours of standardised and defined weight range, preferably less than 1g, and before the onset of significant necrosis. This will obviously depend on the particular tumour model chosen.

In addition to expressing quantitative data in the form of absolute percentage uptake or relative uptake (per gram) a number of other parameters may be usefully applied. The ratio of relative uptake in tumour to the relative uptake in normal tissue, eg blood, muscle or skin may give an indication of specificity of distribution in the animal being studied but changes in this value may be an indication of changes in the overall biodistribution of the injection rather than its specificity for tumour. In order to rule out non-specific effects responsible for tumour localisation of activity, some researchers favour the concurrent injection of a nonspecific, labelled immunoglobulin. In this way the tumour uptake relative to normal tissue can be compared for the test and control materials to give a "localisation index". Thus:

$$\text{Localisation Index (LI)} = \frac{\% \, g^{-1} \, \text{tumour}/\% \, g^{-1} \, \text{muscle (test antibody)}}{\% \, g^{-1} \, \text{tumour}/\% \, g^{-1} \, \text{muscle (control antibody)}}$$

This concept has been taken one step further by Mann et al (32) who, in mice bearing two separate tumours, have compared the localisation indices of two coinjected antibodies each specific for one tumour and non-specific for the other. The resulting figure is termed the "binding advantage". Since, however, the uptake of each antibody in muscle appears in both the numerator and the denominator the index is more simply a comparison of the relative concentration of each antibody in each tumour.

Thus:

$$\text{"Binding Advantage"} = \cfrac{\cfrac{\text{Anti A \% g}^{-1}\text{ tumour A/Anti A \% g}^{-1}\text{ muscle}}{\text{Anti B \% g}^{-1}\text{ tumour A/Anti B \% g}^{-1}\text{ muscle}}}{\cfrac{\text{Anti A \% g}^{-1}\text{ tumour B/Anti A \% g}^{-1}\text{ muscle}}{\text{Anti B \% g}^{-1}\text{ tumour B/Anti B \% g}^{-1}\text{ muscle}}}$$

$$= \cfrac{\text{Anti A \% g}^{-1}\text{ tumour A/Anti B \% g}^{-1}\text{ tumour A}}{\text{Anti B \% g}^{-1}\text{ tumour B/Anti B \% g}^{-1}\text{ tumour B}}$$

As might be expected these authors have shown some specificity of binding of their radiolabelled antibodies to tumours but the tumour to tissue ratios and the "binding advantage" appeared to depend more on tumour type and size than on specificity of the antibody.

This serves to reiterate the point made earlier that animal studies of this type, when used cautiously, enable comparisons between test agents to be made but present many problems to the unwary if direct extrapolation to man is attempted.

As regards the growing interest in the use of radiopharmaceuticals for the labelling of cells this is a product directed research area where I would argue that the use of animal models is not justified. The availability of human blood for in vitro studies renders the use of animal models unnecessary during the research phase. At this stage the questions being asked are whether the potential radiopharmaceutical can efficiently label the blood cells be they erythrocytes, platelets or leucocytes and whether the successfully labelled cells retain their functional characteristics. Answers to these questions can be supplied quickly and reproducibly using in vitro techniques. For all cell types labelling efficiency and retention or elution characteristics can be demonstrated by in vitro incubation of precisely known cell numbers with controlled concentrations of the radiopharmaceutical. A wide range of in vitro techniques are then available to measure the effects, if any, on cellular function. Such tests which are described in more detail elsewhere include for platelets, aggregation in response to suitable stimuli and for leucocytes phagocytic activity or chemotaxis. Note should, however, be taken of the possible influence of functional inhibitors which may be present in the labelling mixture(38). Some animal models, however, may be applicable during the development or regulatory phases of a project and these will be discussed later. The same is true of labelled proteins which can be very well characterised in vitro and such techniques are much more applicable during the research phase where quick and reliable qualitative answers are required to screen potential radiopharmaceuticals or labelling methods.

Thus, during the research phase we need quick, reproducible methods to enable us to select candidate compounds for future development. It is doubtful if animal models play a significant role here except, as I have indicated, in the initial qualitative assessment of biological behaviour using normal animals and possibly the use of tumour models for radiolabelled antibodies to tumour antigens.

3.2 Development

The research and development phases of radiopharmaceuticals projects may overlap. As a result of initial in vitro and in vivo screening a potential radiopharmaceutical may be identified. This may have been as a result of a targetted programme aimed at a specific goal or of a serendipitous observation. Whichever route, the next stage is to formulate the compound or refine the method such that it may be presented as a convenient and effective radiopharmaceutical. Much of the testing during the development phase is repetitive and changes in the performance characteristics in response to formulation modifications or under a variety of storage conditions for example, need to be monitored. For this reason test systems used during the development phase of a project must be simple, reproducible and preferably quantitative. Because the specifications for a product are now much more clearly defined, performance criteria can be more precisely set and studies performed which will quantitatively identify deviations from these criteria. Minor formulation changes, for example the amount of reductant in a Tc-99m-based radiopharmaceutical kit, can fundamentally affect the performance of a radiopharmaceutical. Chromatographic methods are available to enable in vitro assessment of radiochemical purity and in vitro stability but during the development phase, frequent use is made of more specific animal models. These models may have been refined during the research phase such that a model will be used to test for specific parameters. Experience during our researoh into Tc99m-labelled brain agents showed that the percentage of activity excreted in the urine was a sensitive indicator of the presence of less lipophilic complexes and that the brain to muscle ratio (% g^{-1}) provided a good indication of efficacy. A dissection protocol was thus developed to provide accurate quantitative data for these and a number of other parameters whereby trends in efficacy could be related to formulation changes.

Similarly for monoclonal antibodies the experience of the research phase can identify possible variables in the animal model which need controlling to enable the model's use as an indicator of performance during development testing. For example a single time point after injection may be selected as that appropriate for assessing antibodies from different sources, a variety of labelling techniques and storage conditions and the consideration of the use of whole antibody or fragments. The effect of labelling methods and formulation modifications on the immunoreactivity or specificity can be readily assessed in vitro. This is the preferred method when one considers the variability of the quantitative results derived from tumour

bearing animals and the sometimes subtle changes in performance
that need to be measured during formulation optimisation. However, the principal use of animal models during the development
phase of a labelled antibody is in the assessment of in vivo
stability and the possible benefits of interventions to reduce
background activity. For example, Ward et al(39) showed that
intraperitoneally administered metal chelating agents such as
deoferrioxamine, DTPA and EDHPA could affect the biodistribution of In-111 or Ga-67 citrate in normal BALB/c mice but that
similar treatment did not affect the biodistribution of indium
or gallium labelled monoclonal antibody in normal or tumour
bearing mice. However, in similar studies, Goodwin et al(40)
have elegantly demonstrated that daily administration of $CaNa_2$
EDTA i.p. enhances the whole body disappearance of activity
from mice injected with monoclonal antibody labelled with In-
111 via the bisanhydride of DTPA but not antibody labelled via
bromoacetamido benzyl EDTA. Although observations of these authors were statistically significant they concluded that both
labelling methods gave conjugates of sufficient stability for
studies lasting one to three days.

Similar studies are of use in the assessment of other labelled proteins(4). One factor that can be a very useful indicator
of the quality is the clearance rate. Whole body retention has
been used as a limit test for radiopharmaceuticals that are
supposed to be cleared rapidly. For example the USPXX1 monographs for Tc-99m Ferpentetate and Pentetate require that not
more than 5% be retained in mice at 24 hours after injection.
On the other hand, for products such as Tc-99m-HSA clearance
from the blood should be minimal and thus a "not less than"
limit is specified in the blood of rats 30 minutes post injection, determined by dissection. An alternative approach might
be to take sequential blood samples from, for example, the ear
vein of rabbits to compute a clearance half-life. This approach
has been used by Janoki et al(41) to assess factors influencing
the biological properties of labelled proteins.

Analysis of the blood clearance curves in rabbits revealed

marked differences in the clearance of I-125-HSA and of iodinated HSA which had been reacted with the conjugation reagents
carbodi- imide or glutaraldehyde. Similarly, they demonstrated
using the same model, the marked enhancement of the clearance
of I-125 fibrinogen following treatment of the rabbits with
antihuman fibrinogen antibody three minutes after the injection
of the radioactive material.

Blood levels can be measured at two selected time points if,
based on prior experience, it is known that the clearance curve
is essentially monophasic between those times. Calculation of
the zero time intercept may also give information on the radiochemical purity, if an injection standard is also counted and
an assumption made about the animal's blood volume or an internal blood pool marker is used.

For radiolabelled cells a variety of models exist. Having
established that the appropriate cell type can be successfully
labelled and that, in vitro, there is no significant loss of
label or function, this must also be demonstrated in vivo. Unfortunately one cannot guarantee that the in vivo biological
behaviour of radiolabelled animal cells will parallel that seen
in the clinical situation, nor can one expect labelled human
cells to perform comparably when administered to animals. However, models may again be used to compare formulations or techniques against a known standard performance based on previous
experience with that model. The simplest model would be, as we
have discussed, to assess the whole body retention or blood
clearance rates and compare the data with laboratory standards.

As regards biological models to assess the function of labelled cells there are many examples in the literature. Most
are again aimed at understanding fundamental principles rather
than for the evaluation of radiopharmaceuticals during product
research and development. However, one or two may be of use.

For thrombus detection using radiolabelled platelets, in
vitro methods such as the Chandler's loop(42) are of particular
relevance. In spite of the fact that an in vivo thrombus is
not an inactive substance, unaffected by changes in the sur-

rounding blood, there is good general agreement between in vi
tro and in vivo incorporation as noted by Kempi et al(43). They
compared their in vitro data with the in vivo results of Stahlberg et al(44) who used an anaesthetised rabbit model. Carbonyl
iron particles (100 mg) were injected into an ear vein and were
trapped in the external jugular vein by a magnetic field. After
30 minutes the magnet was removed and the fixation of the trapped iron particles was verified by X-ray imaging and by gamma
camera imaging of previously injected I-125-fibrinogen. A study
involving 14 radiopharmaceutical preparations looked at the
thrombus to blood ratio for the test substance normalised to
the thrombus to blood ratio for the I-125-fibrinogen to correct
for differences in thrombi between the experiments. The results
suggested the involvement of non-specific interactions for most
of the substances showing the best thrombus to blood ratios.
Baker et al(45) evaluated this and two other rabbit models for
the comparison of Tc-99m-labelled plasmin with a range of acy-
lated plasmins. Neither the jugular iron particles nor a woollen thread in the abdominal inferior vena cava proved successful in their hands. Dissection showed that the iron particles
appeared to occlude the veins and very little thrombus was present (although they did inject five times as much carbonyl iron
as did Stahlberg et al). The woollen thread produced negligible
thrombus and being adjacent to the spinal column and abdominal
viscera was in a position which interfered with scintigraphic
imaging. However, they did have success with a third model.
This was based on those of Rosenberg(46) and Didishem(47) and
involved exposing and clamping the jugular vein of anaesthetised rabbits. Undiluted formalin solution was carefully applied
to the surface of the vein for 20 minutes avoiding contact with
other tissues. The area was then thoroughly swabbed with saline, the clamp removed and the incision closed. Three hours after thrombus induction the test materials were injected on the
contra lateral side. Uptake was recorded using a gamma camera
or by dissection. Although some difficulty was experienced (the
overall success rate was approximately 70%) thrombus formation

was usually reliable, resulting in a thrombus weighing 30-300 mg. One complication may result from the relatively high uptake of radioactivity per gram found in the intima of the vein in the formalin damaged area. The model was subsequently used however by the same group (48) to study Tc-99-fibrinogen and In-111-labelled autologous platelets. Both were shown to be superior to the previously studied Tc-99m-plasmins. The same model was also successfully used by Spett et al(49) to compare the biological behaviour of fibrinogen labelled directly with iodine-125 or with Tc-99m via three different routes. Not only could the thrombus to blood ratio be determined for each product but when coupled with in vitro data on clottability and in vivo blood clearance and biodistribution data marked differences in thè behaviour of the otherwise similar products could be demonstrated.

In addition to providing a detailed review of the use of In-111-labelled platelets to study platelet function in animals, Mathias and Welch(50) also evaluated four animal models resulting in intravascular platelet deposition. These models were a) an acute arterial endothelium injury produced by an inflated balloon catheter in the abdominal aorta of non-human primates (Macaca) b) atherosclerosis in non-human primates fed a high cholesterol diet for four years c) a canine model of acute coronary artery thrombosis induced by placing a small length of copper wire in the left anterior descending coronary artery and d) small diameter vascular grafts of PTFE or Dacron inserted into the carotid or femoral arteries of dogs. All four methods proved useful in producing platelet deposition as indicated by the uptake of In-111-labelled autologous platelets.

Because of the value of the animals involved in these models they do not lend themselves to study by dissection. Gamma scintigraphy was therefore used but blood pool subtraction techniques were required and quantification was complicated. The models were, however, effectively used to assess antithrombotic and thrombolytic drugs. PTFE vascular grafts have also been used in acute studies in pigs(51). The grafts were inserted into each femoral artery of anaesthetised pigs. About 10 to 15

minutes prior to re-establishing blood flow the animals received autologous platelets labelled with In-111-oxine. The uptake
of activity over the grafts was monitored continuously by external imaging and was reproducibly found to reach a peak at 60
minutes after the re-establishment of bloodflow through the
grafts. Thereafter the activity ratios decreased slowly. These
authors do not, however, report observations when the labelled
platelets were administered after clot formation.

Such methods may also have application in the evaluation of
labelled anti-platelet antibodies(52).

For the evaluation of labelled red blood cells a simple,
reproducible animal model is possible because the principal use
of these cells is to image the normal blood pool. The current
methods of red blood cell labelling with technetium by pretinning appear equally effective in animals and humans and so
straightforward blood clearance measurements provide an accurate quantitative measure of efficacy.

Labelled leucocytes are useful in the localisation of inflammatory lesions and a number of models have been developed.
Again for product development reproducible quantitative methods
are desirable but most enable only a qualitative judgement of
efficacy. A septic abscess model has been successfully used by
Hawker(53) to evaluate the in vivo behaviour of mixed leucocytes labelled via Tc-99m-HMPAO or In-111-oxine. Their model
was an intra-abdominal abscess produced in rats by implantation
of a 1 cm x 2.5 cm cylinder of open-pored polyester sponge impregnated with a 24-hour broth culture of rat faeces.

Studies were performed by imaging or dissection during the
acute phase at seven days post implantation or during the chronic phase after 28 days. The method is simple and reproducible
producing walled-off, pus-filled abscesses. Using the method,
Hawker has demonstrated that during both the acute and chronic
phases, uptake of Tc-99m- or In-111-labelled mixed leucocytes
was equivalent but the more efficient clearance of eluted technetium reduced background levels more effectively such that at
24 hours post injection, target to non-target ratios were better for the Tc-99m-HMPAO labelled cells.

Thus, during the research phase of a radiopharmaceutical project we initially use qualitative or semi-quantitative systems to screen compounds for selected properties. During the development phase we require quantitative methods to compare the performance of the chosen candidate compound or entity in different formulations or under different storage conditions.

3.3 Regulatory

During the regulatory phase the manufacturer must assemble a package of information which should not only describe and fully characterise the product but demonstrate satisfactorily the product's safety and efficacy. This will require a detailed description of pharmacokinetics in normal animals and is probably best derived from dissection studies. At the same time it may also be desirable to determine the biological fate of administered activity in an appropriate model of human disease. Such information is useful in the generation of radiation dose estimate prior to initial human evaluation. Caution must, however, be exercised when extrapolating such data to humans. Note should be taken of possible differences in the rate of the biodistribution process in animals of different sizes or age(8) and differences in body composition. For example, on a weight for weight basis extrapolation from rat to man yields human testes weighing 0.5 kg each or the size of two grapefruits.

Frequently, biodistribution in the normal animal is insufficient evidence of efficacy particularly if the function to be monitored is not present in the normal animal. For this reason some of the models described above can be used but it should be remembered that their prior use was to <u>compare</u> the performance of products or formulations. The inadequacy of animal models for direct extrapolation to humans for the purpose of making a statement of efficacy must be recognised. However, their value in comparing performance in relation to an existing product of known clinical utility will justify their use in certain circumstances.

As regards safety evaluation, it should be borne in mind that diagnostic radiopharmaceuticals are intended for use in a hospital environment by medically qualified staff. They are thus not available to members of the general public. In the majority of cases it is expected that a patient may only receive a single injection. The extent of toxicity testing must therefore reflect this proposed usage rather than be dictated by the criteria normally applied to conventional therapeutic or prophylatic medicinal products. In most cases it should not be necessary to determine an LD_{50} for example but more appropriately to demonstrate safety in laboratory animals at dose levels several orders of magnitude in excess of the proposed human dosage. For products of biological origin there are additional complications. For example, a position paper on polypeptide medicinal products derived from biotechnology, prepared by the European Federation of Pharmaceutical Industries Associations- (54) has stated that "the potential safety risks involved with biotechnologically produced polypeptides can better be ruled out by chemical, biochemical, physical and (in vitro) biological analysis than by extensive toxicological studies such as are usually conducted on conventional medicinal products". It is further stated that "compounds homologous for humans may be expected to induce immune responses when administered to heterologous experimental animals. After repetitive parenteral administration, the resulting symptoms in these animals are not related to the pharmacological and toxicological activity profile of those compounds and, due to the imunogenicity of human proteins in animals, do not provide relevant information about the safety of such products. For this reason, long term animal studies are not meaningful and toxicological investigations can at most be carried out during a restricted time period". In conclusion the position paper emphasises that safety and efficacy should be assured by limited short term animal tests accompanied by physico-chemical and (in vitro) biological methods.

3.4 Production

Once approved for sale, a product must be subject to stringent quality control procedures. For well established radiopharmaceuticals the guidelines set out in the pharmacopoeial monographs indicate tests for product identity, quality and safety. In this context two uses of laboratory animals are relevant - biodistribution tests and general safety (or abnormal toxicity) tests.

In the European, British and United States Pharmacopoeias there are 21 current monographs for Tc-99m-radiopharmaceuticals. In 19 of these a biodistribution test is described or specified. Ten different tests are described but, in general, they all involve the intravenous administration of the product to rats or mice. At a suitable time after injection the fate of the administered activity is determined with respect to specified acceptance criteria. These are quoted in the form of limits for the percentage of the administered activity which must be achieved or not exceeded. Yet again, the tests do not set out to enable a prediction of clinical performance but strive to compare the behaviour of a particular product in relation to pre-determined standards based on a knowledge of the performance of clinically efficacious material. The tests may detect the presence of radiochemical impurities as well as provide an indication of product quality.

The toxicity of conventional radiopharmaceuticals will have been established during research and development. Quality assurance testing using in vitro methods can establish that the identity and quality of the product are the same as that previously studied. However, it is felt that, for products of biological origin there is the possibility for the introduction of extraneous contaminants during manufacture. For this reason tests for abnormal toxicity are prescribed. These involve the intravenous and/or intraperitoneal administration of the test substance to mice and/or guinea pigs. In animals of the correct weight, the daily or weekly weight gain can be a rather sensitive indicator of toxicity. Thus, apart from overt, obvious signs of toxicological response a weight gain over the test period is required to demonstrate lack of toxicity.

4. CONCLUSIONS

Animal models play a valuable role in all phases of a radio-pharmaceuticals research and development project. Moral and legal constraints require that we consider whether our proposed use of laboratory animals is justified and in making these decisions we should be fully aware of the limitations of animal models. The principal advantage to be gained from the use of animal models is that reproducibly, and in a controlled fashion, comparisons may be made between the performance of a test substance and predetermined qualitative or quantitative criteria or against similar products of known clinical utility.

REFERENCES
1. Council Directive of 24 November 1986 on the approximation of laws, regulations and administrative provisions of the Member States regarding the protection of animals used for experimental and other scientific purposes. Official Journal of the European Communities, vol 29 No.L358. 1986.
2. Animals (Scientific Procedures) Act 1986, Her Majesty's Stationery Office, London.
3. Advisory Committee on the administration of the Cruelty to Animals Act 1876, Report to the Secretary of State on the LD_{50} Test. Home Office, London 1979.
4. Kristensen, K. Biodistribution in rats of ^{99m}Tc-labelled human serum albumin. Nucl Med Com 1986; 7: 617-624.
5. Masi, R. et al - Personal Communication.
6. Reid, L.M., Holland, J., Jones, C. et al. Some variables affecting the success of transplantation of human tumours into the athymic (nude) mouse. In Proceedings of the Symposium on the Use of Athymic (Nude) mice in Cancer Research, Houchens, D.P. and Ovejera, A.A. (eds). Stuttgart. Gustav Fischer 1978.
7. Fritzberg, A.R. and Bloedow, D.C. Animal Models in the Study of Hepatobiliary Radiotracers. In: Animal Models in Radiotracer Design. Lambrecht, R.M. and Eckelman, W.C. (Eds) Springer-Verlag 1984.
8. McAfee, J.C. and Subramanian, G. Experimental Models and Evaluation of Animal Data for Renal Radiodiagnostic Agents. In: Animal Models in Radiotracer Design. Lambrecht, R.M. and Eckelman, W.C. (Eds) Springer-Verlag 1984.
9. Ketring, A.R., Deutsch, E. Lisbon, K. and Vanderheyden, J-L. The Noah's Ark experiment. A search for a suitable animal model for the evaluation of cationic Tc-99m Myocardial Imaging agents. J Nucl Med 1983; 24: 9.
10. Moldofsky, P.J., Powe, J. and Hammond, N.D. Monoclonal Antibodies for Radioimmunoimaging: Current Persperctives. Nuclear Medicine Annual 1986: 57-103.
11. Joint Committee of the C.R.C. and N.I.B.S.C. Operation Manual for Control of production, preclinical toxicology and Phase I trials of anti-tumour antibodies and drug antibody conjugates. Br J Cancer 1986; 54: 557-568.

12. Lentle, B. Tumour Detection with Radiolabelled Agents. In: Current Applications in Radiopharmacology. Billinghurst, M.W. (Ed) Pergammon Press 1986.
13. Wiebe, L.I. Small Animal Oncological Models for Screening Diagnostic Radiotracers. In: Animal Models in Radiotracer Design, Lambrecht, R.M. and Eckelman, W.C. (Eds). Springer-Verlag, 1984.
14. Spencer, R.P., Leutzinger, E.E., Spitznagle, L.A. et al. Problem with Mouse Neuroblastoma (C1300) as a Model for Iodine-131 MIBG Uptake. J Nucl Med 1986; 27: 726.
15. Rygaard, J. and Povlsen, C.O. Heterotransplantation of a human malignant tumour to the mouse mutant "nude". Acta Pathol Microbiol Scand 1969; 77: 758-760.
16. Gallagher, B.M. Monoclonal Antibodies: The Design of Appropriate Carrier and Evaluation Systems. In: Animal Models in Radiotracer Design, Lambrecht, R.M. and Eckelman, W.C. (Eds) Springer-Verlag, 1984.
17. Nakamura, T., Sakahara, M., Hosoi, S. et al. In vivo radiolocalisation of antiosteogenic sarcoma monoclonal antibodies in osteogenic sarcoma xenografts. Cancer Res. 1984; 44: 2078-2083.
18. Pimm, M.V. and Baldwin, R.W. Quantitative evaluation of the localisation of a monoclonal antibody (791T/36) in human osteogenic sarcoma xenografts. Eur J Cancer Clin Oncol 1984; 20: 515-524.
19. Keenan, A.M., Colcher, D., Larson, S.M. and Schlom, J. Radioimmunoscintigraphy of human colon cancer xenografts in mice with radioiodinate monoclonal antibody B72.3. J Nucl Med 1984; 25: 1197-1203.
20. Colcher, D., Keenan, A.M., Larson, S.M. and Schlom, J. Prolonged Binding of a radiolabelled monoclonal antibody (B72.3) used for the in situ radioimmunodetection of human colon carcinoma xenografts. Cancer Res 1984; 44: 5744-5751.
21. Brown, J.M., Greager, J.A., Pavel D.G. and Gupta, T.K. Localization of radiolabelled monoclonal antibody in a human soft tissue sarcoma xenograft. 1985; 75: 637-644.
22. Searle, F., Adam, T. and Boden, J.A. Distribution of intact and F(ab') fragments of anti-human chorionic gonadotrophin antibodies in nude mice bearing human choriocarcinoma xenografts. Cancer Immunol Immunother 1986; 21: 205-8.
23. Buckley, R.G., Barnett, P. Searle, F. et al. A comparative distribution study of In-111-labelled DTPA and TTHA monoclonal antibody conjugates in a choriocarcinoma xenograft model. Eur J Nucl Med 1986; 12: 394-396.
24. Duwell, S., Horst, W. and Westera, G. Uptake of a monoclonal antibody against CEA (Tumak 431/31) in a human colon tumour (Co-112) xenografted in the nude mouse. Cancer Immunol Immunother 1986; 23: 101-106.
25. Shani, J., Wolf, W., Chanachai, W. et al. Labelling and Comparative Biodistribution of the Monoclonal Antibody KS 1/4 in Nude Mice Bearing Human Lung Adenocarcinoma. Nucl Med Biol 1986; 13: 379-382.
26. Bubenik, J. Kieler, J., Perlmann, P. et al. Monoclonal an-

tibodies against human urinary bladder carcinomas: selectivity and utilization for gamma scintigraphy. Eur J Cancer Clin Oncol 1985; 21: 701-710.

27. Klapdor, R., Montz, R., Lander, H. et al. Untersuchungen zur intratumoralen Radioimmuntherapie transplantierter Pankreaskarzinome mit 131-J-anti-CA 19-9/CEA. Nuc Compact 1985; 16: 424-427.

28. Senekowitsch, R., Baum, R.P., Maul, F.D. et al. Biokinetische Studien zur szintigraphischen Darstellung xenotransplantierter menschlicker Pankreaskarzinome mit 131 Jod Markierten $F(ab')_2$ - Fragmenten verschiedener monoklonaler Antikorper. Nuc Compact 1985; 16:414-419.

29. Andrew, S.M., Pimm, M.V., Perkins, A.C. and Baldwin, R.W. Comparative imaging and biodistribution studies with an anti-CEA monoclonal antibody and its $F(ab)_2$ and Fab fragments in mice with colon carcinoma xenografts. Eur J Nucl Med 1986; 12: 168-175.

30. Hagan, P., Halpern, S.E., Chen, A. et al. In vivo kinetics of Radiolabelled Monoclonal Anti-CEA Antibodies in Animal Models. J Nucl Med 1985; 26: 1418-1423.

31. Jones, P.L., Gallagher, B.M. and Sands, M. Autoradiographic Analysis of Monoclonal Antibody Distribution in Human Colon and Breast Tumour Xenografts. Cancer Immun 1986; 22: 139-143.

32. Mann, B.D., Cohen, M.B., Saxton, R.E. et al. Imaging of Human Tumour Xenografts in Nude Mice with radiolabelled Monoclonal Antibodies: Limitations of Specificity due to Non-Specific Uptake of Antibody. Cancer 1984; 54: 1318-1327.

33. Rogers, G.T. Limitations Associated with the Use of Labelled Antibodies Against CEA for Potential Tumour Localisation and Therapy. Eur J Cancer Clin Oncol 1986; 22: 1127-1133.

34. Hagan, P.L., Halpern, S.E., Dillman, R.O. et al. Tumor Size: Effect on Monoclonal Antibody Uptake in Tumour Models. J Nucl Med 1986; 27: 422-427.

35. Bullard, D.E., Wikstrand, C.J., Humphrey, P.A. et al. Specific Imaging of Human Brain Tumour Xenografts Utilizing Radiolabelled Monoclonal Antibodies (MAbs). Nucl Med 1986; 25: 210-215.

36. Pimm, M.V. and Baldwin, R.W. Effect of Tumour Size on Monoclonal Antibody Uptake in Tumour Models. J Nucl Med 1986; 27: 1788-1789.

37. Cohen, M.B., Saxton, R.E. and Mann, B. Effect of Tumour Size on Monoclonal Antibody Uptake in Tumour Models. J Nucl Med; 1986: 27: 1789-1790.

38. Peters, A.M., Lavender, J.P. and Hawker, R.J. Correspondence Nucl Med Comm 1987; 8: 183-184.

39. Ward, M.C., Roberts, K.R., Westwood, J.M. et al. The Effect of Chelating Agents on the Distribution of Monoclonal Antibodies in Mice. J. Nucl Med 1986; 27: 1746-1750.

40. Goodwin, D.A., Meares, C.F., McTigne, M. et al. Metal decomposition rates of In-111-DTPA and EDTA conjugates of monoclonal antibodies in vivo. Nucl Med comm 1986; 7: 831-838.

41. Janoki, G.A., Korosi, L. and Spett, B. Factors influencing the Biological Properties of Labelled Protein. In: Current Applications in Radiopharmacology, Billinghurst, M.W. (Ed) Pergamon Press, 1986.

42. Chandler, A.B. In vitro Thrombotic Coagulation of the Blood. A Method for Producing a Thrombus. Laboratory Investigation 1958; 7: 110-114.

43. Kempi, J. and Persson, B.R.R. In vitro interaction between venous Blood Clots and Radiopharmaceuticals. Nuklear Medizin 1985; 24: 173-179.

44. Stahlberg, F., Andersson, L. Edenbrandt, C-M. and Strand, S-E. Quantitative in vivo and in vitro comparison between radiolabelled colloids, biomolecules and blood cells in their ability to diagnose deep venous thrombosis. Nucl Med Comm 1984; 5: 741-762.

45. Baker, R.J., McLaren, A.B. Campell, J., et al. Studies of Tc-99m-Acyl plasmins as agents for thrombus detection. Eur J Nucl Med 1985; 10: 155-159.

46. Rosenberg, N., Moolten, S.E. and Vroman, L.A. calibrated technique for experimental production of venous thrombosis. Surgery 1959; 46: 764-767.

47. Didishem, P. Animal models useful in the study of thrombosis and antithrombotic agents. In: Progress in hemostatis and thrombosis. Greene and Stratton inc., N.Y. 1978; 1: 165-187.

48. Campbell, J., Bellen J.C. Baker, R.J. and McLaren, A.B. A Comparison of Radiolabelled Agent for Thrombus Imaging using a Rabbit Model. Nucl Med Biol 1986; 13: 295-300.

49. Spett, B., Janoki, G.A. and Korosi, L. Comparative Study Between direct labelled and DTPA-chelated Human Fibrinogen. In: Current Applications in Radiopharmacology. Billinghurst, M.W. (Ed). Pergamon Press 1986.

50. Mathias, C.J. and Welch, M.J. In-111-Labelled Platelets for the Detection of Vascular Disorders in Animal Models. In: Animal Models in Radiotracer Design. Lambrecht, R.M. and Eckelman, WE.C. (Eds). Springer-Verlag 1984.

51. Christenson, J.T., Arvidsson, D., Qvarfordt, P. et al. The early platelet uptake and distribution of platelets in small-diameter polytetra fluoroethylene (PTFE) vascular grafts in vivo. Eur J Nucl Med 1985; 10: 160-164.

52. Som, P., Oster, Z.H., Zamora, P.O. et al. Radioimmunoimaging of Experimentatl Thrombi in Dogs Using Technetium-99m-Labelled Monoclonal Antibody Fragments Reactive with Human Platelets. J Nucl Med 1986; 27: 1315-1320.

53. Hawker, R.J. Personal Communication.'

54. European Federation of Pharmaceutical Industries Associations, Working Party No. 1. Position paper on Production and Quality Control of Polypeptide Medicinal Products derived from Biotechnology, March 1986.

7. MODELS FOR SAFETY TESTING OF IMMUNOREACTIVE PHARMACEUTICALS

O. SVENDSEN, H.B. CHRISTENSEN, P. JUUL, J. RYGAARD

1. INTRODUCTION

Pharmaceuticals of different molecular structure and different therapeutic classes may cause immunological reactions (immunostimulation, immunosupression or allergy) either by themselves or by acting as haptens. Also, it is known in some instances as described later in this presentation, - and as may be further supposed - that toxic effects of drugs, in themselves indetectable, may cause release of antigens that seconda-rily can lead to an immune response and subsequent tissue damage. The immunological reaction may not only take place in patients treated with the drug but also in experimental animals used for preclinical safety testing. The topic of the present paper concerns those pharmaceuticals which are species-specific proteins developed in order to be identical or related to human proteins or to interact with human cell membrane receptors or antigens. Since such pharmaceuticals are species-specific for humans, they may accordingly be immunoreactive in experimental animals used for safety testing and animals may lack specific ligands for these substances. Additionally there could be, as briefly mentioned above, autoantigens released due to the primary effect of the pharmaceutical, but not distinguishable as a two step reaction in conventional testing systems. These pharmaceuticals include monoclonal antibodies and products derived by recombinant DNA technology.

The main safety concern with monoclonal antibodies is the possibility that they may interact with antigenic determinants in unintended target tissue or on structurally related proteins. Medical products derived by recombinant DNA technology such as endogenous human proteins (hormones, interferons, enzymes, cytokines and neuroactive peptides) may exert other effects than via receptors in target tissue, i.e. a systemic or exaggerated pharmacological effect. In addition, they are immunologically active in animal models used for safety testing. This may result in formation of neutralizing antibodies or in immune complex deposit disease. The manufactoring process of recombinant DNA products also pose the possibility of toxic contaminants in the final product, and minimal amounts of other potential antigens.

The conventional toxicological studies to be conducted in animals with a new drug before marketing can be summarized as follows:

1. Acute toxicity in two species with at least oral and intravenous dosing.
2. Chronic toxicity (6-12 months) in a rodent and a non-rodent species.
3. Reproductive toxicology and embryotoxicity.
   3.1. Teratogenicity and fetal toxicity in one or two species (rats/rabbits).
   3.2. Reproduction toxicity for two generation in one species (rats).
   3.3. Pre- and postnatal toxicity in one species (rats).
4. Mutagenicity (gene mutation and chromosome aberration) in vitro and in vivo.
5. Carcinogenicity in one or two species (mice and rats).
6. Local toxicity with drugs for parenteral or topical application.

The methods used are generally accepted and also validated for the preclinical safety evaluation of new drugs manufactured by conventional methods. Similar preclinical toxicity studies in animals with monoclonal antibodies and species-specific recombinant DNA products have been performed for some years. The experience accumulated so far with recombinant human interferon shows that routine testing procedures failed to identify side-effects (influenza-like symptons, leucocytopenia and serum transaminase elevation) observed in subsequent clinical trials (Fent and Zbinden, 1987). However, retrospectively some specialized animal studies have identified some known side effects. On the other hand, with interleukines characteristic toxic effect can be studied in laboratory animals.

2. MONOCLONAL ANTIBODIES

The fusion of myeloma cells with B-lymphocytes from immunized animals may result in formation of hybrid cells, so-called hybridomas. They have the cabability of secreting antibodies and they can grow continuously which allows for production of antibodies in large quantities. By means of cloning technique it is possible to select hybridomas with stable secretion of antibodies of defined specificity. The antibodies are homogeneous populations of immunoglobulin molecules having antibody combining sites selected to bind uniformily to descrete antigenic determinants.

This technique has resulted in many new investigational biotechnological products which previously it would not have been possible to produce in adequate quantities for pre-clinical and clinical research. Monoclonal antibodies are available as new drugs for anti-tumour therapy, immunomodulation and passive immunisation. They are also used as carriers to deliver cytotoxics, other xenobiotics and radionuclides to particular tissues or receptors.

General classical toxicological studies in animals may be of only limited relevance to studies of monoclonal antibodies. They are likely to be immunogenic in test animals. However, classical toxicological studies might be relevant with monoclonal antibodies coupled to drugs, toxins, radionuclides or other xenobiotics.

Unintentional reactions of monoclonal antibodies with human tissue are also a matter of concern. Preclinical safety testing ought to include immunohistochemical or cytochemical studies on different human tissues for cross-reactivity of monoclonal antibodies. If cross-reactions are encountered, the resultant hazard or risk for potential recipients should be evaluated. Other control problems with monoclonal antibodies are possible presence of viruses or potentially tumorigenic material for which testing also has to be considered.

The overall extent of testing has to be influenced by the clinical use of the product. A monoclonal antibody for use in otherwise untreatable life-threatening conditions may require less extensive testing.

In addition to toxicity testing, consideration may be given to studies of distribution, metabolism, excretion and kinetics in a relevant animal model.

3. MEDICINAL PRODUCTS DERIVED BY RECOMBINANT DNA TECHNOLOGY

Recombinant DNA techniques have enabled the production of highly purified species-specific proteins. As a result a number of natural endogenous human proteins with considerable biological and pharmacological potency (hormones, interferons, neuroactive peptides, coagulation factors, enzymes and cytokines) have become available for preclinical studies.

These novel molecules have to be tested for toxicity in non-homologous animal species. However, due to their immunogenicity they may cause formation of antibodies in the test animals or the animals may lack specific ligands. This is a new situation in toxicology and it poses a major challenge for toxicologists in universities, industry and regulatory authority.

For a new drug to be used clinically over a longer period preclinical data on the following issues have to be presented: 1) Acute toxicity in two species, 2) chronic toxicity in a rodent and a non-rodent, 3) teratogenicity in a rodent and a non-rodent, 4) reproduction toxicity in a rodent, 5) mutagenicity testing and 6) carcinogenicity in two species. Studies on teratogenicity and reproduction toxicity require short-term dosing. With the new species-specific human proteins there is a substantial risk of antibody formation in the animals especially in those used for chronic toxicity and carcinogenicity testing.

On the testing of such products several documents have recently been released by international and national regulatory authorities. The majority deals with these issues in draft form only. The documents are advisory or discussion documents. New legislation for these products is considered inappropriate as it would probably be out of date when issued and could hinder developments in such a rapidly moving field. At present the review by most regulatory agencies is based on the intended use of the product and is done on a case-by-case basis.

Breefly, the regulatory agencies have taken the following standpoints. If the amino acid sequence is exactly the same as the natural product, and this has been sufficiently tested previously, toxicity testing of the substance may be omitted. However, antigenicity and pyrogenicity data should be provided and also data on toxicity of impurities and contaminants. The pharmacodynamic action should be investigated as for a normal drug unless the product is identical to that occurring naturally. Studies on pharmacokinetics and metabolism should be performed as for conventionally produced drugs. Comprehensive preclinical safety testing, including toxicology would be expected for a product which differs in any way from its natural counterpart, or has an entirely new structure. Certain products, however prepared, would be expected to be intrinsically associated with adverse biological properties. For such products conventional toxicological studies may not be applicable.

An international working group has recently summarized existing experience from the testing of such products and attempted to transfer the resulting knowledge into future testing strategies (Teelmann et al., 1986). Current experience in experimental safety testing of species-specific proteins has largely been gained with human interferon or interleukines.

The efficacy and safety of recombinant DNA products may be compromised by manufacturing procedures. Since in addition safety evaluation based on routine toxicity testing is problematic, strong regulatory requirements for quality control and for detailed description of technical, analytical and biological characterization of these products seems highly justified.

3.1. Repeated dose toxicology

The overall problems related to testing recombinant DNA products produced for clinical use can be divided into two subgroups.

Firstly, the product may in humans or animals exert other effects than via receptors in target tissue. In case this effect is species-specific, experiments in animals would either not predict the effect or the effect would be a false positive response. As a consequence this effect would not be recognized until human exposure takes place or the product will be considered unsuitable for clinical trials and discarded.

Secondly, in preclinical studies the dose levels applied to animals are usually considerably higher than clinical dose levels. The consequence of this fact is two-fold. In repeated dose studies changes secondary to the exaggerated effect on the target tissue may show up. This is well known from testing of human growth hormone in animals. The high dose level may also cause a systemic response elicited from receptors which are not affected at physiological levels of the product.

The risk of this phenomenon does not only take place in animal studies but may also be seen in cases where the product clinically is given in dosages higher than that required to substitute the underlying deficiency. This is in particular a risk in clinical trials with new neuroactive peptides which may affect other than diseased central neurons or normal peripheral neurons.

The above mentioned difficulties have a common denominator namely the selection of appropriate animal species for preclinical testing. Not only should the species be relevant for pharmacodynamic testing and for the identification and understanding of potential side-effects, it should also be immunologically relevant. The two first points of relevance are common for all types of pharmaceuticals except that many of the new products have a molecular structure similar or identical to endogenous molecules.

The third point of relevance is difficult to handle. In repeated dosing studies in animals formation of neutralizing antibodies or functionally inhibiting antibodies may take place in two to three weeks time. In addition, indications of development of immune complex disease or other immunopathological conditions may show up. In case of antibody formation, toxic effects may be masked on the one hand, and immunopathological phenomena have on the other hand to be considered as irrelevant findings.

Neutralizing antibody formation may primarily be a common rate-limiting factor in the study of chronic toxicity of species-specific substance. For this reason analyses for such antibodies should be included regularly in the conduct of the study for termination of the study when present.

The predictive value of animal studies would probably be elevated if homologous products were used for each species of test animals. In this case the development of antibodies would be reduced and the animals carry species-specific ligands.

Contaminants or impurities are another element of concern. However, from the production process they are supposed to be present in such a low level that no effect can be expected to show up in routine toxicity testing. These tests have a rather low sensitivity. The problems related to impurities can best be handled by development of good analytical procedures.

3.2 Reproductive toxicology

It is known from testing of hormonnally active compounds that species-specific proteins may cause reproduction toxicity and fetal toxicity. The absence of immune reactions is a prerequisite for meaningfull reproduction toxicity studies because immunogenicity may interfere with pregnancy or cause malformations. For this reason it is important to analyse for serum antibodies in beforehand or during the course of reproduction toxicity studies in pregnant animals. They may react differently from non-pregnant animals.

Among the three types of reproduction toxicity studies the standard time of dosing is considerably shorter in teratogenicity studies than in multigeneration studies and perinatal studies. Since immunogenicity may increase with duration of dosing, teratogenicity studies should be performed at first. The experience gained from chronic toxicity studies on the likelihood of immunogenic reactions may be helpful for deciding whether there is a rationale for the conduct of multigeneration or perinatal studies.

3.3 Mutagenicity

Mutagenicity testing of high molecular weight substances seems in many cases not worthwhile. There is no clear rationale for the conduct of mutagenicity testing on naturally occurring polypeptides or species-specific human proteins. With novel polypeptides consideration may be given to mutagenicity testing in in vitro systems. However, the uptake mechanisms of such products may lead to negative or misleading results.

4. SECONDARY IMMUNE REACTIONS TO DRUG-INDUCED CELL/TISSUE DAMAGE.

Toxic reactions of drugs, and intended cell/tissue damage induced by antibody-targeted radiotherapy may in themselves be undetectable in ordinay toxicity testing, but observed reactions may occur due to a secondary immune response. This may probably be both cellular and/or humoral.

It is most important to be aware of this fact and to be able to distinguish the primary and secondary phase. The primary phase will in all probability be dosedependent, whereas an immune response, once elicited, may cause a biological "landslide". In our own laboratory we have been able to study this effect in a diabetes model, where we obtain differential responses in normal athymic animals as mentioned below. In our opinion, more investigations should be focused on this point.

5. EPILOGUE

Since the major problem with preclinical safety testing of species-specific human proteins obviously is formation of antibodies in experimental animals, we have speculated whether immunologically incompetent animals could be used as a model for testing. Immunologically incompetent experimental animals are readily available in the form of athymic nude mouse and rat strains. One prerequisite for their usage as test model in toxicology would be that they respond with toxicological manifestations similar to those seen in conventional laboratory mice and rats. Athymic animals are not useful for identification of toxicity mediated through thymus-dependent immunological mechanisms. This seems to be the case for the diabetogenic effect of streptozotocin in mice (Buschard and Rygaard, 1978) or mercury chloride induction of immune complex deposits in certain strains of mice (Hultman and Eneström, 1987).

The mentioned prerequisite was tested in a pilot study in our laboratories where mercury chloride or paracetamol were given to groups of immunologically incompetent and competent mice and rats of both sexes. The animals were killed one or two days after dosing. The liver was examined microscopically from animals given paracetamol and kidneys from animals given mercury chloride.

Mercury chloride caused renal corticomedullary tubular necrosis in most rats and mice. Immunocompetent female mice were most sensitive. In rats the males were most sensitive. Paracetamol caused focal hepatic necrosis in all groups of mice and most marked in immunocompetent females and athymic males. The dose selected (500 mg/kg, i.p.) for the rats was apparently too small to cause hepatic damage or the time span from dosing to sacrifice too short (Poulsen et al., 1981).

Although the results are limited and some variation was seen, they seem encouraging for further evaluation of the suitability of atymic rodent strains as models for single and repeated dose toxicity testing of immunogenic potential drugs.

Acknowledgement

The mice and rats were gifts from Bomholtgaard Breeding and Research Centre, DK-8680 Ry, and Møllegaard Breeding Centre, DK-4623 Lille Skensved, respectively.

REFERENCES
1.   Buschard, K. and Rygaard, J. Is the diabetogenic effect of streptozotocin in part thymus-dependent? Acta path microbiol scand Sect C, 1978; 86: 23-27.

2. Fent, K. and Zbinden, G. Toxicity of interferon and inter-
    leukin. TIPS 1987; 8: 100-105.
3. Hultman, P. and Eneström, S. The induction of immune com-
    plex deposits in mice by oral and parenteral administra-
    tion of mercuri chloride: Strain dependent susceptibility.
    Clin Exp Immunol 1987; 67: 283-292.
4. Poulsen, H.E., Petersen, P. and Vilstrup, H. Quantitative
    liver function and morphology after paracetamol admini-
    stration to rats. Eur J Clin Invest 1981; 11: 161-164.
5. Teelman, K., Hohbach, C., Lehman, H. and The International
    Working Group. Preclinical safety testing of species-speci-
    fic proteins produced with recombinant DNA-techniques. An
    attempt to transfer current experience into future testing
    strategies. Arch Toxicol 1986; 59: 195-200.

8. A MOUSE TUMOR MODEL FOR SCREENING RADIOTRACER UPTAKE INTO PRIMARY NEOPLASMS AND METASTATIC DISEASE

L.I. WIEBE, A. KANCLERZ, K. LUU AND E.E. KNAUS.

1. INTRODUCTION

Tumor progression and the subsequent formation of metastases present theoretical and pratical barriers to successful diagnosis and treatment of neoplastic disease. Metastatic disease still accounts for the majority of cancer related deaths, particularly because of difficulty in early detection and delineation of metastases (4,21). Early detection, a major objective of oncological nuclear medicine, will be achieved only through an understanding of the mechanisms of tumor progression and the response of normal tissues to invasion by neoplastic tissue. The use of radiotracers in diagnostic oncology, and the use of experimental tumor models for radiotracer design have been the subject of previous reviews (6-8,11,15,20).

A large number of radionuclides and radiotracers have been used for both experimental and clinical studies of oncological disease. Of these, the radiotracer of choice for tumor diagnostic scintigraphy is Ga-67 citrate despite its disadvantages which include cost, high radiation dosimetry, low photon flux in the desired energy range, slow clearance through the liver and intestines and its non-specific uptake in abscesses and other damaged tissues (5,8,10,19). The successful clinical use of Ga-67 for imaging pulmonary cancers (15), lymphatic neoplasia (7) and other cancers (8) has been shown to be dependent not only on the type of neoplasm involved, but also on the objectives of the investigator (12). Although the literature is replete with reports of Ga-67-use in clinical nuclear and experimental biodistribution studies (1,2,3,14,16,22), there are only limited data on its biodistribution over the full term of neoplastic disease including spontaneous metastases.

In an attempt to further characterize the process of spontaneous metastasis of the murine Lewis lung carcinoma, we have studied the biodistribution of Ga-67 citrate at various stages of tumor growth. We now report on the influence of the primary tumors of different size, due to different numbers of implanted tumor cells, on the metastases formation in the lungs and in the lymphatic system, and the response of normal tissues as reflected by Ga-67 citrate uptake.

2. MATERIALS AND METHODS

Inbred male $B_6D_2F_1$ mice were purchased from the Charles River Laboratory, Wilmington, Ma, and delivered to the animal facility of the Faculty of Pharmacy when weaned. At the beginning of each experiment they were 8-10 weeks of age and weighed 20-25 g. The Lewis lung carcimona (LLC) used in this study originated from the Institute of Cancer Research, London, England. Tumors were maintained in vivo by serial i.m. transplantation 10 days after inoculation. LLC was used as a source of tumour tissue for animal experimentation. Mechanically isolated cells (10^5 or 10^6 in 25 microliter standard MEM) were injected i.m. into the right thigh. Viability of injected cells, determined by the trypan blue exclusion test, exceeded 85%.

Ga-67 citrate was kindly supplied by Mr. J.R. Scott of the Edmonton Radiopharmaceutical Centre. Animals injected with 10^5 tumor cells were divided into three groups of 6 animals each: 4 mice were used for the Ga-67 uptake study and 2 for scientigraphic imaging, performed on days 16, 24 and 33 after tumor challenge. Studies on mice injected with 10^6 cells were made on days 16 and 24 only. Separate control groups of health animals were used on the same days, 3 for dissection to examine the quantitative biodistribution of Ga-67 and 2 for imaging. In each case Ga-67 citrate was injected into the lateral tail vein 48 hr before dissection or imaging at a dose of 37 kBq and 3.7

MBq, respectively. On a given day mice were sacrificed by as-phyxiation in carbon dioxide followed by partial exsanguination by cardiac punture. Tumors were removed and their outer part separated from the inner, necrotic region. Pulmonary metastases and metastases to the regional lymph nodes were excised, and the remaining pulmonary tissue, liver, spleen, kidneys and bone were dissected. Radioactivity of all the samples was measured by gamma counting in a Beckmann 8000 gamma well counter. The tissue:blood ratios, % of dose/organ and % of dose/g tissue were calculated for each tissue sample. Imaging was carried out with a Searle pho gamma camera and ADAC data system on animals anesthesized with Ketamine and Xylazine. A pinhole collimator was used for imaging (100,000 counts per image) at an animal to crystal distance of 10 cm. After imaging the animals were sa-crificed for quantitative radiometry.

Figures 1 to 7 show the animal tumor model used in the pre-sent study. Figures 9 and 10 are the scintigrams of the animals bearing i.m. LLC. Figure 8, submitted for comparison, shows an image of the healthy control.

Statistical analysis of the data was performed using the Student's t-test. A p value of 0.05 or less was considered sig-nificant.

3. RESULTS AND DISCUSSION

The biodistribution data were expressed as the % of admini-stered dose/weight of the wet organ or the % of administered dose/g of the wet tissue and the relative Ga-67 uptake as the tissue:blood concentration ratio. Ga-67 concentrations in the blood increased during the whole observation period, reaching the highest level on day 24 after implantation in the animals challenged with 10^6 cells (see Figure 11). The radionuclide up-take in the external and inner parts of the primary tumor, ex-pressed per weight of the whole specimen, decreased with time as the tumor volume increased. Consequently, there was a de-crease in the relative uptake (tumor:blood ratio) of the radio-tracer in the whole tumor volume and also in both the outer, viable and inner, necrotic parts of each LLC (see Figure 12).

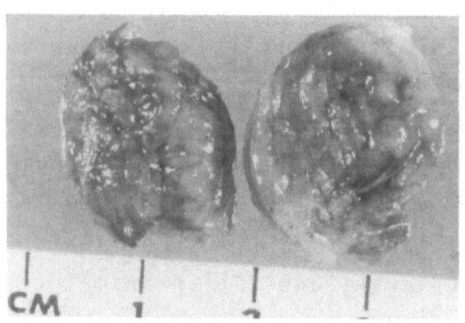

FIGURE 1.Primary Lewis lung carcinoma dissected on day 21 after i.m. implantation (10^5 cells). Note large necrotic center and the narrow outer rim of viable tumor tissue.

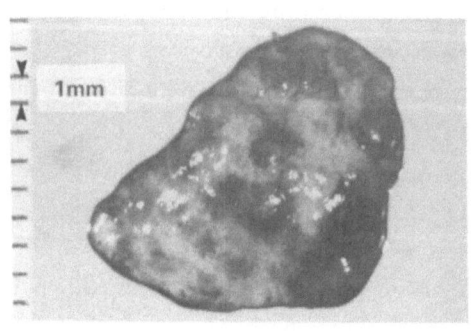

FIGURE 2. Separated lobe of excised lungs from the mouse bearing Lewis lung carcinoma on day 33 after implantation. Metastatic nodules of different size are visible on the surface.

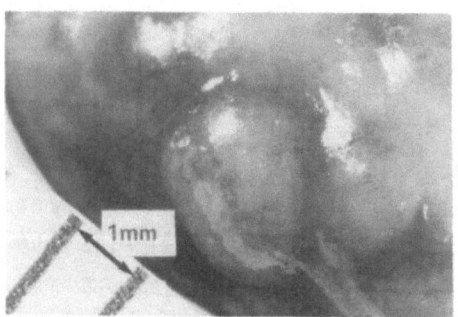

FIGURE 3. Metastatic nodules on the lung surface from the specimen shown on Fig. 2 before dissection for further experimental procedure. Note haemorrhagic foci in the center of the larger lesion.

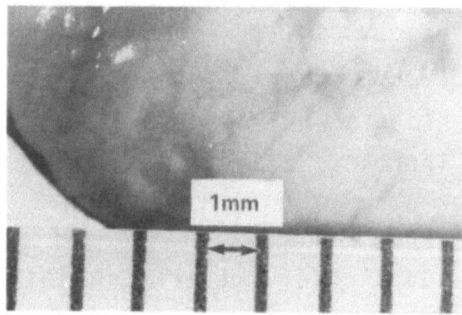

FIGURE 4. Surface of the normal lung from the control mouse as seen under a dissecting microscope.

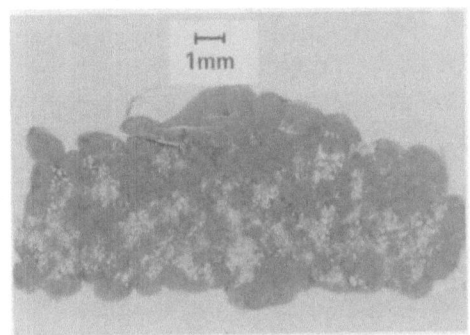

FIGURE 5. Macrophotograph of the lung with advanced metastatic disease. Multiple metastatic nodules infiltrating the whole volume of the organ with massive destruction of the healthy tissue. Hematoxylin and eosin stain.

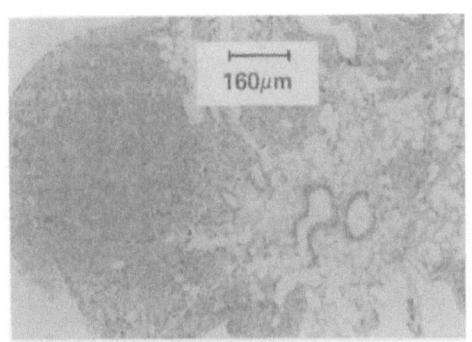

FIGURE 6. Higher-magnification photomicrograph of a selected area form Figure 5.

FIGURE 7. Lewis lung carcinoma cells invading into parenchyma of a lymph node. Fragments of the normal lymphatic tissue are seen in the top of the photomicrograph. Hematoxylin and eosin stain.

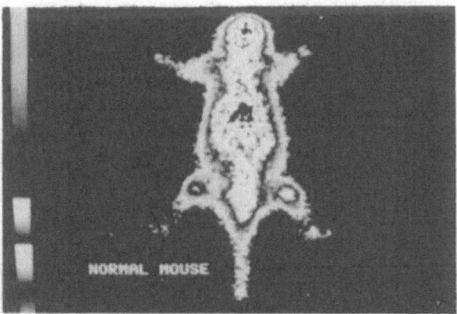

FIGURE 8. Ga-67 distribution in the normal mouse 48 hr after i.v. injection. The scintigrams shows a small blood pool image with the highest concentration in the region of the heart.

120

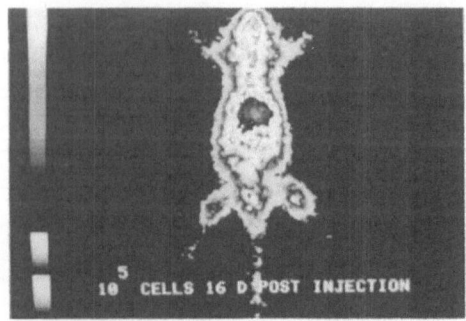

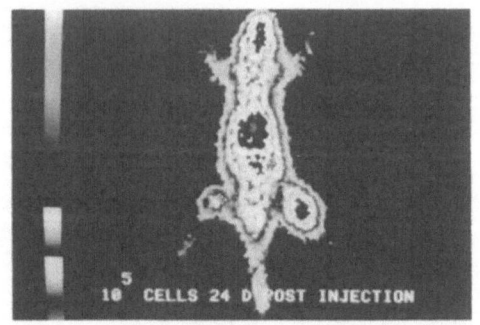

FIGURE 9. 16 days after implantation with 10^5 Lewis lung carcinoma cells there is increased accumulation og Ga-67 in the region of the lungs but very little evidence of Ga-67 in the region of the primary tumor (the right thigh). At autopsy this animal had small visible metastases (total metastatic burden in the lungs estimated at 5-10 mg) and the primary tumor of approximately 200 mg.

FIGURE 10. 24 days after implantation with 10^5 tumor cells there is marked accumulation of Ga-67 in the region of the lungs and also accumulation of the tracer in the region of the primary tumor. Total metastatic burden in the lungs estimated at 20 mg and the primary tumor of approximately 750 mg.

Ga-67 concentrations were highest in the viable portion of small tumors, which were in the rapidly expanding exponential phase of their growth, with only a small proportion of necrotic cells (18). The difference in the radiotracer uptake between viable and necrotic portions of the same tumor demonstrates in-vivo accumulation of the tracer in rapidly growing, metabolically active parts of the primary neoplasia. A high accumulation of the radionuclide was found in the metastatic pulmonary deposits as well, but the concentrations measured were lower than in the primary tumor. The highest Ga-67 uptake was observed in small pulmonary metastatic nodules, but as with the primary tumor, it decreased as the metastatic lesions developed. LLC metastases rapidly increased their volume in the lungs; hypoxia, usually preceding development of necrosis, has been found in nodules as small as 0.5 mm^3 (17).

An increase in the uptake of Ga-67 citrate was observed in the regional (iliac and inguinal) lymph nodes, particularly on the LLC implant side where cells released from the primary tumor are most likely to be entrapped. Larger metastases were formed on the tumor than on the contralateral side. Ga-67 concentration in lymph nodes decreased with time, reaching the lowest values on day 24 after injection of 10^6 cells. A similar decay was observed in metastatic tumor growing in the mediastinal lymphatic tissue (see Figure 12).

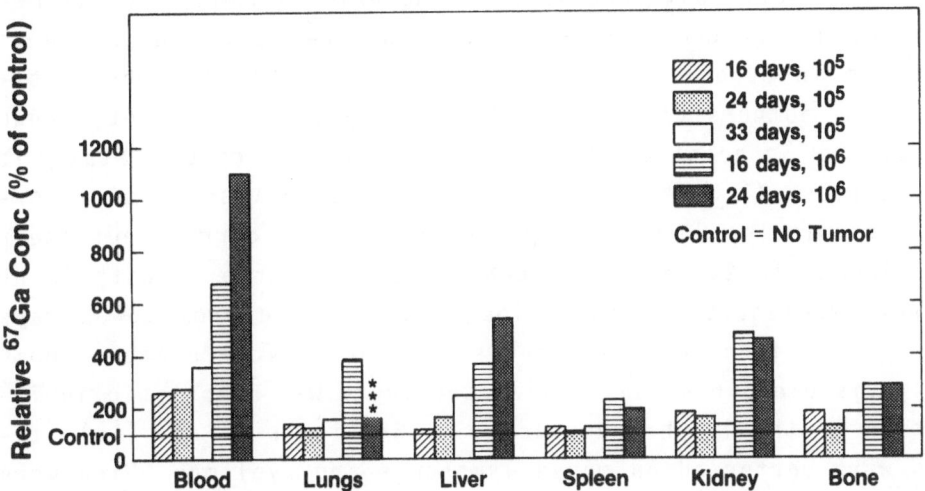

FIGURE 11. Effect of tumor growht and metastasis on the biodistribution of Ga-67 48 hr after i.v. injection of Ga-67 citrate into $B_6D_2F_1$ mice bearing lewis lung carcinoma.

No visible metastases were found in the liver, spleen, kidneys and bone in each experiment. The radionuclide uptake (% of dose/g or % of dose/organ) was higher in these organs excised from tumor-bearing mice than from control animals (see Figure 11). The relative (tissue:blood ratios) Ga-67 concentration, however, decreased in all the organs examined, reaching the lowest values in animals with relatively large tumor burdens, i.e. 24 days after inoculation with 10^6 cells. The decrease in relative values is attributable to greatly elevated blood levels of Ga-67 in tumor-bearing mice. Our results demonstrate that the growing metastatic tumor does affect distribution of

Ga-67 in normal tissues of the host (2,31,14). The growth of the primary and secondary tumors alters accumulation of the radiotracer in the neoplastic tissue as well. Concentrations of the radiopharmaceutical in the tumor and in its metastases are dependent on the tumor volume (mass) and age, thereby implying that Ga-67 uptake can be useful in staging the cancer disease.

The Ga-67 biodistribution in metastases-free organs, excised from animals with disseminated LLC, showed a pattern suggestive of marked changes in normal tissues which usually have low avidity for Ga-67. Host reactions to the primary tumor and its metastases increased the radiocolloid uptake in our experiments which is in opposition to the previously published observations. Some authors claim that the growing tumor does not change radiotracer concentration (2,14,16), whereas others state it can suppress (1,3,14) radionuclide uptake in tissues of tumor-bearing animals. However, Sephton et al. (16) carried out their experiments to 24 hr after Ga-67 injection compared with 48 hr in our studies. Our observation period ranged from 16-33 days after tumor transfer; mestatases in the lungs were macroscopically visible during this time, and there was neoplastic infiltration of the lymph nodes as well. Sephton's et al. (16) studies were performed on mouse lymphomas and myelomas which were 1-2 weeks old. In experiments on rats injected s.c. with mammary adenocarcinomas, Ga-67 distribution showed some variability over a 32 day post-transfer period and presented evidence of changes in concentration as a function of time (2). However, the reported observations were limited to healthy tissues and Ga-67 concentrations were not significantly different in animals bearing metastatic or nonmetastatis tumors. Nelson et al. (13) also stated that diversion of Ga-67 to tumor did not alter its concentration in normal tissues; their clinical data showed considerable variability from case to case. Nelson's et al. patients represented a heterogenous group with respect to type of cancer, tumor stage and clinical complications, wheras our model was homogenous in this respect.

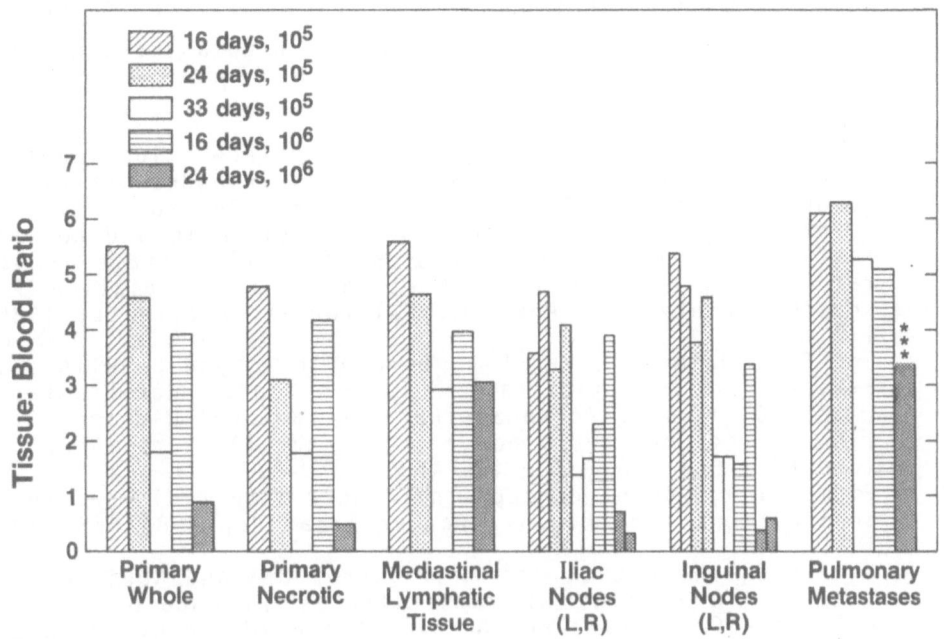

FIGURE 12. Effect of tumor growth and metastasis on the relative uptake of Ga-67 48 hr after i.v. injection of Ga-67 citrate into $B_6D_2F_1$ mice bearing lewis lung carcinoma.
L = left, contralateral. R = right, ipsilateral.

The differences between bibliographical data and our findings require further investigation using a "standardized" animal model in which the transplanted tumor can serve as the paired control for the metastases and gives the opportunity to study quantitative distribution of the radiotracer in transplanted and metastatic tumor in one animal (9). The work using such a model of metastatic disease is in progress in our laboratory.

4. SUMMARY

The combination of advanced primary tumor and extensive pulmonary and lymphatic metastases in the Lewis lung carcinoma/$B_6D_2F_1$ mouse model led progressively to 1) decreasing concentrations of Ga-67 in neoplastic tissues, 2) large increases in Ga-67 blood concentration and 3) increases in the Ga-67 uptake by some tissues which were free of metastatic disease. We can conclude that the presence of metastatic tumor in the host changes Ga-67 biodistribution not only in neoplastic tissue but also in normal tissues not affected by the neoplastic disease.

REFERENCES
1. Boak J L and Agwunobi T C, A study of technetium-labelled sulphide colloid uptake by regional lymph nodes draining a tumor-bearing area. Br J Surg 1978; 65: 374-378.
2. Durakovic A, Effect of two tumors (metastatic and non-metastatic) on tissue distribution of Ga-67 citrate in the rat. Thirty-third Annuale Meeting of the Radiation Reseasch Society, Los Angeles, California, Abstracts. 1985: 112.
3. Ege G N, Nold J B, Eng R R, Durakovic A, and Conklin J J, Effects of a metastatic (13762) and nonmetastatic (R3230AC) mammary adenocarcinoma on radiocolloid localization in regional lymph nodes in Fischer 344 rats. R Reticuloedothel Soc 1983; 34: 449-462.
4. Fidler I J, Recent concepts of cancer metastasis and their implications for therapy. Cancer Treat Rep 1984; 68: 193-198.
5. Gati L J, Wiebe L I, Tse J W, Turner C J and Noujaim A A, Comparative studies of radiocitrates in oncological models. Tc-99m citrate and Ga-67 citrate uptake by EMT-6 tumors in mice. Nucl Med Biol 1986; 13: 253-255.
6. Haynie T P, Konikowski T, and Glemm H J, Experimental models for evaluation of radioactive tumor-localizing agents, Semin Nucl Med 1976; 6: 347-369.
7. Hör G, Munz D L, Brandhorst I, Maul F D, Holtzmann H, Altmeyer P, and Baum R P, Scintigraphy of lymphokinetics and lymphatic neoplasia, In "Nuclear Medicine in Clinical Oncology" C Winkler (Ed.), Springer-Verlag, Heidelberg 1986: 94-107.
8. Johnston G S, Clinical applications of gallium in oncology, Int J Nucl MEd Biol 1981; 8: 249-255.
9. Kanclerz A and Chapman J D, The effectiveness of cis-platinum, cyclophosphanide and melphalan in treating disseminated tumor cells in mice, Clin Expl Metastasis 1987: 5 (in press).
10. Kaplan W D, Mechanisms responsible for radioactive tracer uptake in malignancies, In "Nuclear Medicine in Clinical Oncology", C. Winkler (Ed.), Springer-Verlag, Heidelberg 1986: 14-24.
11. Kim E E and Heynie T P, Role of nuclear medicine in chemotherapy of malignant lesions, Semin Nucl Med 1985; 15: 12-20.
12. Lentle B C, Scott J R, Schmidt R P, Hooper H R and Catz Z, The clinical value of direct tumor scinitigraphy: A new hypothesis, J Nucl MEd 1985; 26: 1215-1217.
13. Nelson B, Hayes R L, Edwards C L, Kniseley R M and Andrews G A, Distribution of gallium in human tissues after intravenous administration, J Nucl. Med 1971; 13: 92-100.

14. Osborne M P, Jeyasingh K, Richardson V J, Vincenti A C, Jewkes R F and Burn J I, The detection of lymph node metastases using radiolabelled colloids, Br J Surg 1978; 65: 354 (Abstract).
15. Schümichen C, Clinical aspects of detection and imaging of lung tumors, In "Nuclear Medicine in Clinical Oncology", C. Winkler (Ed.), Springer-Verlag, Heidelberg 1986: 74-79.
16. Sephton R G, Hodgson G S, DeAbrew S and Harris A W, Ga-67 and Fe-59 distributions in mice, J Nucl Med 1978; 19: 930-935.
17. Stanley J A, Shipley W U and Steel G G, Influence of tumor size on hypoxic fraction and therapeutic sensitivity of Lewis lung tumor, Br J Cancer 1977; 36: 105-113.
18. Steel G G, Growth kinetics of tumors, Clarendon Press, Oxford 1975.
19. Tsan M F and Scheffel U, Mechanism of Gallium-67 accumulation in tumors, J Nucl Med 1986; 27: 1215-1219.
20. Wiebe L I, Small animal oncological models for screening diagnostic radiotracers, In "Animal Models in Radiotracer Design", R M Lambrecht and W C Eckelman (Eds.), Springer-Verlag, New York 1983: 107-147.
21. Weiss L, Principles of Metastasis, Academic Press, Orlando 1985.
22. Zayas F, Olivia J, Lage A, Diaz J W, Alcorta L F, Warder M and Gastra G, Ga-67 citrate distribution in solid hepatoma 22, Eur J Nucl Med 1984; 9: 157-160.

9. MONOCLONAL ANTIBODIES AND THEIR RADIONUCLIDE CONJUGATES: PRACTICAL AND REGULATORY ASPECTS.

Jesper Zeuthen

1. INTRODUCTION

In 1975 Köhler and Milstein (30) published their results establishing a technique for the production of essentially un-limited quantities of homogenous, monospecific antibody of pre-selected specificity. Today, more than a hundred monoclonal antibody based products are available commercially for in vitro diagnostic tests. Moreover, monoclonal antibodies and their de-rivatives are being intensively investigated for the treatment of cancer, autoimmune diseases, allergic conditions, drug over-dose, viral and parasitic infections, and transplant rejection.

The increasing medical applications of monoclonal antibodies has led to the development of more efficient and economical pro-duction methods. With the expected long term use of monoclonal antibodies in humans, attention has now been focused on the re-producibility of the production process and the purity, potency and safety of the final product. This review attempts to pro-vide a conceptual background for understanding the production of monoclonal antibodies and the control methods applicable to define their specifications. The Food and Drug Administration (FDA) in the USA has established criteria which may be develo-ped into guidelines or regulations to be considered in the ma-nufacture of monoclonal antibodies. Similar criteria have re-cently been issued by the Commission of the European Communi-ties.

The production of monoclonal antibodies involves four di-stinct steps (Fig.1):

128

I. First, a mouse is injected with the target antigen. Shortly after injection, the immune system of the mouse starts to produce B lymphocytes capable of antibody production. Each individual B lymphocyte produces only one specific antibody.

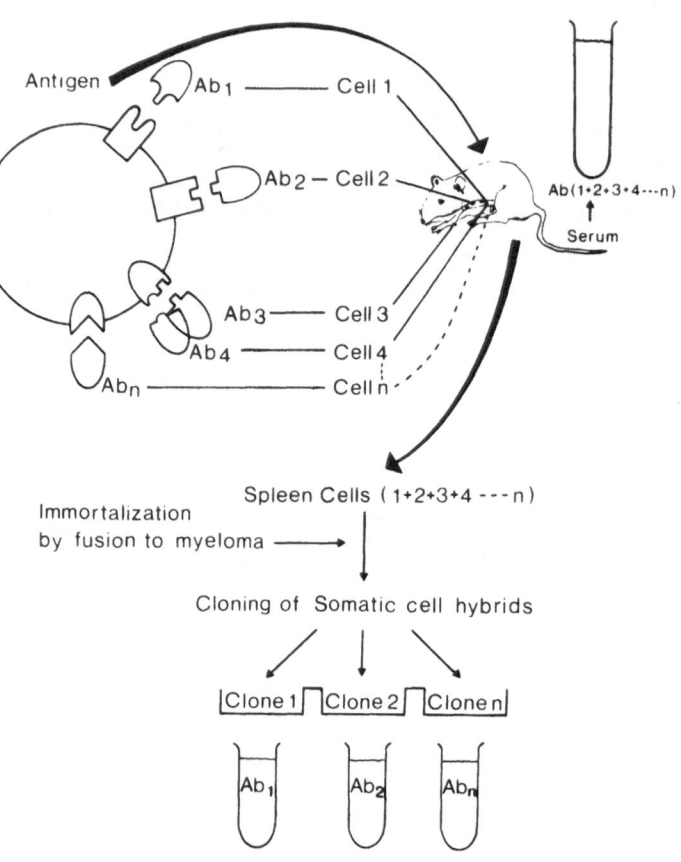

Fig. 1 Principle of the production of monoclonal antibodies by the hybridoma technique. The immune response of an animal to an antigen is very complex. Each antibody is synthesized by cell fusion to provide an inexhaustible supply of monoclonal antibody.

II. The spleen of the mouse is removed from the immunized mouse. Spleen cells, containing the B lymphocytes, are mixed with mouse myeloma cells together with a fusing agent; now polyethylene glycol is commonly used. Some of these cells will fuse and a few of these will form viable hybrid cells which are capable of endless reproduction. For the fusion a mutant myeloma cell line (HPRT-) is used which can only produce purine nucleotides through the folic acid pathway. Such cells will be killed in a medium containing a folic acid analogue, as for instance aminopterin wich is a component in the hypoxanthine-aminopterin-thymidine supplemented medium (HAT medium) used for selection of hybrid cells.

Normal cells will survive by using their hypoxanthine escape pathway, and so will all hybrids that have retained the enzyme hypoxanthine phosphoribosyl transferase (HPRT), brougth in by the lymphocyte partner. Thus, with the myeloma celle killed in the HAT medium and the lymphocytes dying a natural death, the only suvivors will be hybrids.

III. This population of hybrid cells, usually seeded into individual wells of microtitre plates, is screened to identify the hybrids wich secrete antibody against the antigen body for a particular application. For selection of antibodies with putative selectivity for tumor-associated antigens, several of these antibodies my have to be tested in preclinical evaluation.

IV. Finally, the selected hybrid cells are cloned to ensure stability and production of a truly monoclonal antibody. The result of the cloning is a homogenous culture of in principle immortal cells.

These cells may be grown in vitro in tissue culture or in mouse ascites and will secrete the particular monoclonal antibody of interest. Each cloned cell line will produce just one monoclonal antibody. These are all identical proteins with exactly the same amino acid sequences and the same immunoreactive behaviour.

The pioneering work of Köhler and Milstein (30) described methods for production of mouse or murine monoclonal antibodies. Similar systems have now been developed for the production of rat monoclonal antibodies. The progress of development of systems for developing the corresponding human monoclonal antibodies have so far been rather disappointing, but recent progress in this field indicates that development of clinically useful human monoclonal antibodies could be a real possibility.

Further, an exciting recent development is the construction of chimeric antibodies in which the antigenrecognizing variable regions of mouse antibodies are joined with the constant regions of human antibodies (23).

Monoclonal antibodies have a major potential for specific recognition of tumor-associated antigens and several monoclonal antibodies of murine origin have been described that identify antigens on a variety of solid and hematopoietic human tumors. if tumor-associated antigen is present on the tumor cell surface, then monoclonal antibodies specific for this antigen may be of value as targeting agents for delivery of diagnostic or therapeutic agents to the tumor. Current cancer therapy modalities are not highly selective for tumor tissue, but rather deliver therapeutic agents in a generalized fashion to the entire body or groups of organs e.g. radiation therapy or chemotherapy. Monoclonal antibody-targeted therapy has the potential for relatively selective delivery of a toxic agent to the tumor cells, with minimal damage to surrounding tissues or to tissues that are particulary susceptible to the effects of the toxic agent alone, e.g. the bone marrow.

Current cancer diagnostic modalities employ either invasive techniques (e.g. surgery) or depend on characteristics such as density or vascularity in order to aid identification of a tumor. The latter parameters are the basis for CAT scans and lymphangiograms, and as a result these techniques are limited in the size of tumor masses that can be detected. Monoclonal antibody-radionuclide immunoconjugates have the potential for non-invasive specific detection of tumors and metastases of very small size.

Promising preliminary investigations in this field have been carried out and encourage further research efforts. A coordinated program for testing and evaluating monoclonal antibodies and their immunoconjugates of radionuclides is necessary when selecting monoclonal antibodies with the greatest potential for use in clinical trials.

Effective preclinical assesment of monoclonal antibodies and their conjugates is an extensive undertaking involving several different stages. Several questions should be adressed with regards to monoclonal antibodies intendend for in vivo administration (Table 1).The extent and type of evaluation or characterization must be tailored to match the characteristics and extent of existing knowledge of each individual monoclonal antibody as well as the proposed purpose (e.g. therapeutic or diagnostic) for that monoclonal antibody or radionuclide conjugate.

TABLE 1. ASSESMENT OF MONOCLONAL ANTIBODIES

Antibody specificity

     Immunoperoxiddase
     Radiolocalization

Antigen Characterization

     Biochemixal nature
     Topography
     Epitope (different parts of the antigen molecule)
     Heterogeneity

Antibody-Antigen Interaction

     Dose
     Regimen
     Route
     Pharmacokinetics
     Comparison of various agents conjugated to same antibody

---

2. PRODUCTION AF MONOCLONAL ANTIBODIES.

The production of monoclonal antibodies in vivo by harvesting the ascitic fluid from hydbridoma implanted animals is a very common procedure due to the high concentration of monoclonal antibody obtainable. Antibody levels in serum or ascitic fluid can typically reach 5-15 mg/ml. This represents 16 to 30% of the total mouse proteins and 50-70% of the mouse IgG.

In large scale in vivo production of monoclonal antibodies the only limit to the quantity of antibody that can be produced is the number of mice that can be housed in a production facility at any one time. Hybridoma cells have short doubling times in vitro, so the propagation of sufficient numbers of cells for mouse inoculation is not difficult. It is advisable that inoculation of mice is performed with a well controlled culture batch since it is important to ensure that the line maintains its characteristics. Therefore continuous passage of cells in vivo is not recommended.

Growth of hybridomas in vivo is associated with problems such as lack of defined and well controlled conditions, the need for animal housing facilities and adequate attention to animal husbandry. Therefore, in vitro production methods have several distinct advantages which provide a strong impetus for continued improvement of efficient in vitro production methods. Large-scale tissue culture techniques is the most important method of bulk production of monoclonal antibodies. In vitro propagation methods can be better defined and lead to the production of better defined products than growth of hybridomas as ascites cultures in vivo. The scale of in vitro cultures can be expanded by upscaling of culture vessels allowing one to benefit from economies of scale, especially in relation to labor and capital costs. Large quantities of antibody are therefore produced more economically by this route (15). The risk of contamination by extraneous antibodies or adventitious agents of rodent origin is also reduced in cell cultures. Current research to improve tissue culture techniques for monoclonal antibody production has three main aims (4):

a) to increase the yield of antibody produced per cell;
b) the reduction or elimination of extraneous proteins
used for culture;

c) production of monoclonal antibodies in large culture
vessels.

The production of monoclonal antibodies by hybridoma cells is variable ranging from 5 to 100 microgrammes of antibody per 10^6 cells per 24 hours. This corresponds to a mean synthesis of 200-4000 IgG molecules/cell/second. A typical growth medium for large scale culture is RPMl-1640 or Dulbecco's modified Eagle's medium with high glucose, supplemented with 10-15% fetal calf serum. With a monoclonal antibody concentration of the order of 10-50 microgrammes/ml, there will be 6000 microgrammes/ml of total protein and 300 microgrammes/ml of immunoglobulin from the fetal calf serum. The monoclonal antibody may therefore represent only 3 to 15% of the total immunoglobulin in tissue culture fluid. This is obviously a serious impediment to the use of monoclonal antibodies produced in cell cultures since a pure product is desired for many of the applications of mono-clonal antibodies. Even if depletion of fetal calf serum for unwanted bovine immunoglobulin for practical purposes can be achieved by means of Protein A column chromatography (if this is also later used for the purification of the monoclonal antibody) fetal calf serum is a. complex mixture of components which will vary in its suitability for supporting cell growth and antibody production. Each lot of serum must be individually tested and assayed to ensure its suitability before use. In order to eliminate this source of variability and to simplify purification of the monoclonal antibody, efforts have been made to develop serum-free culture media for hybridomas (7; 38).

Cell cultures of hybridomas may be expanded to very large sizes. Up to 200 ml cultures may be grown in tissue culture flasks, but for larger cultures roller bottles are used. Large-scale reactors (1000 liters) have been developed for hy-bridomas as so-called air-lift fermentors (1). Other systems have been designed as perfusion systems in which the depleted medium is constantly removed and fresh medium added. Perfusion systems use special sensors, sampling ports, input and output piping to maintain pH, oxygen, carbon dioxide and nutrients at

the proper level. Such systems permit higher cell densities
which is important as lymphoid cells do not grow well at low
densities. The concentration of secreted monoclonal antibody
is higher in perfusion reactors, typically in the order of 200
microgrammes/ml. The application of microencapsulation technology to the culture of hybridoma cells has gained increasing
recognition as a method for commercial production of monoclonal
antibodies (15). Hybridomas are encapsulated under physiological conditions using mild chemicals and reactions. The micro-
capsules can then be transferred to a reactor and nutrients and
oxygen will diffuse across the capsule membrane while contaminating proteins including the irrelevant bovine immunoglobulins
from the medium are excluded. Using this method very high densities of hybridoma cells can be cultured, resulting in high
concentrations of monoclonal antibodies. To harvest the antibody the capsules are opened physically and these will contain
some 45-80% of total protein being the desired antibody. A
rather similar technique involves entrapment of cells within
agarose microbeads (41). This technique also allows growth at
high cell densities and production of high concentrations of
immunoglobulin. In contrast to the microencapsulation technique, however, purification of the monoclonal antibody from
the medium is required. Growth of hybridoma cells have also
been investigated in hollow fibre or artificial capillary culture systems (52). These porous fibres retain the hybridoma
cells which release secreted monoclonal antibody into the outside fluid. The growth of hybridomas in these systems results
in yields of antibody of 6-8 mg/ml which approaches the yields
of antibody obtained in vivo by harvesting ascitic fluid in
hybridoma-implanted animals. Antibody levels in serum or
ascitic fluid can typically reach 5-15 mg/ml. This represents
in this case 16-30% of the total mouse proteins and 50-70% of
the mouse immunoglobulin.

3. PURIFICATION OF MONOCLONAL ANTIBODIES

For the large-scale purification of monoclonal antibodies

several different procedures may be used (43). The processes used for monoclonal antibody purification can be divided into three stages: 1) initial enrichment; 2) intermediate purification and 3) final purification. The purity and concentration of the starting material and the demands of purity versus yield for the final product will determine how many of these stages are necessary. An enrichment of the starting material is performed if a more concentrated starting material is required. Ultrafiltration (hollow fibre or tangential flow) where a membrane retains larger molecules while smaller molecules (such as water and salts) are removed, can concentrate the products up to 50 times with quantitative recoveries. For the intermediate stage of purification there are currently three basic techniques suitable for the large-scale purification of monoclonal antibodies: Affinity chromatography, ion-exchange chromatography and adsorption chromatography. Affinity chromatography is based on highly specific interactions between an immobilized ligand and the substances of interest. For monoclonal antibodies, either the specific antigen-antibody interaction or the affinity of staphylococcal Protein A for immunoglobulins can be exploited. Affinity chromatography using immobilized Protein A is a well documented method for research scale purification of immunoglobulins (especially IgG) from rodents and other species (17; 22) and has been adapted for monoclonal antibody purification where the purity attained is close to 100% with yields typically between 50 and 80% (36; 50). Protein A does not have an affinity for all immunoglobulins (22) but for murine monoclonal antibodies, all the subclasses of IgG, including IgG1, will bind especially if conditions of high ionic strength are used.

In ion exchange chromatography, the isoelectric point and charge density of the monoclonal antibody should determine the type of ion exchange employed. Anion exchange has been most commonly used and has been adapted to HPLC for preparative processing of monoclonal antibodies with typical recoveries of 95% (3; 21). Anion exchange with FPLC for ascites fluid (10;

11) has been performed at research scale with good results both for IgG and IgM monoclonal antibodies. In cation exchange, the conditions (pH and ionic strength) can be manipulated so all the product and only few contaminants (5) are bound initally. Cation exchange is more suitable than anion exchange when scaling up to gram quantities of the product.

Final purification is only undertaken if the demands for product purity are very high and the desired purity has not already been obtained by the previous purification steps. If this is necessary gel filtration (5) is the most commonly used method and there are several media available commercially which are suitable for scale-up of this purification.

Two variable regions of an antibody can bind to specific antigenic sites, and a constant region interacts with the host immune system. Enzymatic digestion with pepsin removes part of the constant region (F_c) to produce a $F(ab')_2$ fragment, whereas papain splits the antibody molecule into F_c fragment and two Fab fragments. It is on the Fab and $F(ab')_2$ fragments that one finds the sequence of amino acids referred to as the variable antigen-binding site, where true specificity occurs. Fab fragments are monovalent and binding to antigens is weaker than with the divalent $F(ab')_2$. The F_c portion is more likely to trigger allergic reactions than may adversely affect the utility of whole antibodies for in vivo administration. Also, the F_c portion is nonspecifically taken up by the reticuloendothelial system.

Antibodies may be cleaved into these fragments using pepsin or papain (Fig. 2). Generally, $F(ab')_2$ fragments produced after pepsin digestion retain their immunoreactivity, but with Fab or Fab' fragments this is not always the case. The produced fragments can be conveniently purified by means of HPLC or FPLC. These methods also can be used in connection with quality control of labelled and unlabelled antibodies used for in vivo administration. In Fig. 3 the FPLC profiles of intact IgG, $F(ab')_2$ and Fab' fragments analyzed on a TSK 2000 column is illustrated. These methods also provide a useful means of checking for possible aggregation in the antibody preparations.

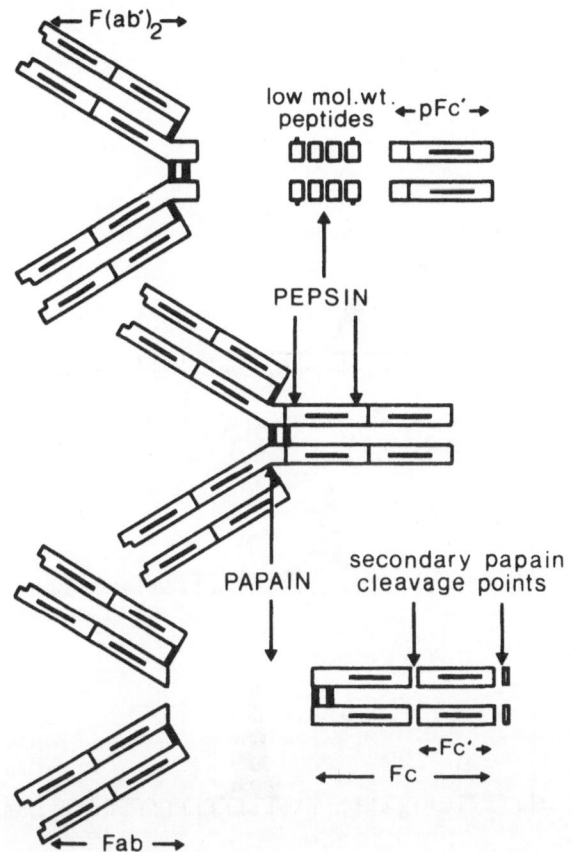

Fig. 2. Enzymatic cleavage of immunoglobin (IgG).
    Pepsin cleaves the IgG heavy chain to yield the F (ab')$_2$ and
pFc' fragments. Further action reduces the central fragment to
low molecular weigh peptides. Papain splits the molecule to low
molecular weight peptides. Papain splits the molecule in the
hinge region yielding two Fab fragments and the F$_c$ fragment.
Secondary action on the F$_c$ fragment produces F$_c$' fragments.

138

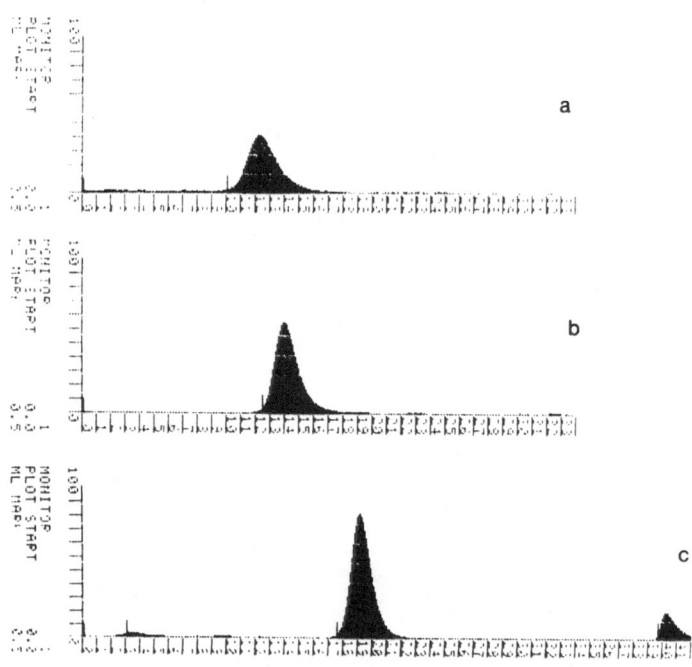

Fig. 3. Examples of analyses of monoclonal antibody preparations by means of FPLC. (a) intact IgG monoclonal antibody; (b)
F(ab')$_2$ fragment of an IgG monoclonal antibody obtained by pepsin digestion; (c) Fab fragment of an IgG monoclonal antibody
obtained by papain digestion. Samples were analyzed on a Pharmacia FPLC system using a TSK 2000 column (loop 100 ul, range
0.05). (Data courtsey of Dr. Arne Agerlin Olsen).

4. RADIOLABELLING OF MONOCLONAL ANTIBODIES

For both radioimmunoimaging and radioimmunotherapy, it is necessary to successfully attach a radioisotope to the antibody so that the resultant product is stable and yet retains the ability to bind to the targeted antigen. Until recently, iodination was the most common method, but the last 10 years have seen the rapid development of a variety of methods which covalently link metal chelating groups to antibodies enabling them to be subsequently labeled with a variety of different radionuclides which are bound tightly by the antibody conjugated chelates.

The iodination of proteins has been a common laboratory practice for over 40 years and while the choice of isotopes is limited, the methods are relatively simple. Most of the inital experiments using radiolabeled antibodies were performed using antibodies iodinated with either I-125 or I-131; and much of the clinical work being performed today still utilized I-131 labelled antibody preparations. The major disadvantages of I-131 labeled antibodies are the relative in vivo instability and the poor imaging and dosimetry characteristics of I-131. Extensive dehalogenation occurs at many sites in the body includinc the tumor and this not only decreases absolute tumor uptake, but also leads to problems with I-131 concentration in the thyroid ands astrointestinal system (primarily stomach). While I-123 is a more ideal radioiodine for imaging purposes because of its more suitable photon energy and lower particulate radiations, it is limited by high cost, short half-life and relative unavailability.

Radioiodine is available as NaI and the I^-, iodide ion, is not in a reactive form for labeling proteins. In order to make iodide reactive for iodination, it must be oxidized to I^+ (active iodine or iodonium ion) and this is accomplished by a variety of oxidizing agents or electrolytic oxidations. Oxidation of iodide to iodine produces H_2OI^+ the "hydrated iodinated ion" in water which in turn reacts with ionized (anionic) tyrosine residues in the protein which results in the stable attachment

of the iodine ion to the phenol ring of tyrosine in the ortho
position (47). Both ortho positions may be iodinated resulting
in two iodine per tyrosine residue. Under conditions of high
iodine concentration, it is possible that some of the iodine
may attach to histidine residues although this attachment is
generally less stable.

The most common oxidizing agent in use is chloramine-T.
Chloramine-T slowly liberates hypochlorous acid in solution and
so oxidizes the iodide present. However, chloramine-T is a very
reactive substance and tends to easily damage antibodies by
both chlorination and the production of aggregates. In addition, the reaction must be terminated by the addition of a reducing agent like metabisulfite. However, by the proper adjust-
ment of concentrations, most antibodies can be efficiently labeled to a high specific activity without significant loss of
immunoreactivity. Iodobeads are a useful alternative to chloramine-T. The oxidant (N-chlorobenzenesulfonamide) is similar to
chloramine-T and attached to solid beads. These beads can be
easily added to a mixture of antibody and iodide and 10-20 minutes later the reaction is terminated by simple removal of the
beads or aspiration of the antibody solution. There is usually
little denaturation of the antibody and yields as high as 95%
have been reported (37).

The most common enzymatic method of oxidizing iodide is the
use of lactoperoxidase in association with small concentrations
of hydrogen peroxide. Hydrogen peroxide oxidizes iodide to iodine and the lactoperoxidase acts as a catalyst. The reaction
proceeds efficiently with little damage to the antibody but on
occasion, self iodination of the lactoperoxidase is a problem.
To faciliate the separation of antibody from the lactoperoxidase, this method most commonly uses the enzyme attached to a
solid support. Beads with lactoperoxidase and glucose oxidase
attached (Enzymobeads) are available commercially and in the
presence of glucose the glucose oxidase produces a constant
supply of hydrogen peroxide for the catalytic reaction. Separation and termination of the reaction is accomplished by
simple removal of the beads.

The electrolytic process is the most gentle method of iodination, but requires special apparatus and may be relatively ineffecient although yields as high as 80% are possible. The iodide and antibody are placed in the anode compartment of the electrolytic cell and current turned on for 30-60 minutes. Electrolysis releases active iodine at a slow rate and this relatively slow rate of reaction causes a fairly uniform distribution of iodine between antibody molecules.

The oxidative method that we and others have found quick and easy is the iodogen method where the oxidative reaction occurs on a solid phase. Iodogen (1,3,4,6-tetrachloro3alfa6alfadiphenylglycoluril) is dried onto the walls of the reaction vessel, the antibody and iodide added and the reaction allowed to proceed for 5-15 minutes. Iodogen is insoluble in water and so the reaction is terminated by removing the solution from the reaction vial. The yield can be as high as 70-80% and generally denaturation of antibody is minimal although labeling may be less uniform than with some other methods.

With all of these oxidative methods, the conditions of iodination need to be individualized for each monoclonal antibody in order to obtain the highest yield with the minimum damage. Factors influencing incorporation include concentration of reactants and protein, pH (6-8), temperature and time. In addition, the presence of contaminating reducing agents will reduce yields although most commercial preparations of radioiodide are relatively free of contaminants. Azide will interfere with lactoperoxidase labeling.

The final method of iodination to consider is the nonoxidative method of Bolton and Hunter. The reagent used is the N-hydroxysuccinimide ester of iodinated p-hydroxyphenyl propionic acid. This reagent available commercially reacts with the lysine groups on antibodies and is especially useful to iodinate antibodies that are easily denatured by oxidative methods due to sensitive tyrosines. However, the reagent is expensive and yields are relatively low.

Some general considerations that apply to most labeled antibody preparations irrespective of method used are the mechanisms of damage to the antibody. Chemical damage due to the effects of the oxidizing agents reacting particularly on sulfhydryl groups and disulfide bonds in common. Aggregates of antibodies can be easily produced particularly at higher concentrations of reactants. Radiolysis occurs over a period of time and refers to both direct damage to chemical bonds by the radiation or indirect damage due to the production of free radicals and hydrogen peroxide by the interaction of radiation with aqueous solutions. Finally, it must be remembered that most methods of labeling are random; that is the attachment of the isotope or conjugate occurs randomly to the appropriate exposed amino acids. That means that when there is an average of 0.5-1.0 iodine atoms per antibody, 39.60% of all iodine is actually attached to antibodies carrying two or more iodine atoms (47).

As mentioned before, there are a large numbers of metallic isotopes that are useful as agents for radioimaging and/or therapy. The major method of attaching metallic isotopes to antibodies involves the use of bifunctional or heterobifunctional chelating agents since metals (with the exception of Tc-99m) cannot be attached directly to anti-bodies. These techniques are rapidly developing and undoubtedly will become the major method of labeling antibodies for in vivo applications in the future. There are a large number of agents currently available with new agents and methods being published almost monthly. The basic concept is the same for all methods. A chelator which has the ability to bind metallic isotopes (like In-III, Ga-67, Ru-97, Pd-109, Y-90 etc.) is attached to the antibody by a reactive functional group. The reactive functional groups primarily used today include isothiocyanate, carboxylic acid derivatives, bromoacetyl groups and the diazonium ion (53). A popular method has been the cyclic anhydride method (25). Chelators in common use are DTPA, EDTA and deferoxamine. While bifunctional chelates can be designed to attach to a variety of

positions on the antibody molecule (amino groups, free sulfhy-
dryls, tyrosine) the majority bind to lysine residues which are
present in abundance in the antibody molecule.

We labeled 17-1A with Indium-111 using the cyclic anhydride
method and found a great deal of loss of immunoreactivity due
to polymerization and intra and intermolecular cross linking of
the antibody molecules, particularly at higher numbers of chelates per antibody (44). Again, the attachment of these chelating groups to the antibody is random with these techniques and
this randomness of conjugation coupled with the high frequency
of amino groups on antibodies means that specific activities
must be kept relatively low to diminish the risk of denaturation. Heterobifunctional chelating agents avoid some of these
problems since they have one specific attachment arm and so
avoid crosslinking (51). On occasion, conjugations can be designed so that only one group is available for conjugation
especially with smaller fragments like Fab' and in this way
conjugation is specific (53). In addition, newer methods of
conjugation can utilize site specific labeling such as methods
which attach by way of the carbohydrate side chains (33).

Once the chelate is conjugated to the antibody, it can be
leisurely examined and tested to ensure preserved immuno reactivity. The final complexing of the metallic ion is accomplished immediately prior to use and can be performed simply
without further loss of antibody activity. Indium-111, while it
hydrolyzes and produces a precipitate or colloid above pH 2.0,
can be raised to pH 6.5 in the appropriate buffer (citrate or
bicarbonate) and then reacted with the conjugated antibody-che-
late in excess. The major hindrance to easy labeling is the
presence of trace metallic comtaminants which can significantly
interfere with chelation of indium by binding to the chelate
first. Meticulous care must be taken to avoid even trace metallic ion contaminants in any of the preparations or glassware.

Antibodies labeled with In-111 are more stable in vivo than
iodinated antibodies, and have more absolute uptake in tumors.
Their major drawback is increased hepatic concentrations of in-

dium activity and are not worked out. It appears that indium is carried to the liver by antibody or fragments of antibodies and that after internalization by the Kupffer cells the indium may be stripped from the chelate and subsequently strongly bound by interacellular proteins that have a very high affinity for metallic ions (9). Attempts to reduce hepatic uptake center about the use of chelates with stronger affinitites for the isotopes being used (29) and the possibility of using a biodegradable functional group or attachment arm.

Regardless of the methods used to label a monoclonal antibody, a number of quality controls are necessary and these controls may vary somewhat from antibody to antibody. For human use, apyrogenicity, sterility, radiochemical purity and specificity of the preparation must be ensured prior to injection although in highly reproducible systems, these controls need not be performed prior to each use of labeled antibody. The radioimmunoreactivity can be tested by incubation of labeled antibody in the presence of excess antigen. When the antigen is available in purified form, binding to antigen as in an affinity column can be examined. For cell surface antigens, incubation with increasing concentrations of cells should yield a suitable measurement of immunoreactivity (28). However, subtle changes in immunereactivity may be missed by these techniques and testing should also include competitive binding assays to demonstrate equal binding of labeled and unlabeled antibdoy to antigen on cell surfaces where practical.

5. HUMAN STUDIES WITH RADIOLABELLED MONOCLONAL ANTIBODIES

The potential of radionuclides for localizing and treating malignant disease has long been recognized. A major challenge has been to localize the radionuclides in tumor but not normal tissue. Diagnostic imaging studies of colorectal cancer were among the first in vivo clinical applications of radiolabelled monoclonal antibodies. Mach (34) reported some improvement with a monoclonal antibody directed against carcinoembryonic antigen (CEA) compared to his earlier work with goat antisera against

CEA. In a series of 28 patients, 14 had positive planar images at 36-48 hrs., 6 were equivocal and 8 were negative. An additional 14 patients were evaluated using single photon emission computed tomography (SPECT); primary tumor sites were correctly identified in 13. The monoclonal anti-CEA was compared with non-specific mouse IgG and an average ratio of specific to non-specific tumor uptake of 4.3 was found. In a subsequent multicentre study using the monoclonal antibody 17-1A, directed against a cell bound colorectal carcinoma antigen, sensitivities of 51% with whole antibody and 61% with $F(ab')_2$ fragments in studies of 52 patients with 63 known tumor sites were reported (35). Ratios of tumor activity to adjacent normal tissue ranged from 3.6 to 6.3. Scans using antibody 17-1A and its $F(ab')_2$ fragment were negative in a group of patients with cancers other than colorectal carcinoma. Other investigators (8) used not only antibody 17-1A and its $F(ab')_2$ fragment for detecting colon cancer but also antibody 19.9, which recognizes a tumorassociated sialoganglioside that is shed into the circulation where it can be detected by radioimmunoasay. Antibody 17-1A and its $F(ab')_2$ fragment had a sensitivity of 59% for documented colon cancer sites and antibody 19.9 and its $F(ab')_2$ fragment had a sensitivity of 66%. When the two antibodies were used together in 12 patients, 10 of 13 tumor sites were identified.

Malignant melanoma has been an important neoplasm in evaluating radiolabelled monoclonal antibodies for diagnostic imaging and therapy. Melanoma has several well-characterized antigens (24). Superficial metastases of melanoma can readily be evaluated to assess radiolabeled antibody localization for imaging and therapy. Disseminated melanoma cannot be cured with presently availabe therapy making an alternative therapy highly desirable. Larson (31; 32) evaluated melanoma imaging using I-131-labelled antibodies 96.5 and 8.2 and their Fab fragments. These antibodies are both specific for the antigen p97, a 97 kilodalton glycoprotein expressed on the melanoma cell surface. In imaging studies of 33 patients using Fab fragments, 20 studies were positive. Ten of the remaining 13 patients had tumors less than 1.5 cm in diameter, 2 had low p97 antigen levels in tumor biopsy specimens and in one patient the Fab iodination was a technical failure. Imaging sensitivity for metastatic sites greater than 1.5 cm in diameter was 88%. Twenty patients received simultaneous isotype matched I-125- labelled Fab fragments not specific for p97; tumor biopsies in 8 of these patients showed specific to nonspecific antibody ratios of approximately 3.5.

The human imaging studies with radiolabelled monoclonal antibody that have been reviewed thus far all used I-131 as the label. Other similar studies have used I-123 (16). Methods for attaching metals such as indium to proteins using bifunctional chelates have also been described (49; 39). Studies using In-111 labelled monoclonal antibodies have been reported in human tumor xenografts in nude mice (48) as well as in human clinical trials (46; 14).

Larson et al. (32) and Carrasquillo et al. (6) first reported their results in treating a series of patients with metastatic melanoma using I-131-labelled Fab fragments of antibodies 96.5 and 8.2, both directed against the p97 melanoma antigen, and 48.7 antibody which is directed against the melanoma high molecular weight p250 antigen (250 kilodaltons). The melanoma patients received 4 to 10 mg of the Fab fragments. Individual doses ranged from 132 to 861 mCi in a series of 10 patients.

Significant toxicity was not observed below cumulative doses of 500 mCi. Above that level, some patients had a 50% drop in neutrophil and platelet count, reaching this level at 3-4 weeks after treatment and then improving.

Radiation dose estimates in the melanoma patients per 100 mCi I-131-Fab were 1040 rad to tumor, 325 rad to liver, and for the most critical organ, the bone marrow 30 rad. A very important conclusion from this study was that I-131-Fab, in properly selected patients, could be repeatedly localized in the tumor.

6. REGULATORY GUIDELINES AND POINTS TO CONSIDER

The Food and Drug Administration (FDA) in the USA is responsible for the regulation of monoclonal antibody products for human use if the products are to be shipped in "interstate commerce". FDA activities have been recently described (27). At this writing, most monoclonal antibody products have been of murine origin. Murine monoclonal antibodies have been licensed for in vitro diagnostic use, and investigational use in man has been permitted. As of now, only one murine monoclonal antibody product Orthoclone OKT-3 has been licensed for human administration in the USA as well as in France, Italy and Switzerland, and is awaitinq approval in the UK and in W.Germany. OKT-3 is a murine monoclonal anti-human T cell antibody developed by Ortho and Janssen and is used therapeutically for the prevention of kidney transplant rejection (42). OKT-3 can be used to inactivate T cells in marrow harvested from normal donors before transplantation into patients and may reduce graft versus-host disease (45).

The comments provided here are based on the litterature and the cited recommendations but do not constitute formal guidelines. The FDA may publish Guidelines or Points to Consider. These may assist the communication between product developers and regulators, but do not have the force of law. A notice regarding "Points to Consider in the Manufacture of Monoclonal Antibody Products for Human Use" was published in the US Federal Register (19) and has been discussed by Merchant (40) and by Hoffman et al. (26).

FDA standards for monoclonal antibodies have not yet been fully established. The draft Points to Consider provides information that can be used in preparation and evaluating material to be submitted to the FDA concerning hybridoma products. Specific considerations will have to evolve with technological advances. In general, it appears that "the use of highly purified products with optimal specificity as established by rigorous and copious experimental data represents the best possibility of ensuring their safe and efficaceous therapeutic use" (26).

For each hybridoma product, the origins of the product will need to be carefully considered in considering the products potential risks (2). This will involve characterization of the fusion partners and their donors and tissues of origin; the immunogen; the immunization procedure; the screening procedure; the cloning procedure; and the seed lot system. The latter should be characterized as to identity, stability and known microbial contaminants. If murine cells have been employed, testing of the manufacturers working cell bank for potential human pathogens such as lymphocytic choromeningitis virus (LCM), polyoma, reoviruses, or murine leukemia viruses is indicated (Tables II and III). If human cells have been employed, tests for Epstein Barr virus (EBV), EBV genomes, cytomegalovirus (CMV), hepatitis B virus and retroviruses, including human T-lymphotropic viruses, are advised. Cell lines that actively produce identifiable virus are discouraged as a source of monoclonal antibody.

TABLE II. LIST OF VIRUS TESTING*

Group	Virus	Species Affected
I	Hantavirus (haemorrhagic fever with renal syndrome)*	M R
	Lymphocytic choriomeningitis virus (LCMV)*	M
	Reovirus type 3 (reo 3)*	M, R
	Sendai*	M, R
II	Ectromelia virus*	M
	Epizootic diarrhoea of infant mice (EDIM)*	M
	K virus (K)	M
	Kilham rat virus (KRV)	R
	Lactic dehydrogenase virus (LDH)	M
	Minute virus of mice (MVM)	M, R
	Mouse adenovirus (MAV)	M
	Mouse cytomegalovirus	M

Mouse encephalomyelitis (MEV, Theiler's
or GDVII)   M

Mouse hepatitis virus (MHV)   M

Pneumonia virus of mice (PVM)   M, R

Polyoma virus   M

Rat coronavirus (RCV)   R

Retroviruses*   M, R

Sialodacryodadenitis virus (SDA)   R

Thymic virus   M

Toolan virus (HI)*   R

M = Mouse

R = Rat

---

* Committee for Proprietary Medicinal Products. Commission of
the European Communities. Draft Notes on Requirements for
the Quality Control of Monoclonal Antibodies of Murine Origin Intended for Use in Man (12).

TABLE III. TESTING SCHEME FOR VIRAL CONTAMINANTS*

	Tests which are applicable
Hybridoma (seed lot)	(a) (b) (c)
Mouse colony	(a)
Ascitic fluid harvest	(a) (b)
In vitro Bulk harvest	(b)
Bulk final processed product	(b)

(a) Tests for detection of viruses listed in table I, for
example Mouse Antibody Production (MAP) and Rat Antibody
Production (RAP) tests or other tests of at least
equivalent sensitivity and reliability. Additional

specific tests need to be carried out for mouse cytomegalo virus, epizootic diarrhoea virus of infant mice, thymic virus and lactic dehydrogenase virus. Tests capable of detecting murine retroviruses should be included, for example the XC plaque assay or the S^+L^- focus assay for the detection of ectropic or xenotropic retroviruses respectively.

(b) Inoculation of cell cultures capable of detecting a wide range of murine, human and bovine viruses. Examples of useful cell types (substrates) are: murine fibroblast cultures eg mouse embryo cultures; human fibroblast cultures, eg human diploid cells such as MRC5; transformed cell lines of human, murine and bovine origin. Tests for retroviruses, as under (a), should be included.

Fertilized eggs may also act as useful substrates. Test material should be injected into eggs by appropriate routes, the chorioallantoic membrane and yolk sack of each of 10 embryonated chicken eggs, 9-11 days old. The embryonated eggs should be examined after not less than 5 days incubation. The allantoic fluids should be tested with guinea-pig and chick or other avian red cells for the presence of haemaolutinins.

(c) Tests in animals for adventitious agents should include the inoculation by the intramuscular route of each of the following groups of animals with the test material or with disrupted cells from the seed lot propagated beyond the maximum level (or population doubling, as appropriate) used for production (WHO Reference):

2 Litters of suckling mice, comprising at least 10 animals less than 24 hours old.
10 adult mice
5 guinea-pigs

Test material should also be injected interacerebrally into each of 10 adult mice.

*   Committee for Proprietary Medicinal Products. Commission
     of the European Communities. Draft Notes on Requirements
     for the Quality Control of Monoclonal Antibodies of
     Murine Origin Intended for Use in Man (12).

It will be necessary to show that the hybridoma products are
not changed in successive production lots by comparison to an
identical, stable reference lot. It is recommended that each
lot should meet criteria for specificity, quantity, stability,
aggregation, denaturation, fragmentation. homogeneity, sterility as well as Mycoplasma and polynucleotide contamination.
Characterization by immunoglobulin class, subclass and isoelectric focusing pattern is currently recommended. If additives
or other modifications of the antibody are being used, these
should be described in the way they are used, and they should
be proven safe.

Specific attention is required to exclude potential viral
contamination. When mouse cells or mice are used, screening is
indicated for LCM virus, by animal or tissue culture inoculation. Mouse antibody production tests are used to detect LCM,
reovirus type 3, polyoma, pneumonia virus of mice, mouse ade-
novirus, minute virus of mice, mouse hepatitis, K. ectromelia,
Sendai and GD VII. Appropriate assays to detect murine cytomegalovirus, EDIM, thymic, LDH viruses or murine leukemia viruses
are currently performed routinely. Serum additives to tissue
cultures need to be shown free of adventitious agents. Preclinical evaluation in animals for toxicity and immunopharmacology
is currently recommended, particularly for products to be administered in vivo in humans. If an animal model exists for testing efficacy, this testing could also be employed. Monoclonal
antibody preprations should be screened for cross-reactivity
with human tissues (Table IV). Blood cells or cell lines might
also be employed. Additional considerations pertain to monoclonal antibody products coupled to radionuclides. Determination
of the stability of the conjugate or the complex is important,
and the activity and specificity of the components need to be
maintained.

Other FDA publications may be useful to developers of monoclonal antibody products. These include refs. (18) and (20).

TABLE IV. Suggested list of human tissues to be used for immunohistochemical or cytochemical investigations of cross-reactivity of monoclonal antibodies.

Tonsil, thymus, lymph node.
Bone marrow, peripheral blood.
Lung, liver, kidney, bladder, spleen,
stomach, intestine.
Pancreas, parotid, thyroid, parathyroid, adrenal,
pituitary.
Brain, peripheral nerve.
Heart, striated muscle.
Ovary, testis.
Skin

---

* Committee for Proprietary Medicinal Products. Commission of the European Communities. Draft Notes on Requirements for the Quality Control of Monoclonal Antibodies of Murine Origin Intended for Use in Man (12).

Although not mentioned explicitly in the recommendations from the FDA several recent scientific developments may be of interest to developers of monoclonal antibody products. Methods for the large-scale purification of monoclonal antibodies have been described by Ostlund (43).

Monoclonal antibodies, like all biological products that are intended for in vivo diagnostic or therapeutic use in man, must be shown to be both safe and effective before they can be licensed in the USA and other countries for marketing. For launching in the USA, two licenses have to be issued to the manufacturer by the Office of Biologics Research and Review: a product license for the product and an establishment license for the manufacturing facility. Efficacy must be demonstrated by well-controlled trials before licensing.

The human safety and efficacy data which are part of the license application are collected by obtaining permission to test the biological product in man. In the USA, such testing of unlicensed biological products (which moves in "interstate commerce") requires submission to the FDA of a Notice of Claimed Investigational Exemption for a New Drug (IND). There must be sufficient preclinical animal and in vitro data described in the IND to warrant investigational use of the biological product in man. This implies that there has to be some reason to believe that the product is more likely to do more good than harm or a favorable "risk-benefit" ratio. A certain amount of flexibility in these safety criteria could be possible where the intended use is in a setting of life threatening disease such as cancer.

The FDA requirements in the USA are considered quite stringent compared to those of many other governments. Satisfying requirements in the USA may be accepted by other oovernments as sufficient for approval to market in their countries. The Commission of European Communities Committee for Proprietary Medicinal Products has issued draft "Notes to Applicants for Marketing Authorizations" on Requirements for the Production and Quality Control of Monoclonal Antibodies of Murine Origin (12) as well as of Medicinal Products derived by Recombinant DNA Technology, respectively (13) which in many aspects show great similarities to the FDA recommendations. In addition to these recommendations a working Party on the Clinical Use of Antibodies in the UK (54) has issued a rather detailed operation manual describing the control of production, preclinical toxicology and phase trials of antitumor antibodies and drug antibody conjugates which is of relevance in the present context.

To cite from this Document: "It is recognized that the requirements of the licensing authority in regard to physicians undertaking a limited trial of a drug in their own patients are less demanding than those required of a drug company seeking a clinical trial certificate. The cost of toxicology, which must be borne by grants from government or charitable sources, would be prohibitive and destructive to the venture if the safety requirements of the licensing authority were set too high. The aim of this document is to establish guidelines for the quality and safety of antibodies and drug antibody conjugates produced in hospitals and university departments and to establish principles on which phase 1 trials of these agents will be conducted." (54).

This brief manual draws on the very reasonable comparison of the use of monoclonal antibodies in vivo with conventional chemotherapeutic agents for cancer patients. It specifically stresses the inadequacy of animal models for assesment of the potential of a monoclonal for imaging or therapeutic use in man and summarizes what is considered the minimal data necessary to satisfy and to assist the clinician contemplating phase 1 testing with all information necessary while at the same time recognizing the cost and feasability of obtaining this information in the laboratory. For in vivo use of radiolabeled antibody the rationale should include 1) evidence of localisation of the monoclonal antibody to the appropriate type of tumor cell by immunocytochemistry; and/or 2) evidence of in vivo localisation of the antibody in a xenograft of the appropriate human tumor in experimental animals (e.g. nude mice); and/or 3) evidence of in vitro binding of the antibody to a purified tumor-associated antigen expressed in the relevant type of human tumor. If the purity and specificity of the monoclonal antibody has been shown to be satisfactory, it is expected that the results of single dose toxicity studies should be available. These studies will normally be conducted in mice and one other species (e.g. guinea pig or rabbit). The number of animals required is in the order of 6-10 animals per dose. The dose should be 10 times that proposed in man (mg per kg body weight). In certain circumstances, a second dose may be advisable, for example in order to cover the possible need for dose escalation in man. The aim of this toxicity study is to identify any untoward or unexpected effect of the antibody. As concerns a radiolabeled conjugate of such an antibody it might be advisable to carry out the studies using a cold product prepared in the same way a the radiolabeled product, but for example substituting I-127 instead of I-131. If this is not possible, then toxicity studies should be carried out using the unconjugated monoclonal antibody only.

7. CONCLUSION

At present, monoclonal antibody imaging and radioimmunotherapy faces an uncertain future although these approaches offer great promise. The methods of producing, purifying and labelling antibodies discussed above have yielded antibody preparations suitable for initial investigations and further clinical studies which have been encouraging enough to stimulate further trials. However, it seems probable that further improvements both in the specificity and affinity of the antibodies to be used as well as in the technology used for labelling of these antibodies with radionuclides will be necessary for studies of this nature to be widely utilized. In connection with all further work necessary to develop radionuclide conjugated monoclonal antibodies for monoclonal antbody imaging and radioimmunotherapy it will be necessary to adhere to certain standards as regards safety requirements and quality control which have been presented here. In order to stimulate further developments in this area it will be necessary to contiunally to revise the guidelines proposed for such work based on the accumulated experience. In line with further recent recommendations it will be important to clearly distinguish the requirements for a radiopharmaceutical used in phase 1 trials and that of a final radiopharmaceutical product based on monoclonal antibodies.

Acknowledgement
The author wishes to thank Ms. Gerd Zachariassen for unfailing secretarial assistance and moral support during the preparation of this review.

156

References

1. Birch J R, Boraston R, Wood L. Bulk production of monoclonal antibodies in fermenters. Trends in Biotechnol, 1985; 3: 162-166.
2. Bozeman M H. The regulation of hybridoma products. In: The impact of Hybridoma Technology on the Device and Diagnostic Product Industry. Proceeding of the Educational Seminar, Arlington, VA June 14-15, (1982). Health Industry Manufacturers Association Reports, Report 82-1 1982: 63-82.
3. Burgoyne R F. HPLC techniques advance monoclonal antibody isolation. Res Dev 1985; 27: 82-85.
4. Bussard A E. How pure are monoclonal antibodies? Dev Biol Stand 1984; 57: 13-15.
5. Carlsson M, Hedin A, Inganäs M, Härfast B, Blomberg F. Purification of in vitro produced mouse monoclonal antibodies. A two-step procedure utilizing cation exchange chromatography and gel filtration. J Immunol Methods 1985; 79: 89-98.
6. Carrasquillo J A, Krohn K A, Beaumier P, McGuffin R W, Brown J P, Hellström K E, Hellström I, Larson S M. Diagnosis of and therapy for solid tumors with radiolabeled antibodies and immune fragments. Cancer Treat. Rep 1984; 39: 317-328.
7. Chang T H, Steplewski Z, Koprowski H. Production of monclonal antibodies in serum free medium. J Immunol Methods 1980; 39: 369-375.
8. Chatal J F, Saccavini J C, Fumoleau P, Doulliard J Y, Curtet C, Kremer K, Lemevel B, Koprowski H. Immunoscintigraphy of colon carcinoma. J Nucl Med 1984; 25: 307-314.
9. Chatal J.F, Powe, J. Radioimmunoimaging. Hybridoma 1980; 5: 166-170.
10. Clezardin P, McGregor J L, Manach M, Boukerche H, Dechavanne M. One-step procedure for the rapid isolation of mouse monoclonal antibodies and their antigen binding fragments by fast protein liquid chromatography on a Mono Q anion-exchange column. J Chromatogr 1985; 319: 67-77.
11. Clezardin P, Bougro G, McGregor J L. Tandem purification of IgM monoclonal antibodies from mouse ascites fluids by anion-exchange and fast protein liquid chromatography. J Chromatogr 1986; 354: 425-433.
12. Committee for Proprietary Medicinal Products. Commision of the European Communities.: Notes to Applicants for Marketing Authorizations On Requirements for the Production and Quality Control of Monoclonal Antibodies of Murine Origin Intended for Use in Man. Commission of the European Communities III/859/86-EN (in draft form, rev 6) March 1987.
13. Committee for Proprietary Medicinal Products. Commision of the European Communities.: Notes to Applicants for Marketing Authorizations On Requirements for the Production and Quality Control of Medicinal Products. Derived by Recombinant DNA Technology. Commission of the European Communities III/860/86-EN (in draft form, rev 7) March 1987.

14. Dillman R O, Beauregard J C, Sobol R E, Royston I, Bartholomew R M, Hagan P S, Halpern S E. Lack of radioimmunodetection and complications associated with monoclonal anticarcinoembryonic antigen antibody crossreactivity with an antigen on circulation cells. Cancer Res 1984; 44: 2213-2218.

15. Duff R G. Microencapsulation technology. A novel method for monoclonal antibody production. Trends in Biotechnol. 1985; 3: 167-170.

16. Epenetos A, Mather S, Granowska M, Ninnom C C, Hawkins L R, Britton K E, Shepherd J, Taylor-Papadimitriou J, Durbin H, Maplas J S, Bodmer W F. Targeting of iodine-123-labelled tumour-associated monoclonal antibodies to ovarian, breast, and gastrointestinal tumours. Lancet 1982; 2: 999-1006.

17. Ey P L, Prowse S J, Jenkin C R. Isolation of pure IgG1, IgG2a and IgG2b immunoglobulins from mouse serum using protein A-Sepharose. Immunochemistry 1978; 15: 429-436.

18. Federal Register, Docket No. 83N-0070, Licensing of a Biological Monoclonal Antibody Product Prepared by Hybridoma Technology. Fed Register 48, 50795, Nov. 3, 1983.

19. Federal Register, Docket No. 83N-0363, Biological Products; in Vitro or in Vivo Monoclonal Antibodies, ... Availability of Draft Criteria for New Technologies; Requests for Comments, Data, and Recommendations. Notice. Fed. Register 49, 1138, Jan. 9, 1984.

20. Federal Register, Docket No. 84N-0154, Open Meeting; Public workshop on Cell Substrates; Availability of Points to Consider; Requests for Comments. Fed. Register 49, 23456, June 6, 1984.

21. Gemski M J, Doctor B P, Gentry M K, Strickler M P. Single step purification of monoclonal antibody from murine ascites and tissues culture fluids by anion exchange high performance liquid chromatography, BioTechniques 1985; 3: 378-384.

22. Goding J W. Use of staphylococcal protein A as an immuno logical reagent. J Immunol Methods 1978; 20: 241-253.

23. Gritzmacher C A. Expression of recombinant immunoglobin genes to reproduce novel molecules with specific functions. Immunol Res 1986; 5: 210-220.

24. Hellström K E, Hellström I, Brown J P, Monoclonal antibodies to melanoma-associated antigens. In: Wright, G.L. (ed.) Monoclonal antibodies and cancer (Immunology series 23). Marcel Dekker, New York 1984: 31-48.

25. Hnatowich D J, Layne W W, Childs R L, Lanteigne D, Davis M A, Griffin T W, Doherty P W. Radioactive labeling of antibody: A simple and efficient method. Science 1983; 220: 613-615.

26. Hoffman T, Kenimer J, Stein J E. Regulatory issues surrounding therapeutic use of monoclonal antibodies: Points to consider in the manufacture of injectable products intended for human use. In: Monoclonal Antibodies and Cancer Therapy (Reisberg, R.A., Sell, S. eds., ed.). Alan R. Liss, Inc. New York 1985: 431-440.

27. JAMA Medical News. FDA prepares to meet regulatory challenges of the 21st century. JAMA 1985; 254: 2189-2193, 2199-2201.

28. Kennel S J, Foote L J, Lankford P K, Johnson M, Mitchell T, Braslawsky G R. Direct binding of radioiodinated monoclonal antibody to tumor cells: Significance of antibody purity and affinity for drug targeting or tumor imaging. Hybridoma 1983; 2: 297-310.

29. Kozak R W, Waldmann T A, Atcher R W, Gansow O A. Radionuclide-conjugated monoclonal antibodies: A synthesis of immunology, inorganic chemistry and nuclear science. Trends in Biotechnol 1986; 4: 259-263.

30. Köhler G, Milstein C. Continuous cultures of fused cells secreting antibody of predefined specificity. Nature 1975; 256: 495-497.

31. Larson S M, Brown J P, Wright P W, Carrasquillo J A, Hellström I, Hellström K E. Imaging of melanoma with I-131-labeled monoclonal antibodies. J Nucl Med 1983; 24: 123-129.

32. Larson S M, Carrasquillo J A, Krohn K A, Brown J P, McGuffin R W, Ferens J M, Graham M M, Hill L D, Beaumier P L, Hellestöm K E, Hellström I. Localization of I-131-labeled p97-specific Fab fragments in humans as a basis for radiotherapy. J Clin Invest 1983; 72: 2101-2114.

33. Lee C, McKearn T J, Rodwell J D, Hiles B L, Alvarez V L. Radioimmunoimaging with site-specifically modified monoclonal antibodies. Fed Proc 1984; 43: 1932.

34. Mach J P, Buchegger F, Forni M, Ritschard J, Berche C M, Lumbroso J D, Schreyer M, Giradet F, Accolla R S, Carrel S. Use of radiolabeled monoclonal anti-CEA antibodies for the detection of human carinomas by external photoscanning and tomocintigraphy. Immunology Today 1981; 2: 239-249.

35. Mach j P, Chartal J F, Lumbroso J D, Buchegger F, Forni M, Ritschard J, Berche C, Douilliard J Y, Carrel S, Herlyn M, Steplewski Z, Koprowski H. Tumor localization in patients by radiolabeled monoclonal antibodies against colon carcinoma. Cancer Res 1983; 43: 5593-5600.

36. Manil L, Motte P, Pernal P, Troalen F, Bohuon C, Bellet. Evauation of protocols for purifaction of mouse monoclonal antibodies. Yield and purity in two dimensional gel electrophoresis. J Immunol Methods 1984; 90: 25-37.

37. Markwell M A K. A new solid-state reagent to iodinate proteins. 1. Conditions for the efficient labeling of antiserum. Anal Biochem 1982; 125: 427-432.

38. Murakami H, Steplewski Z, Koprowski H. Production of monoclonal antibodies in serum free medium. J Immunol Methods 1980; 39: 369-375.

39. Meares C F, Goodwin D A, Leung C S-H, Giris A Y, Silvester D J, Nuun A D, Lavender P J. Covalent attachment of metal chelates to proteins: The stability In vivo and in vitro of the conjugate of albumin with a chelate of 111 indium. Proc Natl Acad Sci USA 1976; 73: 3803-3806.

40. Merchant E B. Points to consider during monoclonal antibody production. In: The Impact of Hybridoma Tech-

nology in the Medical Device and Diagnostic Product
Industry. Proceedings of the Educational Seminar, Arling-
ton, VA June 14-15, (1982). Health Industry Manufactures
Association Reports, Report 82-1. 1982: 83-92.

41. Nilsson K, Scheirer W, Merten O W, Ostberg L, Liehl E,
Katinger H W D, Mosbach K. Entrapment of animal cells for
production of monoclonal and other biomolecules. Nature
1983; 302: 629-630.

42. Ortho Multicenter Transplant Study Group: A randomized
clinical trial of OKT3 monoclonal antibody for acute rejection of cadaveric renal transplats. N Eng J Med 1985;
313: 337-342.

43. Ostlund C, Large-scale purification of monoclonal
antibodies. Trends in Biotechnol 1986; 4: 288-293.

44. Paik C H, Ebbert M A, Murphy P R, Lassman C R, Reba R C,
Eckelman W C, Pak K Y, Powe J, Steplewski Z, Koprowski H.
Factors influencing DTPA conjugation with antibodies by
cyclic DTPA anhydride. J Nucl Med 1983; 24: 1158-1163.

45. Prentice H G, Janossy G, Skeggs D, Blacklock H A,
Bradstock K F, Goldstein G, Hoffbrand A V. Use of anti-T
cell monoclonal antibody OKT3 to prevent acute graft-
versus-host disease in allogeneic bone marrow transplantation for acute leukeamia. Lancet 1982; 1: 700-703.

46. Reinsbury R M, Westwood J H, Goombes R C, Neville A M,
Ott R J, Kalirai T S, McCready V R, Gazet J C. Location of
metastatic breast carcinoma by a monoclonal antibody chelate labelled with indium-111. Lancet 1983; 2: 934-938.

47. Saha G B. Radioiodination of antibodies for tumor imaging.
In: Burchiel, S.W. and Rhodes, B.A. (eds.). Radioimmunoimaging and radio-immunotherapy. Elsevier, New York
1983: 171-184.

48. Scheinberg D A, Strand M, Gansow OA. Tumor imaging with
radioactive metal chelates conjugated to monoclonal antibodies. Science 1982; 218: 1511-1513.

49. Sundberg M W, Meares C F, Goodwin D A, Diamenti D I.
Selective binding of metal ions to macromolecules using
bifunctional analogs of EDTA. J Med Chem 1974; 17:
1304-1307.

50. Stephenson J R, Lee J W, Wilton-Smith P D. Production and
purification of murine monoclonal antibodies: Aberrant
elution from protein A-Sepharose. Anal Biochem 1984; 142:
189-195.

51. Wang T S T, Ng A K, Fawwaz R A, Alderson P O.
Heterobifunctional reagents: A new approach to radiolabeling of monoclonal antibodies. Proceedings of the 32nd
Annual Meeting of the Society of Nuclear Medicine, Hou-
ston, Texas, USA, June, 2-5, (1985). J Nucl Med 1985; 26:
46.

52. Weimann M L Ball E D, Fanger M W, Dexter D L, McIntyre O
R, Berneier G, Calabresi P. Human and murine hubridoma
antibody production in the artificial capillary culture
system, Clin Res 1983; 31 (2): 511A.

53. Wensel T G, Meares D F. Bifunctional chelating agents for
binding metal ions to proteins. In: Burchiel, S.W. and

160

Rhodes, B.A. (eds.). Radioimmunoimaging and radioimmunotherapy. Elsevier, New York. 1983: 185-196.

54.   "Working Party on Clinical Use of Antibodies": Operation
Manual for control of production, preclinical toxicology
and phase I trials of anti-tumour antibodies and drug
antibody conjugates. Prepared by a Joint Committee of the
Cancer Research Campaign National Institute for Biological
Standards and Control. Br J Cancer 1986; 54: 557-568.

10. SPECIFICATIONS AND QUALITY CONTROL METHODS FOR LABELLED CELLS

H.J. DANPURE AND S. OSMAN

1. INTRODUCTION

Radiolabelled blood cells are used to carry radiopharmaceuticals to specific sites in the body; for example labelled granolocytes and mixed leucocytes are used to detect sites of infection and inflammation (1) labelled platelets accumulate in thromboses (2) and rejected renal transplants (3) and labelled lymphocytes accumulate in lymph nodes (4). Labelled platelets (5), granulocytes (6) and lymphocytes (7) are also used for cell kinetic studies. For all these studies it is essential that the presence of the radiopharmaceutical on the blood cells does not alter their _in vivo_ behaviour. Cell damage may arise from three sources, radiation from the delay of the radionuclide, chemical toxicity from the cell labelling agents and mechanical damage due the extensive manipulations that are often required when labelling cells (8).

Since the introduction of In-111-oxine as a cell labelling agent in 1976 (9), a number of other cell labelling agents have been used in Nuclear Medicine, such as the lipid-soluble complexes. In-111 tropolonate (10) and Tc-99m HM-PAO (11), radiolabelled colloids (12) and cell-specific monoclonal antibodies (13). With most of these agents it is necessary to radiolabel the cells _in vitro_, which is labour intensive and therefore prone to error if the personnel involved are not adequetly instructed as to how to carry out the procedures. But before a method is introduced into clinical use it must be thoroughly tested in the laboratory to ensure its safety and reproducibility. If the cell labelling method has been carefully developed with these aims in mind and the people who are to carry out these studies on patients are well trained, it should not be necessary to carry out extensive quality control measurements on individual labelled cell preparations. In any case it is not advisable to delay the return of the labelled cells to the patient while quality control tests are being performed as this may reduce their viability.

2. ENVIRONMENT FOR THE HANDLING OF BLOOD

Blood should always be handled with great care because of the risk of contracting viral infections such as hepatitis or AIDS. Blood is usually screened for the Hepatitis B antigen before the cell labelling study is undertaken, but at present blood is not routinely screened for AIDS. To protect the operator and the cells, British regulations (14) stipulate that the cell labelling should be carried out in a work station providing air filtered to Class I (British standard 5295) and also complying with the requirements of a Class II or Class III microbiological safety cabinet (British standard 5726). The work station should be reserved for handling blood and only one patients' blood must be labelled at a time using aseptic techniques. All solutions must be sterile and pyrogen-free. Sharps should be avoided. After use, the work station, gloves and all apparatus must be disinfected.

3. QUALITY CONTROL ON LABELLED CELLS

The method for quality control of radiolabelled blood cells will be considered in two parts. First the steps that are taken to develop a safe, reproducible method for labelling cells with a particular radiopharmaceutical, and second the day to day procedures that should be carried out on each batch of cells after they have been labelled.

4. DEVELOPMENT OF THE CELL LABELLING METHOD

Blood cells can be labelled with either a non-selective or

selective agent; a non-selective compound labels all types of
blood cells indiscriminantly whereas a selective compound labels only one, or maybe two, types of cells when added to whole
blood.

Radiolabelling blood cells with a non-selective agent is a
two-step process: the first is to separate the required cells
from whole blood and the second is to radiolabel them. The methods of separating the individual types of cells from whole
blood will be considered first.

5. CELL SEPARATION

Granulocytes, mixed leucocytes as a source of granulocytes
and platelets can all be separated from whole blood by differential centrifugation. The methods are labour intensive and
require a high level of competence by the personnel involved if
they are to be successful. It is therefore essential that the
people involved are fully trained, given time to practice the
techniques and are made aware of the reasons why various steps
are important. Work sheets outlining the various steps in the
cell separation and labelling procedure should be prepared and
clearly displayed close to the work station.

Although many different methods have, and will continue to
be used (15,16) they all aim to produce cells which will function normally when returned to the patient. Mechanical damage
to the cells is the main problem during the cell separation and
carelessness may result in the cells becoming damaged even before they are radiolabelled. The procedures given in the appendix are designed to keep the amount of mechanical damage to a
minimum, for example, by centrifuging the cells at the lowest
possible speed for the shortest time to achieve the required
result and by minimising the sheer forces on the cells by not
shaking them or sucking them through a syringe needle.

5.1. Separation of mixed leucocytes and granulocytes

The method we use to isolate mixed ("crude") leucocytes from
whole blood are shown in Figure 1 and described in the appendix. Variations in this method are given by Hardeman and Feuger

164

(15). There is still a debate as to whether it is better to label granulocytes or mixtures of leucocytes. The choice depends on the clinical study, the patients granulocyte count and the facilities that are available (17). If quantitative studies are required, such as measurements of the extent faecal excretion, then pure granulocytes must be used. If the patient is neutrophilic, i.e. has a granulocyte count greater than 9 million/ml, mixed leucocytes are usually satisfactory but for low-grade infection granulocytes are usually better. If the patient is neutropenic, i.e. has a granulocyte count less than 1.5 million/ml, donor granulocytes may be necessary.

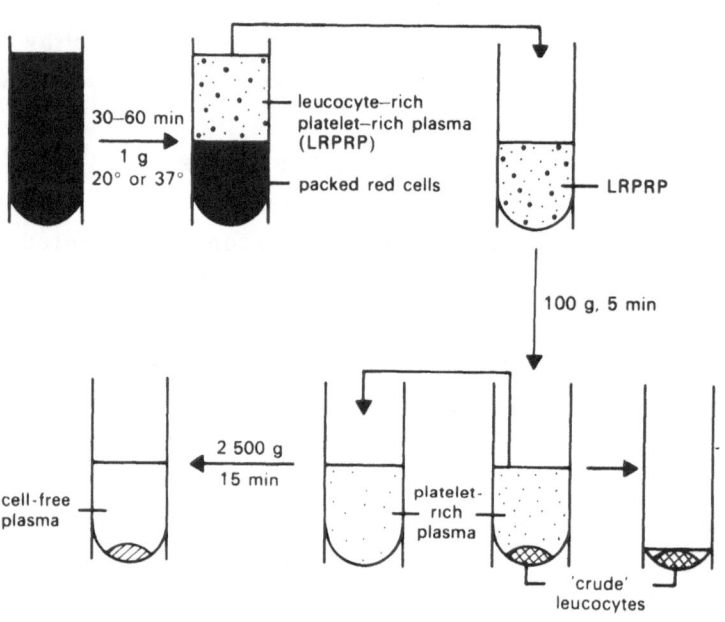

FIGURE 1. Method of isolating "crude" leucocytes from whole blood. From A.E. Theobald (8). Reproduced by kind permission of Taylor and Francis Ltd, London.

The main argument against the use of granulocytes is the possible damage that the cells may receive as a result of the extra manipulations required to separate them from mixed leucocytes. We have shown that no harm is done if the cells are separated on a gradient that contains plasma (18). In the Nether-

lands they insist that pure granulocytes are used because of
the risks of injecting sub-lethally damaged lymphocytes which
might result in the production of tumours.

Granulocytes can be separated from other leucocytes by using
isopycnic density gradients of Percoll (10) or metrizamide (19)
mixed with autologous plasma. The presence of plasma is important to prevent metabollic activation of the granulocytes. Granulocytes isolated by this method contain 15-20% red cells, but
as the red cells incorporate less than 5% of the total cell-
bound In-111 (19) the mixture can be considered as a "pure" population of granulocytes once it has been labelled.

5.2. Methods of separating platelets

The method we use to isolate platelets from whole blood is
shown in Figure 2 and described in the appendix. Variations in
the methods used are documented by Mathias and Welch (16). The
important points for successful separation of platelets from
whole blood are; the use of ACD not heparin to anticoagulate

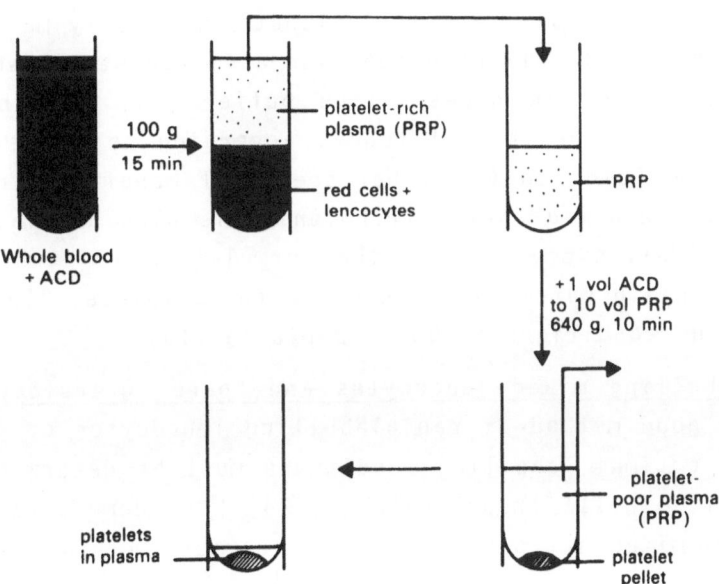

FIGURE 2. Method of isolating platelets from whole blood. From
A.E. Theobald (8). Reproduced by kind permission of Taylor and
Francis Ltd, London.

the blood, the inhibition of spontaneous aggregation of platelets by lowering the pH with ACD (20) or adding prostaglandin (21) and handling the cells as gently as possible. Once again there seems to be general agreement that keeping the cells in plasma during their separation and labelling is better than removing them from plasma (16).

5.3. Methods of isolating lymphocytes from whole blood

Lymphocytes can be isolated from whole blood using Ficoll density gradients (21). If large numbers of cells are required they can be isolated on a cell separator.

6. CELL LABELLING

6.1. With In-111 complexes

The most well known non-selective In-111 complexes used to label blood cells are In-111 oxine and In-111 tropolonate. The former is commercially available as a preformed complex in a-queous solution with detergent (Amersham International plc) or without (Mallinkrodt). It is also available in ethanol (Mediphysics). In contrast In-111 tropolonate is usually made as required by mixing In-111-chloride with a filter-sterilised solution of tropolone in Hepes-saline buffer (10) that has been prepared in the hospital pharmacy, according to the standards given in the Guide to Good Pharmaceutical Manufacturing Practice (23). Preformed In-111 tropolonate is also available commercially (Mallinkcrodt), but the formulation is such that it does not contain sufficient tropolone to radiolabel blood cells under optium conditions in 90% ACD-plasma (10).

6.1.1. Labelling mixed leucocytes and "pure" granulocytes. To

develop a good method of radiolabelling leucocytes or granulocytes the optimum labelling conditions must be determined. Our studies with In-111 tropolonate (10,24) have demonstrated that incubating mixed leucocytes or granulocytes in 1 ml cell-free plasma containing acid-citrate-dextrose (ACD) at a leucocyte concentration greater than 50 million per ml with In-111 tropolonate containing 0.4 mM tropolone for 5 min. at room temperature gives optimal results. The above conditions were chosen as being optimal because they gave maximum uptake of the In-111 complex i.e. a high labelling effiency, maximum stability of the In-111 on the cells and more importantly minimal damage or alteration to the labelled cells. As a result the labelled cells were able to behave in the same way as their unlabelled counterparts when reinjected into the patient. The specific conditions which were important to maintain the functional integrety of the labelled cells were:

1. The use of ACD, not heparin in the labelling medium.
2. The precense of plasma on the cells throughout their cell separation and labelling.
3. The use of the correct amount of tropolone.

ACD was important for two reasons; it inhibited spontaneous aggregation of granulocytes (20) and reduced the optimum amount of tropolene required to label cells (24). Plasma was very important because it inhibited metabolic activation of the granulocytes and resulted in rapid uptake of labelled cells into inflammatory lesions (19), whereas if cells were labelled in a plasma-free medium, with for example In-111 acetylacetone, the cells became sticky and were retained in the lungs for several hours before being released to migrate to other parts of the body (21). The use of the optimum amount of tropolone, which for labelling leucocytes in 90% ACD-plasma is 0.4 mM was very important because this concentration gives maximum incorporation of In-111 and the greatest stability of the radionuclide in the labelled cells.

6.1.2. _Labelling platelets with non-selective agents_. The most widely used agents are In-111 oxine and In-111 tropolonate and using both compounds there have been many studies to develop methods of labelling platelets, and as a result many different methods have been adopted (16). The same criteria apply to the development of methods of labelling platelets as they do for labelling leucocytes, namely the radiolabel must remain firmly attached to the cells for the period of the clinical study and must not alter or damage the cells. Platelets are non-nucleated cells which are radiation resistant and can tolerate 37 MBq (1mCi) on 1000 million platelets (25), but very readily aggregate when subjected to mechanical forces.

Our procedure for labelling platelets with In-111 tropolonate is the same as that given in the appendix for mixed leucocytes and granulocytes except that the platelets are labelled, washed and resuspended in ACD-plasma pH 6.5 not pH 7.2 to prevent spontaneous aggregation. If the platelets are to be used for measurement of platelet life-span the amount of In-111 can be reduced from approximately 10 to 4 MBq provided that imaging is not required.

6.1.3. Labelling lymphocytes with non-selective agents. Human lymphocytes have been labelled with In-111 oxine and used in patients (4) but, unlike granulocytes, lymphocytes can divide and are therefore much more sensitive to radiation than granulocytes. Animal (26) and in vitro (27) studies have shown that lymphocytes are damaged by doses of In-111 in excess of 20 microcurie (0.74 MBq) per 100 million lymphocytes due to the low energy Auger electrons that the In-111 emits when it decays, whereas granulocytes show no signs of damage with fifty times that dose. To image a patient a minimum of 100 microcurie of In-111 is required.

Although normal lymphocyte migration patterns have been achieved with lymphocytes labelled with In-111 (4,28) there is still concern that radiolabelled lymphocytes which have received a sub-lethal dose of radiation might be transformed into malignant cells and produce a tumour (27,29). There is a similar concern about lymphocytes that become labelled when mixed leucocytes are labelled with the In-111 complexes (27).

The procedure given at the end of the chapter for labelling blood cells with In-111 tropolonate could also be used to label lymphocytes provided that the amount of In-111 did not exceed 20 microcurie (0.74 MBq) per 100 million cells.

6.2. Cell labelling with Tc-99m-HM-PAO

Recently the lipid-soluble complex Tc-99m HM-PAO was also introduced as a non-selective leucocyte-labelling agent (11). It is commercially available as a kit from Amersham International. It does not have a product licence in the UK and therefore must be used on named patients only. The method we recently introduced for clinical studies (30) is given in the appendix at the end of the chapter.

7. SELECTIVE CELL LABELLING AGENTS

To date there are very few selective agents for radiolabelling blood cells although considerable effort is being expended on developing new ones. The advantages of a simpler, quicker method would be considerable and might encourage the procedure to be more widely used.

Colloidal substances, such as Tc-99m tin colloid, which are phagocytosed by granulocytes and monocytes, but are not incorporated by the other blood cells, erythrocytes, lymphocytes and platelets have been used for the selective in vitro labelling of phagocytic cells in whole blood (12). Tc-99m tin colloid is available as a commercial kit (Amerscan, Amersham International plc) for liver scintigraphy but needs modification before it will label cells. The size of the colloidal particles in the freshly prepared kit is too small for phagocytosis so the colloid is mixed by rotation for one hour to increase the particle size. Schroth et al (12), found that the colloid that they produced from Amersham's kit labelled predominantly monocytes, whereas Hanna and Lomas (31), who prepared their own colloid using the same formulation, found their radio-colloid principally labelled granulocytes. The notable difference between the two preparations was in the mean size of the colloidal particles, it was 1,5 micrometer using Amersham's kit and between 1.7 and 2.1 micrometer using Hanna and Lomas' preparation. Hanna and Lomas (31) also listed other variables which affected the ability of Tc-99m tin colloid to radiolabel granulocytes. These include the purity of the starting materials, the speed at which the colloid was rotated, the heparin concentration, the type of membrane filter used to sterilise the mixture of stannous fluoride and sodium fluoride and the time the blood was incubated with the colloid. Difficulty in controlling these factors and the reduced viability of the labelled cells with concomitant release of Tc-99m observed by some users (32) has prevented this method from becoming widely used. But recent success with Tc-99m tin colloid by Pulmann et al (33) may encourage others to try this method.

The recent demonstration that monoclonal antibodies (mabs) specific for platelets (34), granulocytes (13) and granulocytes labelling agents in man is of considerable interest. The mabs have either been labelled with I-123 using Iodogen (13,35) or with In-111 using cyclic DTPA (34). Lymphocytes labelled with In-111-anti-lymphocyte mabs have been successfully used to visualise lymph nodes in mice (36), but there are no reports as yet of the clinical use of lymphocytes tagged with labelled mabs. This method could be a good alternative to the liphophilic complexes for labelling lymphocytes because radiolabelled mabs on the surface of the cell will produce less radiation damage to the cells than the In-111 complexes which are found predominantly in the cell nucleus (7). Details of how monoclonal antibodies are produced, radiolabelled and tested are given in the chapters by Zeuthen and Mather and by Goding (37) and will not be dealt with here. Specific information relating to the use of Mabs for labelling blood cells are given in several recent reviews (36,38,39). Although the use of cell-specific mabs is an exciting development the techniques using mabs are still in their infancy and are unlikely to be widely used for some time because careful investigations into the effect that mab has on cell function are required.

8. QUALITY CONTROL ON CELLS AFTER LABELLING

8.1. Granulocytes and mixed leucocytes

There are many in vitro methods of measuring the viability and behaveour of granulocytes after they have been radiolabelled, such as uptake of the dye Trypan blue, phagocytosis of bacteria or other particles such as Zymosan and chemotaxis in response to a chemoattractant. Using these methods the effect of radiation, chemical and mechanical damage to cells have been measured (40,41). The method for measuring phagocytosis is clearly described by Babior and Cohen (42) and for chemotaxis by Territo (43). But how good are these tests in predicting the behaviour of the labelled cells when they are returned to the patient? At Hammersmith hospital we compared the random migration and phagocytosis of granulocytes that had been labelled with In-111 acetylacetone in buffer with those labelled with In-111 tropolonate in plasma and found no differences, nor any differences from unlabelled cells. But when the two sets of labelled cells were reinjected into patients there was a striking difference (18). The cells which had been labelled in buffer were retained in the lungs for several hours whereas those labelled in plasma were not. The _in vitro_ tests had therefore not predicted these differences. An example such as this is used to illustrate that _in vitro_ tests do not necessarily indicate how labelled cells will behave _in vivo_ and care should be excercised in their use. Another problem with using tests such as these is that they take 2 to 3 hours to perform, which added to the 2 hours that it takes to separate and label the cells means that the cells are out of the body for a length of time which approaches the 5 to 6 hour half-life of granulocytes. One would therefore expect to see a deterioration in the cells simply as a result of the time factor. If the labelled blood cells was not returned to the patient for 5 hours there might also be problems in the Nuclear Medicine department in imaging the patient 3 to 4 hours post-injection. A third consideration is that misleading results can be obtained with the tests such as chemotaxis and phagocytosis if they are not carried out by properly trained staff. Therefore it is not really sensible or worthwhile to delay the reinjection of labelled cells in order to get the result from some lengthy _in vitro_ test which may give a misleading answer. In some centres these _in vitro_ tests are performed retrospectively on random samples. Again they are subject to the same shortcomings outlined above. We would like to repeat at this point our belief that training of staff is much more likely to provide a satisfactory "product" than some lengthy _in vitro_ functional tests.

There are however several quick and simple quality control measurements that can, and should, be made on labelled granulocytes or mixed leucocytes before they are reinjected into the patient. The first is to measure the labelling efficiency (LE), which is the proportion of the total radionuclide added to the cells that becomes cell bound. This is not applicable to cells labelled with monoclonal antibodies for the reasons given below. A high LE is usually considered a sign that everything has gone satisfactory, whereas a low LE is considered a sign that something has gone wrong. Generally this is true, but not always. The LE is determined by many factors some of which are (or should be) constant in all preparations, for example the consideration of ligand (e.g. oxine, tropolone or HM-PAO) that is mixed with the In-111 or Tc-99m, the concentration of plasma and the anticoagulant. But some factors vary, especially the number of cells available for labelling. This may occur because of variations in the volume of blood, blood count or cell recoveries. The amount of In-111 or Tc-99m incorporated by cells i.e. the LE is directly proportional to the cell concentration (10), for example, 100 million granulocytes labelled in 1 ml plasma with In-111 tropolonate gave a LE of 90% (24), but only 31% when the cell concentration was reduced ten-fold (10). Thus the lower LE was obtained simply as a result of the lower cell concentration, not because the procedure has been performed incorrectly.

A high LE is not generally obtained with monoclonal antibodies because the cells are usually incubated with an excess of the mab. For example, a 100 million granulocytes, with 20,000 receptors per cell, could bind a maximum of 2×10^{12} molecules of antibody, which for an IgG antibody of molecular weight 150,000 Daltons is equivalent to only 0.5 microgrammes of an IgG antibody. Such low amounts of protein are rarely used.

Another simple test is to look for clumps or aggregates of cells in the final labelled cell preparation, if present the cells should not be reinjected into the patient as this is an indication that they are damaged.

The most useful measure of the functional integrety of the labelled cells is to observe the biodistribution of the labelled cells for the first 20-30 minutes after the labelled cells have been reinjected into the patient. This is usually referred to as dynamic imaging. Undamaged granulocytes rapidly pass through the lungs and accumulate in the spleen and inflammatory lesions, whereas damaged granulocytes are retained by the lungs, show irreversible uptake into the liver and a slow uptake into inflammatory lesions (18).

8.2. Platelets

The most common in vitro method of testing platelet function is aggregometry. By this method platelets are stimulated to aggregate by agents such as adenosine diphosphate (ADP) and collagen and the effect is measured photometrically as a progressive increase in the transmission of light through a suspension of platelets as the single cells become clumps. A trace of the changes in optical density against time is plotted on a chart recorder (44). Unfortunately, platelets that have been separated and radiolabelled by methods such as that outlined above cannot be used for aggregometry because their ability to aggregate has been inhibited by ACD or prostaglandin. Platelet-rich plasma prepared from blood anticoagulated with citrate must be used instead. But platelets prepared in this way have not been subjected to the same treatment as those that have been radiolabelled and therefore their response to ADP is unlikely to be the same. If the labelled platelets are washed free of ACD and then tested this again results in a platelet population that is different from the one that has been prepared for injection into the patient. Thus aggregometry is not a suitable method of assessing the function of radiolabelled platelets.

Peters et al (45) have devised a simple, rapid quantitative method that does measure the function of radiolabelled platelets. A small aliquot (less than 0.1 ml) of the labelled platelets are mixed with a fresh sample of un-anticoagulated blood and passed through a filter paper in a filter funnel. The retention of radioactivity from the labelled platelets is then compared to that of the total platelets which is measured by counting the number of platelets before and after passage through the filter paper. This test can be used on platelets before and after injection.

It is also recommended that the labelling efficiency is measured as described for leucocytes and that the labelled platelets are checked to ensure that they do not contain any clumped cells.

Dynamic imaging of the patient is the method of choice for assessing the behaviour of the labelled platelets. Undamaged platelets rapidly leave the circulation and accumulate in the spleen whereas damaged platelets show a reversible uptake by the liver (46).

8.3. Lymphocytes

Tests that measure the behaviour of labelled lymphocytes, for example, the amount of DNA synthesied after stimulation with a mitogenic agent such as phytohaemagglutanin (PHA), take several days to give a result and cannot be used to assess the viability of the lymphocytes before they are returned to the patient, but can be used retrospectively. Other tests such as measurement of chromosome abberations (27) are also useful in assessing the safety of a method at the developmental stage but not for assessing the viability of the labelled cells before reinjection into the patient.

Measurement of LE and a check that the final suspension of labelled lymphocytes does not contain any clumps of cells are worthwhile QC procedures.

Dynamic imaging of labelled lymphocytes showed rapid uptake of "normal" cells into the spleen whereas heat-damaged cells were initially sequestered by the lung and later migrated to the liver, with very few cells travelling to the spleen (28).

9. CONCLUSION

The procedures currently involved in radiolabelling blood cells are generally complicated and may be carried out by people from widely differing backgrounds. We have met chemists, biochemists, heamatologists, radiopharmacists, radiographers, physicists and clinicians. To ensure that the cells that they label are "safe" to reinject into a patient and are going to give a meaningful result the people involved must be carefully instructed in how to carry out the procedures. Practical training by people who are experienced in the methods, which often seem very complicated to a newcomer, is the only way to be certain that someone is competent to do the clinical cell labelling. Following published methods is not always satisfactory because the trend for concise papers does not allow the inclusion of the practical details which are important for success. The lack of a unified method with a particular radiopharmaceutical also add to the confusion. It seems unlikely that a single procedure will ever be adopted with the In-111 complexes, but this need not be a problem if the methods are fully documented. The methods we use to isolate and label granulocytes, mixed leucocytes and platelets with In-111 tropolonate and mixed leucocytes with Tc-99m HM-PAO are given in full at the end of this chapter.

Practice is also essential; a person who is going to label cells only once a month is likely to have more problems than someone who labels cells every day. Ideally if the studies only occur occasionally then the person should practice the technique regularly to maintain their competence, but with limited time and resources this is not always possible.

It should also be mentioned that equivocal and incorrect clinical results may be obtained through no fault of the person carrying out the technique, but may occur because the cells that were taken from the patient were abnormal, perhaps as a result of the treatment that the patient was receiving. For example, drugs such as asprin cause platelet dysfunction and should not be administered for 7-10 days before a platelet function test is performed (44).

The future trends of cell labelling are towards much simpler methods which will hopefully make the techniques more widely used. At present the most promising compounds are the monoclonal antibodies, which ideally will be available in kit form for easy radiolabelling, then administered intravenously to the patient to selectively label the cells of interest in vivo. Although this procedure has been used (13,34) it is still a new modality which must be thoroughly investigated for its safety before it is used extensively in man.

REFERENCES
1. Segal AW, Arnot RN, Thakur ML, Lavender JP, Indium-111 labelled leucocytes for localisation of abscesses. Lancet 1976; ii: 1556.
2. Goodwin DA, Bushberg JT, Doherty PW, Lipton MJ, Conley FK, Diamanti DI, Meares CF, Indium-111-labelled autologous platelets for localisation of vascular thrombi in humans. J Nucl Med 1978; 19: 626.
3. Smith N, Chandler S, Hawker RJ, Hawker LM, Barnes AD, Indium autologous platelets as a diagnostic aid after renal transplantation. Lancet 1979; 2: 1241.
4. Lavender JP, Goldman JM, Arnot RN, et al. Kinetics of Indium-111-labelled lymphocytes in normal subjects and patients with Hodgkins disease. Brit Med J 1977; 2: 797.
5. Peters AM, Saverymuttu SH, Malik F, Ind PW, Lavender JP. Intrahepatic kinetics of Indium-111-platelets. Thromb and Haemostasis 1985; 54: 595.
6. Peters AM, Saverymuttu SH, Lavender JP, Granulocyte kinetics In: Radiolabelled cellular blood elements. Thakur ML (ed), Plenum Press, New York 1984; 285-303.
7. Goodwin DA, Heckman JR, Fajardo LF, Calin A, Propst SJ, Diamanti CI, Kinetics and migration of Indium-111-labelled human lymphocytes. In: Medical Radionuclide Imaging. International Atomic Agency 1981; Vol.1: 487-497.
8. Danpure HJ. Cell labelling with In-111 complexes. In Radiopharmacy and Radiopharmaceuticals. Theobald AE, (ed) Taylor and Francis, London 1985; 51-87.
9. McAfee JG, Thakur ML, Survey of radioactive agents for in vitro labelling of phagocytic leucocytes, I. Soluble agents. J Nucl Med 1976; 17: 480.
10. Danpure HJ, Osman S, Brady F. The labelling of blood cells in plasma with In-111 tropolonate. Br J Radiol 1982; 55: 247.
11. Peters AM, Danpure HJ, Osman S, Hawker RJ, Henderson BL, Hodgson HJ, Kelly JD, Neirinckx RD, Lavender JP. Clinical experience with Tc-99m-hexamethylpropylene amine oxime for labelling leucocytes and imaging inflammation. Lancet 1986; ii: 946.
12. Schroth HJ, Oberhausen E., Berberich R, Cell labelling with colloidal substances in whole blood. Eur J Nucl Med 1981; 6: 469.
13. Locher JT-H, Seybold K, Anders RY, Schubiger PA, Mach JP, Buchegger F. Imaging of inflammatory and infectious lesions after injection of radiolabelled monoclonal anti-granulocyte antibodies. Nucl Med Commun 1986; 7: 659.

14. Guidance notes for hospitals on the premises and environment for the preparation of radiopharmaceuticals. Department of Health and Social Security, London, 1982.

15. Hardeman MR, Fueger GF. Comparative evaluation of separation and labelling methods of migratory blood cells. In: Blood cells in nuclear medicine Part II Migratory blood cells. Fueger FG (ed) Nijhoff, Amsterdam 1984; 369-392.

16. Mathias CJ, Welch MJ. Radiolabelling of platelets. Seminars in Nucl Med 1984; XIV: 118.

17. Peters AM, Saverymuttu SH. The value of Indium-labelled leucocytes in clinical practice. Blood Reviews 1987; 1: 65.

18. Saverymuttu SH, Peters AM, Danpure HJ, Reavy HJ, Osman S, Lavender JP. Lung transit of labelled granulocytes, Relationship to labelling techniques. Scand J Haematol 1983; 30: 151.

19. Peters AM, Saverymuttu SH, Reavy HJ, Danpure HJ, Osman S, Lavender JP. Imaging of inflammation with Indium-111 tropolonate labelled leucocytes. J Nucl Med 1983; 24: 39.

20. Peters AM, Saverymuttu SH, Danpure HJ, Osman S. Cell labelling. In: Methods i Haematology, Lewis SM, Bayly RJ (eds) 1986; Vol. 14: 79-109.

21. Hawker RJ, Hawker LM, Wilkinson AR. Indium (In-111)-labelled human platelets: optimal method. Clin Sci 1980; 58: 243.

22. Boyum A. Isolation of mononuclear cells and granulocytes from human blood. Scand J Clin Lab Invest 1968; 21: 77.

23. Guide to good pharmaceutical manufacturing practice. Her Majesty's Stationary Office, London. ISBN 0 11 320662 3, 1977.

24. Danpure HJ, Osman S. The importance of radiolabelling human granulocytes with In-111 tropolonate or In-111 2-mercaptopyridine-N-oxide in plasma containing acid-citrate-dextrose. Br J Radiol 1986; 59: 907.

25. Bernard P, Bazan M, Foa C, Mountaz K, Juhan-vague I. Functional and ultrastructural alterations of autologous platelets labelled with In-111 oxine. Eur J Nucl Med 1983; 8: 172.

26. Chisholm PM, Peters AM. The effect of 111-indium labelling on the recirculation of rat lymphocytes. In: In-111-labelled neutrophils, platelets and lymphocytes. Thakur MK, Gottschalk A (eds) Trivirum, New York 1980; 205-211.

27. ten Berge, Natarajan AT, Hardeman MR, van Royen, Schellekens, Labelling with Indium-111 has detrimental effects on human lymphocytes: Concise communication. J Nucl Med 1983; 24: 615.

28. Wagstaff J, Gibson C, Thatcher N, Ford WL, Sharma H, Benson W, Crowther D. A method for following human lymphocyte traffic using Indium-111 oxine labelling. Clin Exp Immunol 1981; 43: 435.

29. Frost P, Frost H. Recirculation of lymphocytes and the use of Indium-111. J Nucl Med 1978; 20: 169.

30. Danpure HJ, Osman S, Carroll MK. In vitro studies to develop a clinical protocol for radiolabelling mixed leucocy-

tes with Tc-99m HM-PAO. Nucl Med Commun 1987; 8: 280.

31. Hanna RW, Lomas FE. Identification of factors affecting technetium 99m leucocyte labelling by phagocytic engulfment and development of an optimal technique. Eur J Nucl Med 1986; 12: 159.

32. Peters AM, Lavender JP, Danpure HJ, Osman S, Saverymuttu SH. Technetium-99m autologous phagocyte scanning: a new imaging technique for inflammatory bowel. Br Med J 1986; 293: 450.

33. Pullman W, Hanna R, Sullivan P, Booth JA, Lomas F, Doe WF, Technetium-99m autologous phagocyte scanning: a new imaging technique for inflammatory bowel disease. Br Med J 1986; 293: 171.

34. Peters AM, Lavender JP, Needham SG, Loufti I, Snook D, Epenetos AA, Lumley P, Keery RJ, Hoog N. Imaging thrombus with radiolabelled monoclonal antibody to platelets. Br Med J 1986; 293: 1525.

35. Danpure HJ, Osman S, Hogg N, Cliff E, Epenetos AA, Lavender JP. Preliminary clinical studies to detect inflammatory lesions using leucocytes labelled in whole blood with an I-123-leucocyte-specific monoclonal antibody. Nucl Med 1986; 25: A53.

36. Goodwinn DA, Meares CF, Indium-111 labelled cells: New approaches and radiation dosimetry. In: Radiolabelled cellular blood elements. Pathophysiology, Techniques and Scintigraphic applications. Thakur ML (ed), Nato ASI Series A. Life Sciences. Plenum Press, New York 1985; Vol. 88: 343-362.

37. Goding JW. Monoclonal antibodies: Principles and practice. Academic Press, London 1983.

38. McAfee JG, Subramanian G, Gagne. Technique of leukocyte harvesting and labelling: Problems and perspectives. Sem Nucl Med 1984; 14: 83.

39. Danpure HJ, Osman S. Iodine-labelled monoclonal antibodies for cell labelling: Principles and prospects. Appl Radiat Isotop 1986; 37: 735.

40. Segal AW, Deteix P, Garcia R, Tooth P, Zanelli GD, Allison AC. Indium-111 labelling of leukocytes: A detrimental effect on neutrophil and lymphocyte function and an improved method of cell labelling. J Nucl Med 1978; 19: 1238.

41. Mortelmans L, Verbruggen A, Bogaerts M, Heynen WJ, de Bakker, De Roo M. Evaluation of granulocyte labelling with In-111 chelated to three different agents by functional tests and electronic microscopy. Nucl Med 1986; 25: 125.

42. Babior BM, Cohen HJ. Measurement of neutrophil function: phagocytosis, degranulation, the respiratory burst and bacterial killing. In: Methods in Haematology, Cline MJ, (ed), Churchill Livingstone, London 1981; Vol.3: 1-38.

43. Territo MC, Chemotaxis. In: Methods in haematology, Cline MJ, (ed), Churchill Livingstone, London 1981; Vol. 3: 39-52.

44. Yardumian DA, Mackie IJ, Machin SJ, Laboratory investigation of platelet function: a review of methodology. J Clin Pathol 1986; 39: 701.

45. Peters AM, Porta M, Reavy HJ, Cousins S, Wardle J, Lewis

SM. A simple quantitative estimate of the function of radiolabelled platelets. Haemostasis 1984; 14: 333.

46. Peters AM, Saverymuttu SH, Malik F, Ind PW, Lavender JP. Intrahepatic kinetics of Indium-111-labelled platelets. Thromb. Haemostasis 1985; 54: 595.

APPENDIX

1. PROCEDURE FOR THE ISOLATION OF MIXED LEUCOCYTES FROM WHOLE BLOOD

1.1. Materials

Anticoagulant acid-citrate-dextrose (ACD) NIH formula A from Travenol. Add 18 ml to 102 ml fresh whole blood. (Do not use heparin).

Sedimenting agent Hespan (6% w/v hydroxyethyl starch from the American Hospital UK). 2 ml aliquots dispensed into 5 Sterilin universal tubes.

1.2. Method

All procedures must be carried out using aseptic techniques.

1. Attach a label to two 60 ml polythene syringes giving the patients' name, case number and date of birth.

2. Dispense 9 ml aliquots of ACD into each syringe.

3. Arrange the collection of 51 ml of fresh venous blood into each syringe using a 19G butterfly neddle infusion set. Close the syringes with sterile hubs.

4. Without attaching a needle to the syringe, dispense 4x20ml aliquots of blood containing ACD into four 30 ml sterile polystyrene Universal tubes each containing 2 ml Hespan by gently running the blood down the wall of the tube to avoid bubble formation and frothing. Close the tubes and gently invert once to mix, then open each tube and burst any bubbles that may have formed with a sterile needle.

5. Allow the blood to stand for 30-60 min. at room temperature (RT) to sediment the erythrocytes. The rate of sedimentation will depend on the patients' condition.

6. Transfer the remaining 2 x 20 ml aliquots of the blood to 30 ml Universal tubes. Centrifuge at RT for 2000 g for 10

min. Carefully collect the supernatant of cell-free ACD-plasma (CFD) and discard the buffy-coat and settled erythrocytes. Use this plasma to make up the Percoll-plasma density-gradients, to suspend the cells for labelling with In-111 tropolonate and for resuspending labelled cells for reinjection into the patient.

7. When the blood has sedimented to give approximately half the volume as sedimented erythrocytes remove the cloudy, straw-coloured upper layer of leucocyte-rich platelet-rich plasma (LRPRP) from the sedimented red cells.

8. Carefully dispense 15 ml aliquots of LRPRP into universal tubes and centrifuge at 150 g for 5 min. Separate the supernatant of platelet-rich plasma, (PRP), from the pellet of mixed leucocytes.

9. Transfer the PRP into universal tubes and centrifuge at 2000 g for 10 min. Collect the supernatant of cell-free plasma containing Hespan and discard the pellet of platelets. Use this plasma to wash cells after Percoll density-gradient separation and after labelling.

10. Loosen the pellets of mixed leucocytes from step 8 by very gently swirling and tapping the tubes.

11. If the cells are to be labelled as mixed leucocytes with In-111 tropolonate resuspend the cell pellet with cell-free ACD-plasma from step 6 so that the volume of cells and plasma is 1 ml. If the cells are to be labelled with Tc-99m HM-PAO add 1 ml ACD-plasma to the cell pellet. If "pure" granulocytes are to be isolated from the mixed leucocytes add 4 ml of PRP to the cell pellet.

The method described above is illustrated in Figure 1.

2. PROTOCOL FOR THE ISOLATION OF "PURE" GRANULOCYTES FROM MIXED LEUCOCYTES

2.1. Materials
Density gradient medium Percoll (Pharmacia) at a specific gravity of 1.13 g/ml.

2.2. Method

1. Prepare iso-osmotic Percoll (IOP = 100%) by mixing 9 parts of Percoll (specific gravity 1.13 g/ml) with 1 part of 1.5 M sodium chloride (9%).

2. Dilute IOP with patient's cell-free ACD-plasma to obtain 65%, 60% and 50% v/v solutions of Percoll in plasma.

3. Prepare three-step discontinuous density-gradients by carefully layering 2 ml of each solution in order of decreasing density into a sterile 10 ml polystyrene centrifuge tube.

4. Carefully overlay about 2 ml of mixed leucocytes in plasma. Use cells from no more than 25-30 ml blood per gradient.

5. Centrifuge the gradient at 150 g for 5 min.

6. Sample the granulocytes from the 50-60% interface.

7. Add 5-10 volumes of cell-free plasma, centrifuge at 150 g for 5 min. and resuspend the cells pellet with ACD-plasma so that the volume of cells and plasma is 1 ml.

3. PROTOCOL FOR THE ISOLATION OF PLATELETS FROM WHOLE BLOOD

3.1. Materials
Anticoagulant Acid-citrate-dextrose (ACD) as above.

3.2. Method

1. Dispense 7.5 ml aliquots of ACD into two 60 ml polythene syringes.

2. Arrange for the collection of 42.5 ml of blood into each syringe according to the instructions given for leucocytes.

3. Dispense 2 x 15 ml of blood containing ACD into polystyrene universals and centrifuge at 2000 g for 10 min. Collect the supernatant of cell-free plasma (CFP) and discard the cells. Add one volume of ACD to ten volumes of CFP to reduce the pH to 6.5. Use this plasma to suspend the cells for labelling and for washing and resuspending the labelled cells for reinjection.

4. Without attaching a needle, dispense the remaining 60 ml

of blood into three polystyrene universals each containing
2 ml Hespan by running the blood gently down the wall of
the tube to avoid frothing. Close the tubes and gently invert them once to mix, then open each tube and burst any
bubbles that have formed with a sterile needle.

5. Immediately centrifuge the blood at 150 g for 15 min. to
obtain a supernatant of platelet-rich-plasma (PRP) and a
loosely packed pellet of leucocytes and red cells.

6. Using a 10 ml syringe without a needle carefully collect
the PRP and transfer to another universal. Add one volume
of ACD to 10 volumes of PRP to lower the pH to 6.5. This
step is very important, if omitted the cells will aggregate and will have to be discarded.

7. Centrifuge the acidified PRP at 640 g for 10 min.

8. Discard the supernatant of plasma, gently loosen the pellet of platelets and resuspend the cells in 1 ml cell-free
plasma containing ACD, pH 6.5, for radiolabelling with In-
111 tropolonate.
   The method is illustrated in figure 2.

4. PROCEDURE FOR THE LABELLING OF MIXED LEUCOCYTES AND "PURE" GRANULOCYTES WITH IN-111 TROPOLONATE

4.1. Materials

Ligand Tropolone (Fluka) at 4.4 mM (0.55 mg/ml) in 20 mM Hepes-saline buffer prepared as a sterile pyrogen-free solution
by the hospital pharmacy and stored at $4^{o}C$ in the dark. It
should be used within 6 months.

Radionuclide In-111-chloride at 370 MBq/ml in 0.04M HCl
(INS.1P Amersham International). If necessary it must be diluted with 0.04M HCl.

4.2. Method

1. Prepare In-111 tropolonate immediately before use by dispensing 10-15 MBq In-111-chloride in less than 50 microliter 0.04M HCl into a universal tube and add 100 microliter tropolone at 4.4 mM in Hepes-saline buffer pH 7.6.

2. Gently add the mixed leucocytes, "pure" granulocytes or

platelets in 1 ml cell-free ACD-plasma, pH 7.2, using a syringe without neddle. This will give a final volume of 1.1 ml and a tropolene concentration of 0.4 mM which is the optimum concentration for labelling cells with In-111 tropolonate in 90% ACD-plasma.

3. Gently mix the cells and incubate at room temperature for 5 min.

4. Add 10 ml plasma containing Hespan, pH 7.2, and centrifuge at 150 g for 5 min.

5. Remove as much of the supernatant as possible from the cells and put on one side, then resuspend the pellet of labelled cells in 5-10 ml cell-free plasma, pH 7.2.

6. Measure the radioactivity in the cells and plasma supernatant and use it to calculate the labelling efficiency (LE), which is the percentage of the total radioactivity bound to the cells.

$$\%LE = \frac{\text{Radioactivity in the cells}}{\text{Total radioactivity in the cells and plasma}} \times 100$$

7. Without attaching a neddle, carefully draw up the labelled cells into a syringe, close with a hub and measure the radioactivity. If necessary discard any excess labelled cells (Between 7.5 and 12 MBq In-111 is the normal adult dose for mixed leucocytes or granulocytes if the patient is to be imaged).

8. Attach a label to the syringe recording the patients name, case number, time of labelling cells and the radioactivity on the cells.

9. Arrange for the intravenous administration of the labelled cells into the patient. This should take place as soon as possible after labelling has finished, but not later than one hour.

If >50 microliter In-111-chloride has to be used the total volume of the reaction mixture must be increased in proportion to the amount of acid used. With low numbers of cells eg for paediatric patients or adults who are neutropenic or thrombocytopenic the cells can be labelled in 0.55 ml instead of 1.1 ml.

5. PROCEDURE FOR LABELLING MIXED LEUCOCYTES WITH TC-99M HM-PAO

5.1. Materials

HM-PAO supplied as a kit from Amersham International (Ceretec).

Tc-99m from a Tc-99m sterile generator (Amertec 11, Amersham International). If necessary dilute in 0.9% W/v sodium chloride for injection.

5.2. Method

1. Take 100 ml blood and anticoagulate it with ACD. Isolate mixed leucocytes from 85 ml and cell-free plasma from 15 ml as outlined earlier.

2. Resuspend the pellet of mixed leucocytes in 1 ml ACD-plasma.

3. Form the Tc-99m-HM-PAO by adding 450-600 MBq Tc-99m in 5 ml saline to a vial of Ceretec containing 0.5 mg HM-PAO, 7.6 microgrammes stannous chloride and 4.5 mg sodium chloride.

4. Immediately add four millilitres of the Tc-99m HM-PAO to the cells and incubate them for 10 min. at room temperature.

5. Wash the cells with 10 ml plasma and resuspend in 5-10 ml plasma for reinjection into the patient.

6. Measure the radiochemical purity of each batch of TC-99m HM-PAO chromatographically according to the manufacturers instructions.

This method results in the mixed leucocytes being labelled at a high cell concentration with 80 microgrammes/ml of HM-PAO in 20% v/v ACD-plasma.

11. RADIOCHEMICAL PURITY DETERMINATIONS OF LABELLED PROTEINS

GY. A. JANOKI

1. INTRODUCTION

Biologically relevant proteins labelled by different isotopes are widely used in nuclear medicine and in many fields of
biological research. Proteins most frequently applied in nuclear medicine are listed in Table 1 while the labelling isotopes are shown in Table 2. For the labelling of proteins
various methods have been introduced. The oldest one is the
direct iodination technique with the use of different oxidizing
agents (1, 2, 3, 4, 5, 6, 7). If the protein contains no tyrosine group or the tyrosine component plays an important role in
the biological activity of the molecule then labeling is performed by conjugation technique (e.g. Bolton and Hunter reagents) (8). Most experiences have been obtained with the preparation, control and clinical administration of proteins directly labelled with Tc-99m. In spite of the longest application, the majority of analytical problems have arisen with
technetium labelling following reduction with Sn(II) -chloride.
As most of the proteins do not contains specific metal binding
groups, stability of the radioisotope-protein complex is usually low. To overcome this disadvantage Sundberg (9) has introduced the conjugation of a chelating agent, like DTPA, to the
protein to improve complex stability. Bifunctional chelates
used for stable protein labelling are presented in Table 3.
In-vivo applicability of labelled proteins prepared from biologically important macromolecules and from the great variety
of available isotopes can be predicted by the level of radiochemical purity of the preparation.

Development of methods for the determination of radiochemical purity is a complex task.

2. PROCEDURE

2.1. Analytical problems

Quality control aspects of labelled proteins designed for clinical use as radioactive drugs were first summarized by B. Rhodes (10). Control data for radiolabelled proteins are shown in Table 4. There are various methods available for the determination of the ratio of protein bound and nonprotein bound activity. However, with proteins labelled by Tc-99m using Sn (II) as a reducing agent, which is most often the case, beside unbound activity other radiochemical contaminations must also be taken into account. These can be summarized as follows:
- unbound pertechnetate,
- labelled complex of low molecular weight,
- Sn-Tc colloid,
- labelled components of high molecular weight arising from labelling of denaturated, polymerized proteins (11).

A special aspect in the determination of radiochemical purity of radioactive protein drugs is to assess also the distribution of activity belonging to different protein fractions. Important information is obtained also by a method suitable to determine the stability of labelled proteins in the blood. There is no single technique to answer all these questions. In many cases parallel use of different methods, which yield different informations, is inevitable. Procedures applied in the everyday routine are usually inadequate to reveal the real radiochemical state of labelled protein. According to our laboratory experiences the following methods seem to be the most suitable for the determination of radiochemical purity of labelled proteins:

TABLE 1.   PROTEINS USED IN NUCLEAR MEDICINE

Native form:	- Human Serum Albumin, transferrin
	- Fibrinogen, plasmin, streptokinase, heparin
	- Human Immunoglobulins
	- Monoclonal antibodies and their fragments /F(ab'), Fab', Fab, HC, LC/
Particulate form:	- Macroaggregated albumin (MAA)
	- Human Albumin microspheres (HAM)
	- Microaggregated Albymin (MiAA)
	- Albumin nanocolloid (ANC)

TABLE 2.   THE MOST IMPORTANT RADIOISOTOPES USED FOR PROTEIN LABELING

Nuclide	1/2		Principal gamma keV
Cr-51	27,7	d	325
Ga-67	78	h	90, 184, 296
Br-77	57	h	245, 521
Tc-99m	6	h	140
In-111	2,8	h	173, 247
In-113m	104	min	390
I-123	13	h	159
I-125	60	d	27, 35
I-131	8,1	d	364

TABLE 3.   PROTEIN-BASED RADIOPHARMACEUTICALS HAVE BEEN
           DEVELOPED BY INTRODUCING STRONG, METAL-CHELATING
           GROUPS INTO BIOLOGICALLY ACTIVE MOLECULES

Biologically active molecules	Chelators	Radiometals
HSA	EDTA	In-111
Fibrinogen	DTPA	Ga-67
Transferrin	Desferrioxamine (DF)	Tc-99m
	iminodiacetic (IDA)	Cu-67
Antibodies	di-thiosemicalasone (DTS)	Ru-97
Polyclonal or	macrocyclic TETA	
monoclonal antibodies	(tetraazacyclotetra-	
and their fragments	decanetetraacetate)	

TABLE 4.   CONTROL DATA FOR RADIOLABELLED PROTEINS

A. Radionuclides
   1. Purity
   2. Quality
   3. Concentration
B. Radiochemicals
   1. Percentage insoluble radioactivity
   2. Percentage unbound radioactivity
   3. Labelling yield
   4. Specific activity
   5. Biodistribution
C. Radiopharmaceuticals
   1. Sterility
   2. Pyrogens
   3. Particles
   4. Toxins

- Polyacrylamide gel electrophoresis (PAGE)
- High performance liquid chromatography (HPLC)
- Electroimmunoassay (EIA)
- Organ distribution studies

In the present work, beside a short survey of literature on the routinely used techniques, we demonstrate also their analytical applicability.

2.2 Survey of the conventional methods used for the determination of radiochemical purity of labelled proteins

The majority of the methods used in the quality control of labelled proteins is aimed at determining protein bound and non-protein bound activity. Thin layer chromatography (12), paper chromatography (13), precipitation with trichloracetic acid or with saturated ammonium sulphate solution (14, 15), electrophoressis (16, 17, 18) and column chromatography (19-25) are the methods most frequently applied.

2.2.1 Thin layer chromatography (TLC) and paper chromatography

(PC). TLC and PC belong to methods most widely applied in practice. Usually Whatman chromatographic paper (20 to 30 cm length) or a layer covered by silica gel (20 cm length) are used as stationary phase. Chromatograms are run by different solvent.

As both methods are time consuming, the so called "miniaturized" version was introduced. In this miniaturized method the carrier layer is not longer than 5-8 cm and thus development of the chromatogram requires 1-2 minutes only.

Acetone, methyl-ethyl ketone, physiological saline or water can be used as developers. Double development permits even the simultaneous determination of free pertechnetate and TcSn-colloid. The necessary minichromatographic kits are now commercially available. According to USP XXI radiochemical purity of Tc-99m-Albumin Injection must be determined as follows. Free technetate is measured by thin layer chromatography (with acetone, on silica gel) and reduced, unbound Tc by paper chromatography.

Chromatographic paper is impregnated with 1% human serum albumin solution, development is performed by N_2-bubbled saline.

2.2.2 Electrophoresis and column chromatography.

Electrophoresis has been used for the study of radiochemical purity of labelled proteins since the sixties. Höye (18) was the first to publish a method for the separation of I-131 iodide and I-131 iodate from I-131 HSA.

Paper electrophoretic techniques, in spite of their early application, did not get widely used. This may be due to fact that electrophoresis does not always yield reproducible result and the non-specific protein binding capacity of chromatographic grade paper causes tailing on the chromatographic band. Resolving power of the method lags behind that of other chromatographic procedures.

Electroosmosis, another unfavourable effect, can be reduced by the use of high voltage but this is accompanied by a rise in the temperature of the system. Pauwels et al (19) have successfully used paper electrophoresis, in connection with Tc-99m-HSA, to determine free pertechnetate and the activity which remained at the start point. Column chromatography offers numerous variations of medium, column size and eluent for analytical purposes.

Separation of the labelled protein from the unbound isotope is usually performed with short columns filled with Sephadex G-25 or 50 (24). High molecular weight contaminants and artifacts can be detected on longer (80-90 cm) columns filled with Sephadex G-200 or Sephacryl S-200, S-300. Phospate buffer (0.04 M, pH 7.4) and 0.9 % NaCl solution are most frequently used as eluents.

2.3 Polyacrylamide gel electrophoresis (PAGE)

Proteins migrate in the gel obtained by the polymerization of acrylamide and N,N'-methylene-bis-acrylamide. Due to its three-dimensional structure, it behaves like a molecular sieving. The method is suitable for the electrophoretic fractionation of proteins, and for the control of their homogeneity. By the use of PAGE human serum can be separated to some 20 distinct fractions. One of its variety, "disc" electrophoresis, is especially useful to analyzę as small amounts of protein as 50 microgrammes and after slicing it permits also activity measurements. In our laboratory Human Serum Albumin Labelled with Tc-99m has been controlled with PAGE as follows. Forty microliters of the labelled compound were applied to a 7.5% gel using 0.2 M phospahate buffer (pH 7.2) as electrode buffer. Electrophoresis was performed for 24 hours at +4°C and at a current intensity of 4 mA per tube. Every sample was tested on two parallel gels. One of the gels was submitted to staining (Coomassie brillant Blue R-250) and scanning, the other was cut to 2 mm sections after freezing and was used for activity measurement. A typical result of "radio-PAGE" testing of Tc-99m-HSA is shown in Fig. 1. Activity distributed between the separated protein polymers is clearly visible.

We have tested Tc-99m-fibrinogen with SDS-PAGE method according to Weber and Osborn (26). Activity distribution of different chans of fibrinogen is shown in Fig. 2.

2.4 High performance liquid chromatography (HPLC)

HPLC combines the high resolution capacity of PAGE with the speed of ITLC methods (27). This technique can separate the radiolabelled protein from the different radioactive contaminants so quickly that it can be successfully applied as a final quality control test prior to injection the preparation to the patient.

Whallabhajosula (28) Müller (29) and Kristensen (30) have used this technique to determine the radiochemical purity of Tc-99m-HSA. Hnatowich (27) has also succesfully applied this procedure for testing the radiochemical purity of labelled antibodies.

In our experiments we have performed HPLC analysis of Tc-99m-HSA and the F(ab')$_2$ fragment of Tc-99m-anti melanoma monoclonal antibody. We have been working with a BIO-RAD HPLC system, using a 300 x 7.5 mm BI-SIL TSK250 molecular weight, sizing column to which a 75 x 7.5 mm BIOSIL TSK guard column was connected. Samples of 20 microliter volume were eluted with

0.02 M NAH$_2$PO$_4$ and 0.05 M Na$_2$SO$_4$ buffer (pH 6.8) at flow rate
of 1 ml/min. Absorption of the protein was measured at 280 nm
and radioactivity was measured by a flow-through scintillation
detector. Result obtained during the testing of the radiochemical purity of Tc-99m-HSA and the serum stability of the compounds are shown in Fig. 3. Radiochromatogram of the F(ab')$_2$
fragment of Tc-99m anti melanoma antibody is demonstrated by
Fig. 4.

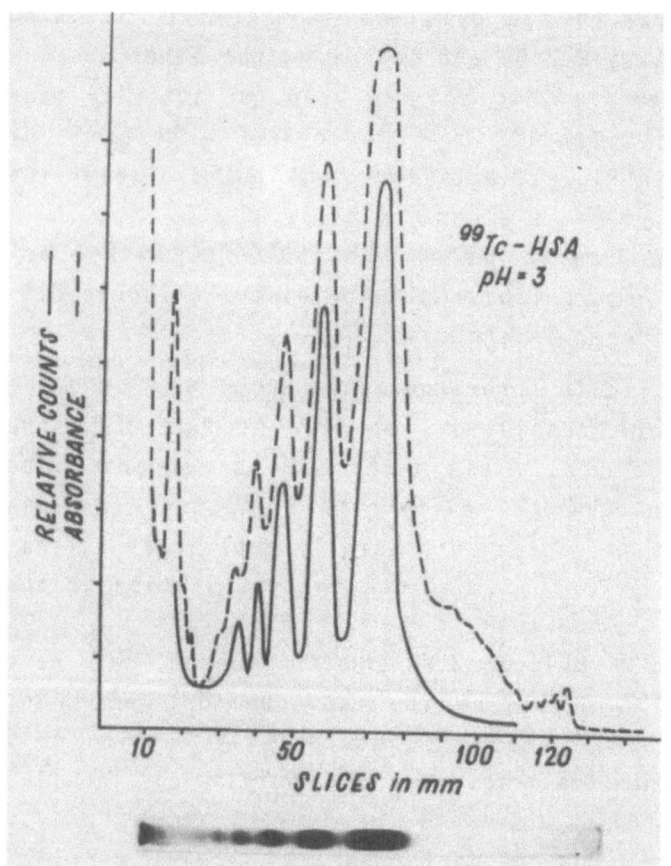

FIGURE 1.

Electrophoretic
patterns and
radioactivity
distribution of
Tc-99m-HSA in
polyacrylamide gel.
Radioactivity
recovered in
protein bound:
monomer   37 %
dimer   27 %
trimer   13 %
high polymers
about   20 %.

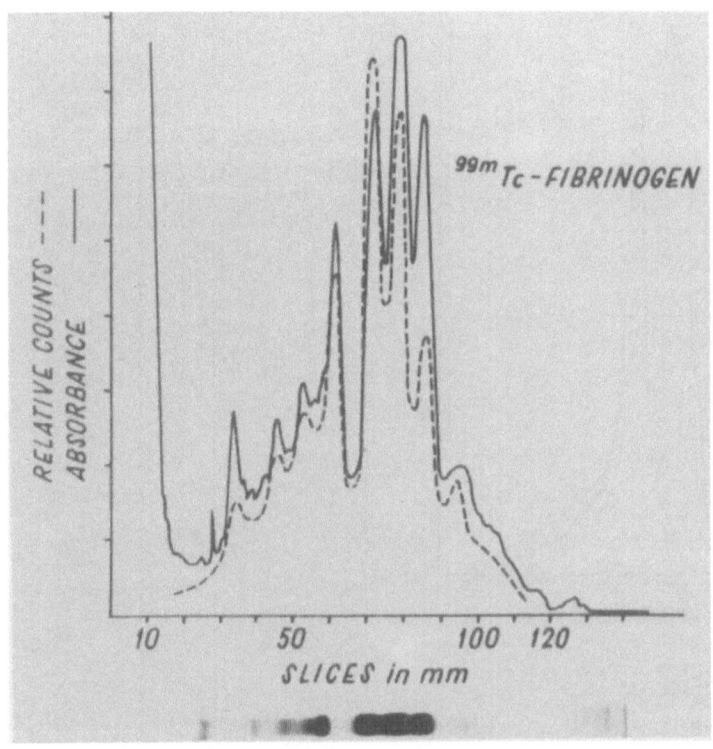

FIGURE 2.
Electrotphoretic patterns vand radioactivity distribuion of Tc-99m-Fibrinogen in SDS polyacrilamide gel. Radioactiity recovered in Alpha, Beta and Gamma chain: about 60%.

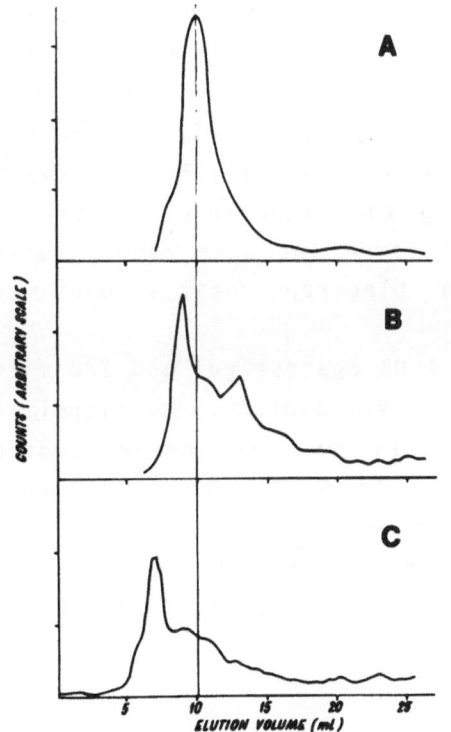

FIGURE 3.
A/ HPLC Radiochromatograms obtained by the analysis of Tc-99m-HSA

B/ Radioactivity tracers of serum sample from rabbits Tc-99m-HSA was injected 60 minutes previously

C/ Radioactivity tracers of serum sample from rabbits Tc-99m-HSA was injected 4 hours previously

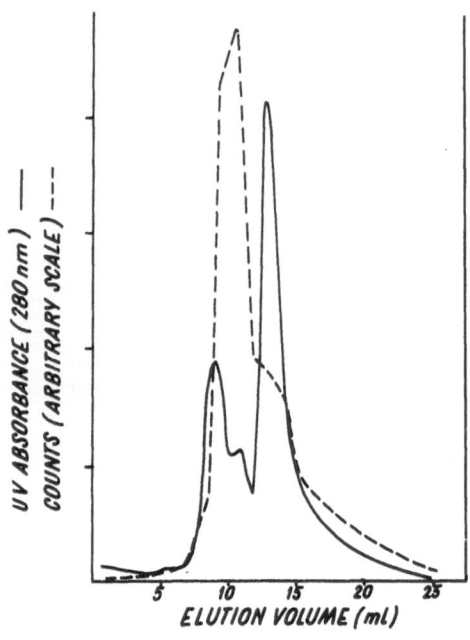

FIGURE 4.

HPLC radiochromatograms obtained by analysis of anti-melanoma monoclonal antibody F(ab')$_2$ fragment, labelled with Tc-99.

2.5 Electroimmunoassay (EIA)

During electrophoresis in an antibody containing agarose gel the protein antigen under study gives a precipitation peak.

Height of the peak is proportional to the antigen concentration. From known concentrations of the protein antigen a calibration curve is constructed from which the concentration of the protein tested can be read off. In our experiments the following labelled proteins have been analyzed: I-125-HSA, Tc-99m-HSA and Ga-67-DF-HSA (31). During the preparation of all the three compounds the same 25% HSA (from the same manufacturing series of the same firm) was used. Electrophoretic studies were performed as follows.

To plates prepared from 12 ml 1.0% agarose gel and 120 microliter anti-HSA goat IgG (Phylaxia Vet.Biol.Co.) 5 microliter sample or 5 microliter standard solution were added. Electrophoresis was performed for 2 hours at 6 mA per plate current intensity (15 V/cm) by the use of 0.1 M barbital buffer (pH 8.4). The standards used contained 10, 15, 20, 25 microgrammes/ml. Plates were stained with Coomassie Brillant Blue R-250.

Human serum almumin prepared from the same protein source, but labelled in different ways, were injected intravenously to rabbits and 2, 5, 10, 30 and 60 minutes after injection blood samples were taken. Activity of 5 microliter serum aliquots obtained from the blood samples was measured and then the human albumin content of the same rabbit sera was determined by electroimmunoassay. Prior to the organ distribution studies, cross reaction of the sera of different species was checked with the available anti-HSA IgG. The following animal sera were tested: mouse, rat, dog and rabbit.

As the rabbit serum gave no cross reaction with the antibody, the test compounds were checked in the rabbit. Electrophoretic profile of the standard series, run together with the serum samples, is shown in Fig. 6. The control rabbit serum gives no precipitation peak; HSA content of serum samples containing the different radio-HSA preparations, injected to the rabbits, are shown in Fig. 6. The control rabbit serum gives no precipitation peak; HSA content of serum samples taken from 2 to 60 min shows practically no change with the time. This is especially conspicuous when compared to the decrease of activity of the same samples.

Analysis of the 60 min serum sample of Tc-99m-HSA revealed that 97% of the HSA content of the injected sample was still in the circulation. The same sample, however, carried only 53% of the original activity. In the cases of Ga-67-DF-HSA and I-125-HSA the HSA content of the 60 min rabbit serum sample did not differ significantly from that of the Tc-99m labelled one. (95-97 % was found in circulation).

In contrast to the homogenous HSA contents, activity contents of the three serum samples were quite different. In the case of Ga-67-DF-HSA 73% and in the case of I-125-HSA 87% of the injected activity, which were significantly higher than the values obtained with Tc-HSA.

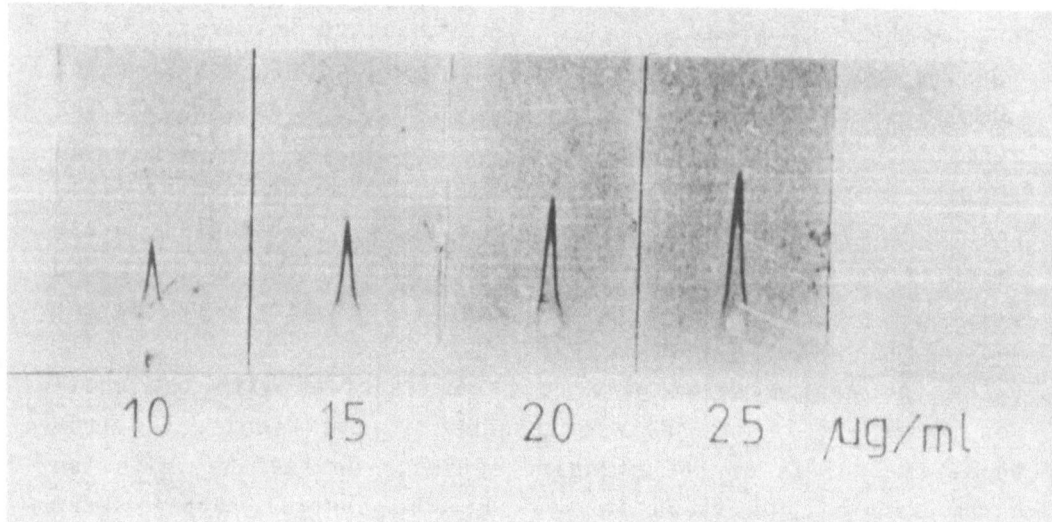

FIGURE 5. Electroimmunoassay pattern of standard HSA series of 10, 15, 20, 25 microgrammes/ml concentration.

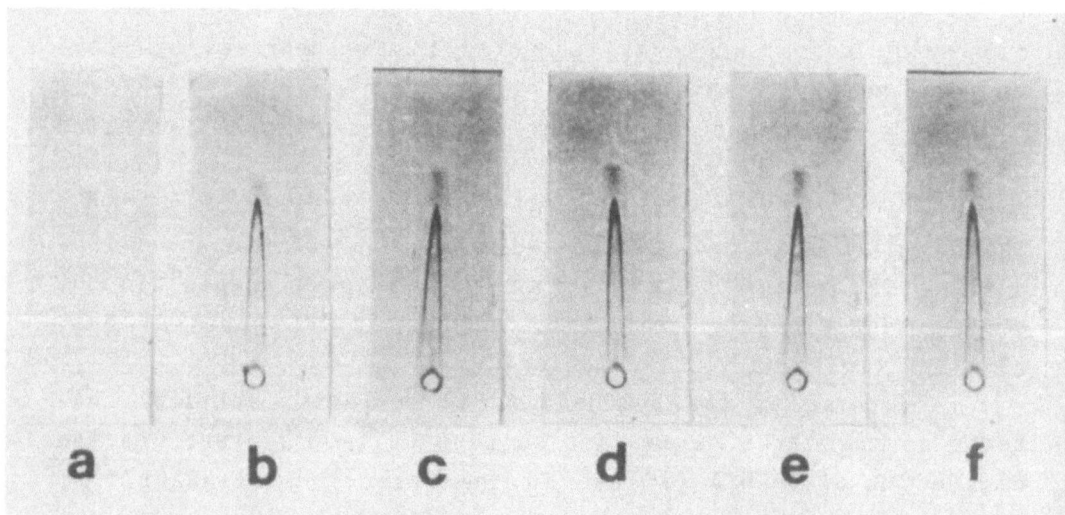

FIGURE 6. Electroimmunoassay of serum samples taken at different points of time after injection of Tc-99m-HSA. a/Control rabbits serum   b/ 2 min,   c/ 5 min, d/ 10 min,   e/ 30 min,   f/ 60 min.

The autoradiogram of the electroimmunoassay of the sera
containing I-125-HSA, as shown in Fig. 7, clearly demonstrates
even distribution of protein content and activity. Data on the
in vivo serum stability of the three labelled proteins are
summarized in Fig. 8. The values shown on the figure clearly
demonstrate that HSA is eliminated from the blood at the same
rate in all the three cases. Differences in the activity of
three serum samples are unequivocally due to labeling and binding differences.

Isotope detachment values are the followings: Tc-99m-HSA:
53%, Ga-67-DF-HSA: 27%, I-125-HSA: 13%.

Instability of Tc-HSA has been discussed in many papers (30,
32, 33, 35).

2.6 Organ distribution and clearance from the blood

Data on organ distribution and clearance from the blood of
labelled proteins may give information on their radiochemical
purity (36). This is because different radiochemical impurities
show different organ distribution patterns and the different
labelled polymers and fragments are eliminated from the blood
by different kinetics (37). For testing of Tc-99m-HSA several
species have been used, like mouse, rat, rabbit and dog. In the
different experiments animals were killed 30 to 60 minutes
after injection and activity of the following organs were
usually measured liver, stomach and blood. According to the
different authors a Tc-HSA preparation of appropriate quality
must follow the biological distribution shown in Table 5.
Experiments were performed, in all the three cases in the mice.
The animals were killed 30 minutes after injection.

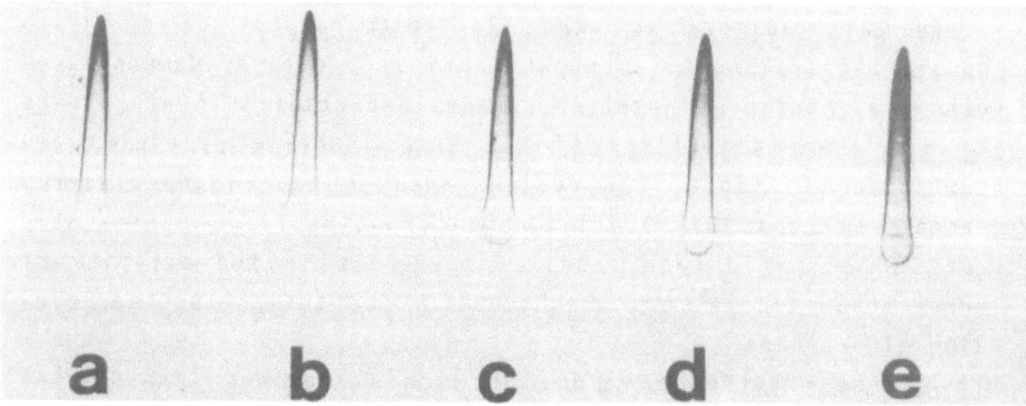

FIGURE 7. Autoradiogram of the electroimmunoassay of I-125-HSA containing serum samples.
a/ 2 min, b/ 5 min, c/ 10 min, d/30 min, e/60 min.

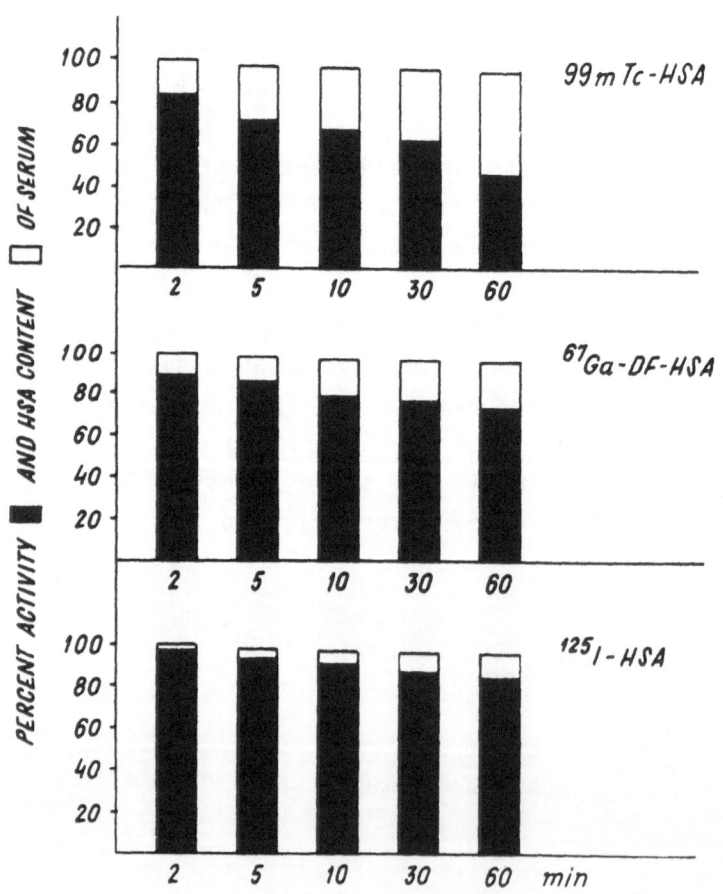

FIGURE 8. Serum stability values of Tc-99m- HSA, Ga-67-DF-HSA and I-125-HSA determined by EIA:

Detachment values:
Tc-99m-HSA   53%
I-125-HSA   13%
Ga-67-DF-HSA 27%

TABLE 5 Organ distribution criteria of Tc-99m-HSA according to different authors

	blood %	liver %	stomach %	max.amount of radiochemical contaminants %
Buck A.Rodes(10)	45-65	10-15	0,5-1,0	-
J.R. McLeen et.al. (36)	greater than 35	less than 15	less than 1	TcO_4 less than 10 TcO_2 not more than 15 ($TcO_4 + TcO_2$ max 20)
USP XXI.Official Monography (38)	not less than 30	not more than 15	not more than 1	not more than 10 (TcO_4+red Tc)

Data of Table 5 clearly show that while activity values of the liver and stomach are practically identical, activity levels in the blood show wide variations.

In vitro analyses of Tc-99m-HSA preparations, performed prior to injection, frequently showed no correlation with the data of biological distribution and clearance from the blood. In our laboratory we have tested the organ distribution and blood clearances of different labelled HSA preparation also in rabbits. Figure 9 compares distribution of Tc-99m-HSA and Tc-99m-RBC.

The figure gives a clear visual image of the different distribution in the blood and liver. Significant differences can be detected also between the clearance values of different preparations. In our studies we have compared various radioactive derivatives of HSA. The blood clearance characteristics of Tc-99m-HSA, Tc-99m-RBC and Ga-67-DF-HSA were compared with the standard radioiodinated derivative (I-125-HSA) with Ga-67-citrate and Ga-67 desferrioxamine which may be formed in vivo during decomposition of conjugate.

Result of these experiments are shown in Figure 10. The significant difference between the clearance values of derivatives prepared from the same protein batch is clearly visible.

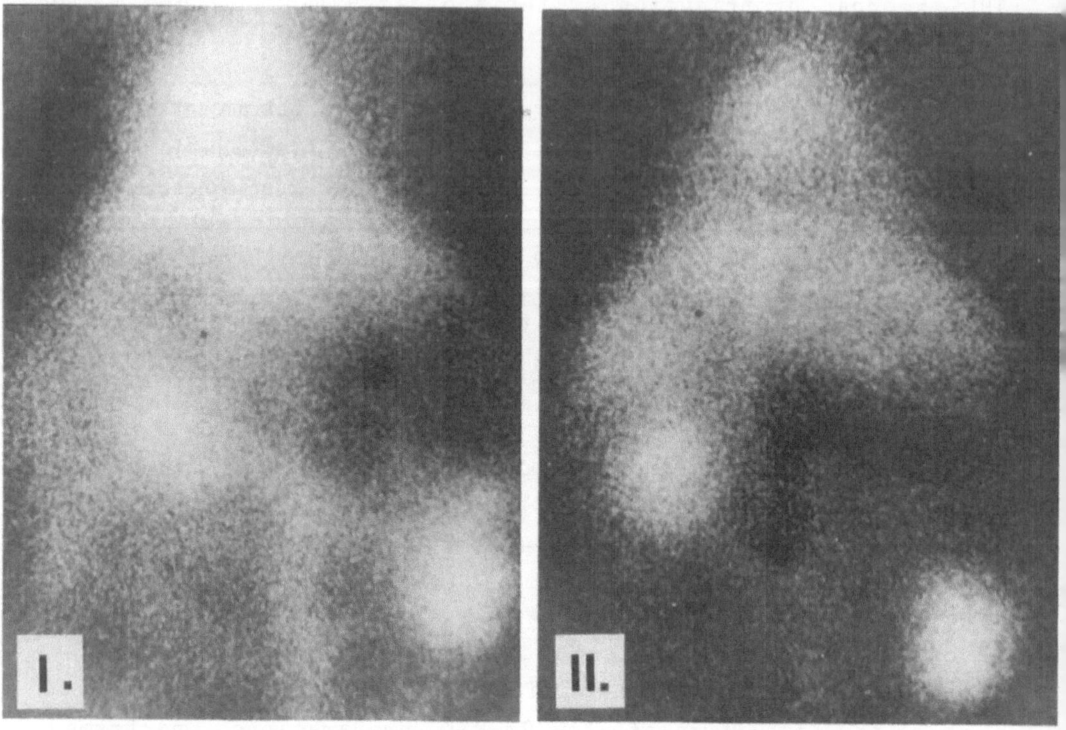

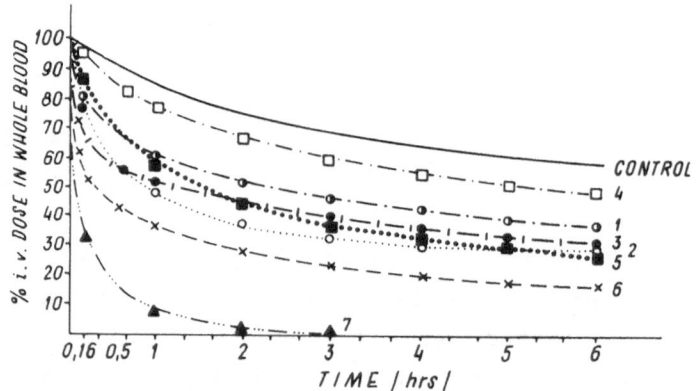

FIGURE 9. Gamma camera images of Tc-99m-HSA (II) and Tc-99m-RBC (I) in rabbits after 60 minutes of i.v. injection.
Note the relative decrease in radiac blood pool activity of Tc-99m-HSA with time. In the Tc-99m-RBC study the relative cardiac blood pool radioactivity remains high compared to the liver.

FIGURE 10. Blood clearence curves of various radiolabelled HSA preparation in rabbits (Data from Reference 36).
Control: I-125-HSA, Curves 1,2,3: Ga-67-DF-HSA (prepared at different conditions (33). 4: Tc-99m-RBC (in vivo labeled) 5: Tc-99m-HSA, 6: Ga-67-citrate, 7: Ga-67-DF (desferrioxamine).

3. DISCUSSION

One of the most important data characteristic of the quality of labelled proteins, -beside vital biological parameters like sterility, apyrogenity, freedom from hepatitis and AIDS viruses- is their radiochemical purity. An appropriate level of purity and its exact determination renders considerable help to assess the experiences obtained during clinical application. Determination of radiochemical purity of proteins is therefore an important task. Both literature data and our own experiences suggest that routine methods (e.g. TLC, PC) have no adequate predictive value concerning biological applicability. This has prompted the evaluation and application of new methods, with higher resolving capacity. These techniques may be of help in clinical investigations, particularly in finding an explanation for radioactivity detected at unexpected sites, when commercial and developmental radiopharmaceutical based on protein are applied. Based on our more than 10 years experience in protein labelling and quality control we are convinced that there is no single technique presently available which could yield all the necessary informations on the quality of a labelled protein.

Satisfactory amount of information can be expected only from the combination of methods with high resolution capacity. Manufacturing and control of labelled protein preparations can be divided into three steps:
- Selection and determination of the composition of initial proteins,
- formulation (pretinning, conjugation, freez-drying etc.) of the selected protein, control of the effect of labelling.
- determination of in-vitro and in-vivo stability (measurement of decomposition or translabelling).

Ranking of the 4 methods discussed, as to their successful application in the 3 main areas, is shown in Table 6.

TABLE 6. Qualification of the applied methods for the complex
radiochemical examination of labeled proteins.

Methods	for initial composition and selection	for composition after formulation and labelling	for in vivo stability determination
PAGE	+++	++	+
HPLC	++	+++	++
EIA	-	+	+++
Standard Biodistribution	-	+	++

According to our opinion the resolving capacity of the above
methods makes them suitable to yield the necessary information
on the radiochemical purity of the various radiolabelled protein.

ACKNOWLEDGEMENT

Helpful discussions of this work Drs. B. Spett, G. Klivényi
and L. Kőrösi are deeply appreciated.

The author wish to thank Mrs. R. Káldi, Mrs. M. Lakner for
skillful technical assistance and Mrs. M. Horváth for the ty-
ping of the manuscript.

The author also wish to thank BIO-RAD Laboratories Ges.mbH.
(Wien) for their generous gift of HPLC column and Sorin- Bio-
medica for making Technemab-1 kit available for this work.

This work is supported by the Scientific Council, Ministry
of Health, Hungary 14/6-16/283.

REFERENCES
1.   McFarlane AS. Efficient trace-labelling of protein with
     iodine. Nature, 1958; 182: 53.
2.   Hunter WM, Greenwood FC. Prereparation of Iodine-131 la-
     belled human growth hormone of high specific activity Na-
     ture, 1962; 194: 495-496.

3. Redshaw MR, Lynch SS. An improved method for the preparation of iodinated antigens for radioimmunoassay. J. Endocrino. 1974; 60: 527-528.
4. Pennisi F, Rosa U. Preparation of radioiodinated insulin by constant current electrolysis.
    J Nucl Biol Med 1969; 13: 64-70.
5. Marchalonis JJ. An enzymatic method for the trace iodination of immunoglobulins and other proteins.
    Biochem J 1969; 113: 299-305.
6. Fraker PS, Speck KI. Protein and Cell Membrane Iodinations with a sparingly soluble chloramide 1, 3, 4 6-Tetrachloro-3a, 6a-diphenylglycouril.
    Biochem Biophys Res Commun 1978; 80: 849.
7. Iodo-Beads TM Pierce Chemical Company Bio-Research Products. Technical Bulleting, 1983.
8. Bolton AE, Hunter WM. Labelling of protein to high specific radioactivities by conjugation for a I-125-containing acylating agent.
    Bichem J 1973; 133: 529.
9. Sundberg MW Ph D Dissertation, Stanford University 1973.
10. Rhodes A. Conciderations in the radiolabeling of Albumin. Seminars in Nucl Med 1974; 4: 281-293.
11. Pettit WA, Deland FH, Blanton L. Labeled proteins: Criteria for quality.
    Radiopharmaceuticals II. The Soc of Nucl Med Inc New York 1979; 33-42.
12. Billinghurst MW. Chromatographic quality control of Tc-99m-labelled compounds.
    J of Nucl Med 1973; Vol. 14. 11: 793-797.
13. Lin MS, Kruse SL, Goodwin DA et al. Albumin-loading effect: A pitfall in saline paper analysis of Tc-99m-albumin.
    J Nucl Med 1974; 15: 1018-1020.
14. McLean JR, Welch WJ. Measurement of unbound Tc-99m in Tc-99m-labeled human serum albumin.
    J Nucl Med 1976; 17: 758-759.
15. Lamson M III, Callahan RJ, Castronovo FP, et al. A rapit index of free activity in preparations of Tc-99m-albumin.
    J Nucl Med 1974; 15: 1060-1062.
16. Meinken G, Srivastava SC, Smith TD, et al. Is there a "good" Tc-99m albumin?
    J Nucl Med 1976; 17: 537 (abst)
17. Patterson HS, Mayron WL, Kaplan E. Analysis of Protein-Labeling Solutions (Tc-99m) by Zonal electrophoresis.
    Int J of Nucl Med and Biol 1976; Vol. 4: 80-83.
18. Höye A. Determination of radiochemical purity of some radiochemicals and pharmaceuticals by paper chromatography, thin layer chromatography and high voltage electrophoresis.
    J. Chromatogr. 1967; 28: 279.
19. Pauwerls EKJ, Feitsma RIJ. Radiochemical Quality Control of Tc-99m-Labeled Radiopharmaceuticals.
    Eur J Nucl Med 1977; 2: 97-103.

20. Eckelman WC, Richards P. Analytical pitfalls with
    Tc-99m-labeled compounds.
    J Nucl Med 1972; 13: 202-204.
21. Billinghurst MW, Rempel S, Westendor BA.
    An investigation of the effect of the quality of stannous
    ion on the quality of technetium-99m labelled albumin. J
    of Labelled Comp. and Radioph 1981; Vol. XVIII.5: 651-662.
22. Dekker BG, Arts CJM, DeLigny CL. Gel-chromatographic
    Analysis of TC-99m labeled Human Serum Albumin Prepared
    with Sn(II) as the Reductant Int J Appl Radiat Isot 1982;
    Vol.33: 1351-1357.
23. DeLigny CL, Gelsema WJ, Beums MH. The influence of
    experimental conditions on the efficiency of labeling
    human serum albumin with Tc-99m, using Sn(II) as the reduc-
    tant.
    Int J Appl Radiat Isot 1976; 20: 241-248.
24. Pettit Wa, DeLand FH, Pepper GH, et al. Characterization
    of tin-technetium colloid in technetium-labelled albumin
    preparations.
    J Nucl Med 1978; 19: 387-392.
25. Persson RBR, Strand SE, Knoos T. Radioanalytical studies
    of Tc-99m-labeled colloids and macro-molecules with gel
    chromatography column scanning technique.
    J Radioanal Chem 1978; 43: 275-286.
26. Weber K, Osborn M. The reliability of molecular weight
    determination by dodecyl sulphate-poliacrylemide gel-elec-
    trophoresis.
    J Biol Chem 1969; 244: 4406-4412.
27. Hnatowich DJ. HPLC of Radiolabeled Antibodies in
    Analytical and Chromatographic Techniques in Radiopharma-
    ceutical Chemistry. Springer Verlag 1986; 14: 279-293.
28. Vallabhajosula S, Goldsmith SJ, Pollina R, Lipazyc H.
    Radiochemical analysis of Tc-99m human serum albumin with
    high pressure liquid chromatography: Concise communication
    J Nucl Med 1982; 23. 326-329.
29. Müller T. Quality control of commercial Tc-99m human
    albumin kits.
    Eur J Nucl Med 1985; 10: 551-553.
30. Kristensen K. Biodistribution in rats of Tc-99m-labeled
    human serum albumin.
    Nucl Med Communications 1986; 7: 617-624.
31. Jánoki GyA, Kőrösi L. Use of electroimmunoassay for the
    determination of in vivo stability of labelled proteins
    (submitted to Nucl Med Comm.)
32. Atkins HL, Klopper JF, Ansari AN, Meinken G, Richards P.
    Srivastava SC. A Comparison of Tc-99m-labeled Human Serum
    Albumin and In Vitro Labeled Red Blood Cells for Blood
    Poos Studies
    Clin Nucl Med 1980; Vol.5. 4: 166-169.
33. Meares CF, Goodwin DA. Linking Radiometals to Proteins
    with Bifunctional Chelating Agents
    J of Protein Chem 1984; Vol.3, 2.215-228.

34. Jánoki GyA, Harwig JF, Chanachal W. Wolf W. (Ga-67)
    Desferrioxamine-HSA: Synthesis of Chelon Protein Conjugates
    Using Carbodiimide as a Coupling Agent
    Int J Appl Radiat Isot 1983; Vol. 34. 6: 871-877.
35. Millar AM, Hannan WJ, Sapru RP, Muir AL. An Evaluation of
    Six Kits of Technetium 99m Human Serum Albumin Injection
    for Cardiac Blood Pool Imaging.
    Eur J Nucl Med 1979; 4: 91-94.
36. McLean JR, Rockwell LJ, Welsh WJ. Comparison of the rat
    and mouse model for monitoring the radiochemical purity of
    Tc-99m Human Serum Albumin
    In Radiopharmaceuticals II Soc of Nucl Med Inc 1979, pp.
    25-31.
37. Jánoki GyA, Harwig JF, Wolf W. Labeling studies of
    proteins using bifunctional chelates: The desferrioxamine-
    Human Serum Albumin (DF-HSA) conjugate.
    J of Lab Comp Radiopharm 1982; 11-12: 1405-1407.
38. Technetium Tc-99m Albumin Injection Monographs pp.
    1012-1013.
    U.S. Pharmacopeia XXI Nat. Formulary XVI. 1985. US Pharma-
    copeial Convention Inc.

12. SAFETY ASPECTS OF HUMAN USE OF LABELLED CELLS.

HARRIET DIGE-PETERSEN

1. INTRODUCTION

It has been questioned whether radioactive labelling of human cells is safe enough to be recommended for clinical use because of very high radiation doses delivered to the labelled cells. Commonly used activities of In-111 or Tc-99m for clinical studies may deliver some 10 to 100 Gy to the cells carrying the intracellular label, mainly from selfirradiation due to Auger electrons (1,2,3,4). Organ and whole body doses, however, are of the same order of magnitude as commonly accepted in diagnostic studies (e.g. 3,5,6,7). The very high cellular doses have been documented from theoretical calculations as well as measurements of functional disturbances, decreased cell viability and finally chromosome aberrations in lymphocytes (8). Although there is no clear relation between chromosome damage and oncogenesis the main concern has been the possible transformation and oncogenetic potential of these heavily irradiated lymphocytes, of which a small fraction may survive and proliferate.

The interest in cell labelling may be traced back to the beginning of nuclear medicine (9). Red blood cell kinetics was studied by isotopes of iron (Fe-55 and Fe-59) since the 1940's. Glycine and diisofluoropropyl labelled with e.g. C-14, H-2, or P-32 were classical methods of cohort labelling. Cr-51 and later In-111, Ga-67 and Tc-99m were used for random labelling procedures - in vivo or in vitro. The era of white cell and platelet labelling started some ten years ago, in the 70'es, the principal radionuclides being In-111 and Tc-99m (5) though others have been employed or proposed (Ga-67, Hg-197, P-32, Ru-97). So far only in vitro labelling methods have been in widespread use, because the affinity of labelling agents used has been nonselective, demanding isolation of the type of cell wanted.

Cell damage during the labelling procedure may be caused by mechanical handling or chemical and radiation toxicity. Not all cell types are equally sensitive to toxic agents including radiation, so any variation of method should be controlled as to cell function. The effects may be direct, causing morphological and functional disturbances and cell killing, and thus potentially invalidating the nuclear medicine study. Late effects - best known from radiation effects on human health - such as oncogenesis and possibly depressed immunocompetence may be related to chromosome damage. Only cells containing a nucleus are of interest in this respect, and only if their lifespan is relatively long and/or some capacity to divide is preserved. Therefore only leucocytes and specifically the rather radiation sensitive lymphocytes will be considered in any detail in the following survey.

2. DOSIMETRY

The most important radionuclides use for white cell labelling are In-111 (20 MBq) and Tc-99m (750 MBq). Generally some 30-50 ml of blood is taken containing 100-400 mill leucocytes (70-80% neutrophils and 20-30% lymphocytes). Every blood sample contains a small fraction of circulating stemcells, <1%. It is assumed that all cells are equally labelled. Most of the label binds irreversibly to intracellular components, cytoplasmic as well as nuclear.

2.1 Cellular absorbed doses

The absorbed dose to the labelled cells is due mainly to low range Auger electrons less than 15 micrometer - emitted from both In-111 and Tc-99m and almost completely absorbed within the single cell. It can be assumed that the dose caused by decays outside the cell or in neighbouring cells can be ignored for at least In-111 in vitro as well as in vivo. It has been calculated (10) that the radiation dose to a cell from a single decay of In-111 is 1,35 mGy. As each of 100 mill leucocytes labelled with 740 kBq (4) recieves 2600 In-111 atoms, the dose is 2600 x 1.35 mGy or 3.5 Gy for this dose. At higher concentrations, assuming uniform distribution of the label, the absorbed dose will increase proportionately. In table 1 the doses from In-111 and Tc-99m are given, per unit activity and per clinical dose.

Table 1. RADIATION DOSES

Leucocytes labelled with In-111 or Tc-99m

	mGy/MBq (mGy/admin. dose)			mSv/MBq (mSv/admin. dose)
	Spleen	bone marrow	labelled cells	Effective dose equivalent
In-111 leuco-cytes (20 MBq)	5 (100)	0,1 (2)	2-5000 (40000-100000)	0.5 (10)
Tc-99m leuco-cytes (750 MBq)	0.04 (30)	- -	100 (75000)	0.005 (4)

2.2 Organ and whole body absorbed doses

There seems to be some variation as to organ distribution for different individuals and for different labelling procedures (7). The cell killing effect of radiation will liberate a fraction of the label which is not readily reincorporated into cells (3). It has been proposed that some In-111 may be transported by transferrin to the bone marrow adding to the radiation dose of stem cells. However, using available information and conventional calculations of effective dose equivalent according to the ICRP recommendations, organ and wholebody doses are of the same order of magnitude as in most diagnostic radiological studies (table 1).

3. PARAMETERS OF CELL DAMAGE.

Studies of leucocyte functions after different labelling procedures and different doses of chemical and/or radioactive label are imperative, partly for quality assurance of the diagnostic study and partly for studying the safety of cell labelling. Ideally each type and subgroup of cells should be studied separately. This is , however, not always possible because of insufficient isolation methods prior to labelling, non-specific labelling methods, and lack of knowledge about certain subgroups of leucocytes and their function. Some examples of commonly used methods will be mentioned, based on today's scientific status of cellular in vivo and in vitro function (5).

Migration pattern, exposure to chemotactic factors and subsequent adherence and morphological changes. Both in vivo and in vitro examinations are relevant.

Viability may be tested by Trypan blue dye exclusion or spontaneous release of label (indium or pertechnetate). Also cell kinetics and in vivo distribution should be compared for different amounts of chelating and radioactive labels and control studies.

Proliferative capacity may be studied by stimulation by different mitogens or antigens followed by measurement of H-3 thymidine incorporation. Cellular proliferation and differentiation are specific responses of different subgroups of lymphocytes, monocytes etc. Dose-response curves (8) may be constructed for different amounts of label and to different stimuli. There may be discrepanses between the responses to different stimuli. Also other methods (11) as mitotic index or the so called Harlequin staining method have been described. This technique is able to demonstrate the number of cells in first, second,or third division at certain labelling levels and after different culture times.

Chromosomal damage in In-111 labelled human lymphocytes has been shown by ten Berge et al. (8) and seems to be associated with impaired proliferative capacity. Chromosome preparations revealed several aberrations such as gaps, breaks and exchanges, and were In-111 dose dependent. The authors estimated that when labelling with 330 kBq/107 cells, the frequency of chromosome aberrations in cells corresponded to the frequency seen after 2-3,5 Gy of X-rays. Edwards and Lloyd (3) using radiation absorbed dose calibration curves of their own laboratory and the results of ten Berge et al. (8) estimated that 560 kBq/107 cells (corresponding to 20 MBq/3.5 x 108 cells) gives a dose to the labelled cells of about 15 Gy. The calculated dose, 30 Gy, is only about a factor of two higher (table 1) than estimated by this biological dosemeter.

It seems that there is a reasonable agreement between physical and biological dosimetry, thus confirming the very high absorbed radiation dose to the cells binding the label.

4. CYTOTOXICITY - RADIO - AND/OR CHEMICAL TOXICITY.

Cytotoxic effects depend on several factors:
The radiosensitivity of different cell types vary. It is generally aggreed that lymphocytes are sensitive whereas neutrophils are not. This corresponds to the conclusions drawn as to all parameters mentioned: lymphocytes exibit functional and proliferative impairment, decreased viability and chromosomal aberrations at radiation doses usually given in clinical studies. Neutrophils seem not to be affected, or to a much more limited degree.

Choice of radiolabel may affect the degree of toxicity. Commonly used doses of Tc99m have been shown to be cytotoxic to lymphocytes, though possibly less seriously than In-111. Merz et al. (11) found a biological effect on Tc-99m labelled lymphocytes (about 1000 MBq/10^9 cells) corresponding to about 4 times less than caused by a clinically relevant In-111 dose. The calculated absorbed doses to cells from the two radionuclides, when estimated to give equal countrates after 24 hours, probably do not differ by more than a factor of about two.

Location of the tracer is important for the toxic effect. Intracellular labelling gives much higher dose than surface labelling by the conventional radionuclides. The latter has so far not been successful (5).

Isolation and incubation procedures are important and should be tested by control experiments able to illustrate mechanical damage as well as chemical toxicity. Segal et al. (12) concluded that oxine had a toxic effect on the function of both neutrophils and lymphocytes, depending on the labelling procedure. ten Berge et al. (8), however demonstrated a radiation dose dependent impairment of lymphocyte function after In-111 oxine labelling, whereas the same amounts of oxine with decayed In-111 had no deletereous effect. Nor did Chisholm et al. (13) find any toxic effect of oxine. Tropolone, another chelator in widespread use, has been shown to have toxic effects (14,15). In addition these authors (14) demonstrated a metal-to-cell-effect of cadmium, which is the decay product of In-111. Also chromosomal changes may be produced by cadmium. The overall toxic effect on cells is ascribed to all three factors: the chelator, the metal cadmium and the radiobiologic exposure.

5. THE SIGNIFICANCE OF CELLULAR TOXICITY.

The direct effects on the labelled cells may as described above decrease cell viability, cause liberation of the label and a variety of functional abnormalities including abnormal cell migration in vivo, and abnormal chemotactic and mitogenic responses. There is no doubt that such changes in cell function may seriously compromise the diagnostic study whether scintigraphic or applied in cellular kinetic studies. On the other hand, such effects are probably without any immediate health effects. The small fraction of cells labelled and eventually killed or removed from the normal circulation in the body may - at most - correspond to 30 or 50 ml of blood removed. As shown in table 1 the organ doses and effective dose equivalent exclude any direct radiation effect apart from the labelled cells themselves.

The significance of chromosomal damage is harder to interpretate. Late effects such as oncogenesis and impaired immunocompetence have been discussed. The significance is, however, not clear.

Thakur et al. (4) point out that the number of aberrations caused by a simple clinical study adds little to the number of aberrations caused by other factors in our environment. There are no long term studies in animals or humans, so it is not known how long the chromosomal aberrations will persist. Nor is it exactly known how many of the heavily irradiated cells will survive. Therefore only theoretical considerations based on certain assumptions can be given.

Circulating mature blood cells have little or no capacity to divide and therefore may be assumed to have a negligible chance of causing cancer. Chronic lymphocytic leukemia is not known to be radiation induced.

It may be suspected that the very small fraction of circulating stemcells ($< 1\%$) should be of some concern, because they may have preserved some capacity to divide after returning to the bone marrow. These cells may theoretically present the major or the only risk caused by irradiation of the blood. Edwards & Lloyd (3) convincingly point out that with 50 Gy internal radiation dose the carcinogenic effect can be practically ignored on cell killing grounds. After a radiation dose to the labelled cells of about 50 Gy the authors find that there is a maximum probability of a single stemcell surviving of 3×10^{-4}. Even with all the surviving stemcells having a potential to become malignant the chance of cancer would not exceed this figure. Furthermore the authors calculate the malignant risk from lower doses, about 5 Gy, ignoring the cell killing effect of high radiation doses, and they conclude that a reasonable risk of fatal cancer in blood forming or lymphatic tissue is 2×10^{-6}. This should be compared to the calculated lifetime risk based on effective dose equivalent: 1.5×10^{-4} for 20 MBq In-111 (3).

There is no medical experience to elucidate the carcinogenic risk of chromosome damage in circulating lymphocytes caused by irradiation of circulating mature cells. Some A-bomb survivors do have chromosome aberrations some 40 years after very high wholebody doses (16). There is, however, no doubt that they had solid bone marrow doses and they are therefore in no way comparable to patients studied by white cell labelling.

6. CONCLUSION.

White cell labelling with chelates and commonly used radio-nuclides as Tc-99m and In-111 deliver very high radiation doses to the labelled cells.

Functional disturbances, decreased viability and chromosome aberrations have been demonstrated in lymphocytes but probably not in neutrophils. The effects may be radiogenic as well as chemical.

There is no solid scientific basis for estimating the oncogenic risk caused by irradiation of a small fraction of white cells. There is a lack of knowledge concerning several factors:

The relation between chromosome damage in circulating cells and lifetime cancer risk is unknown. Likewise the persistance of chromosome aberrations in these patients is not known.

The significance of the much higher age-related "normal" frequency of chromosome damage is not known.

Irradiation of circulating mature cells may not be carcinogenic due to the fact that such cells lack the ability to devide. The cell killing effect of high doses may be protective as to long term effects.

The theory has been put forward, that a very small fraction of labelled stemcells may survive the cell killing effect of high radiation doses - and that this may add to the carcinogenic risk in proportion to their number. This risk is estimated to be lower than the calculated cancer risk based on effective dose equivalent.

Cadmium may add to cell and chromosome damage - and this may be a factor adding to long term risk.

To day it is generally agreed that the dominant risk is due to the effective dose equivalent, and that this risk is in the same range as accepted for diagnostic studies in general. It is also accepted, however, that there is a need for nontoxic chelators, surface labelling methods, and radionuclides which do not deliver very high local doses.

References:
1. Bassano DA, McAfee G. Cellular radiation doses of labeled neutrophils and Platelets. J Nucl Med 1979; 20: 255-259.
2. Baverstock KF. Forum on microdosimetry of radiopharmaceuticals: Committee on effects of ionizing radiation. Int J Rad Biol 1986; 50: 555-68.
3. Edwards AA, Lloyd DC. An assessment of the risk to patients from the labelling of leucocytes with Indium-111. Proceedings of the fourth International Radiopharmaceutical dosimetry Symposium 1985, Oak Ridge, USA. 661-72.
4. Thakur ML, McAfee JG. The Significance of chromosomal aberrations in Indium-111-labeled lymphocytes. J Nucl Med 1984; 25: 922-27.
5. McAfee JG, Subramanian G, Gagne G. Technique of leukocyte harvesting and labeling: Problems and perspectives. Sem Nucl Med 1984; 14: 83-106.
6. Thakur ML, Seifert CL, Madsen MT, Mc Kenney SM, Desai AG, Park CH. Neutrophil labeling: Problems and pitfalls. Sem Nucl Med 1984; 14: 107-17.
7. Goodwin DA, Finston RA, Smith SI. The distribution and dosimetry of In-111 labeled leukocytes and platelets in humans. Proceedings of the third international radiopharmaceutical dosimetry symposium. FDA 81-8166. 1980; 88-101.
8. ten Berge RJM, Natarajan AT, Hardeman MR, van Royen EA, Schellekens PThA. Labeling with Indium-111 has detrimental effects on human lymphocytes: Concise Communication. J Nucl Med 1983; 24: 615-620.
9. Srivastava SC, Chervu LR. Radionuclide-labeled red blood cells: Current status and future prospects. Sem Nucl Med 1984; 14: 68 82.
10. Silvester DJ, Waters SL. Dosimetry of radiolabeled blood cells. Int J Nucl Biol 1983; 10: 141-4.
11. Merz T, Tatum J, Hirsch J. Technetium-99m-labeled lymphocytes: A radiotoxicity study. J Nucl Med 1986; 27: 105-10.
12. Segal AW, Deteix P, Garcia R, Tooth P, Zanelli GD, Allison AC. Indium-111 Labeling of Leukocytes: A detrimental effect on neutrophil and lymphocyte function and an improved method of cell labeling. J Nucl Med 1978; 19: 1238-44.
13. Chisholm PM, Danpure HJ, Healey G, Osman S. Cell damage resulting from the labeling of rat lymphocytes and HeLa S3 cells with In-111 oxine. J Nucl Med 1979; 20: 1308-11.
14. Balaban EP, Simon TR, Frenkel EP. Toxicity of Indium-111 on the radiolabeled lymphocyte. J Nucl Med 1987; 28: 229-33.

15. Balaban ET, Simon TR, Sheean RG et al. The effect of the radiolabel mediator tropolone on lymphocyte structure and function. J Lab Clin Med 1986; 107: 306-14.
16. Awa AA, Honda T, Sofuni T, Neriishi S, Yoshida MC, Matsui T. Chromosome-aberration frequency in cultured blood-cells in relation to radiation dose of A-bomb survivors. Lancet 1971; oct. 23: 903-5.

13. THE BASIS FOR PRELIMINARY CLINICAL TRIALS OF MONOCLONAL ANTIBODIES FOR DIAGNOSIS AND THERAPY

H. HVID HANSEN

1. INTRODUCTION

Since 1940 - 1950 it has been attempted to label different antibodies with radioactive isotopes for use in diagnosis and therapy of special malignant diseases. Today we know why there have been little success. The use of radioactively labelled polyclonal antibodies can only to some extent label a tumour. The detectable signal will be too low and there will not be much difference with respect to the surrounding tissue. With the possibility to produce monoclonal antibodies a unique step was taken foreward because of the highly sensitive reaction with the antigen from which it was developed. At the same time the equipment was developed in direction of higher sensitivity, higher resolution and better selection between different energies from the radionuclides. Thus better separation resulted when different isotopes was used in the same experiment. Imaging methods with labelled antibodies has several unique features in comparison with other methods because they give a "biochemical answer".

Detection with monoclonal antibodies against malignant melanoma seems to be the most promising at present, even though most work so far have been done with CEA antibodies. Also, at present most work have been done with antibodies of murine origin but work with antibodies of human origin may soon be possible.

The application of monoclonal antibodies in both diagnosis and therapy is dependent on:

1. Systems which can label antibodies in a predictable manner without affecting the binding to its corresponding antigen and at the same time give a stable labelled antibody in vivo.
2. Results from monoclonal scintigraphy must rely on exact information about the in vivo distribution of the radiopharmaceutical and exact information of the methods used for optimal localisation in e.g. humans.
3. The information obtained must go in direction of primary diagnosis and based on this background later for therapy.

2. THE RADIOPHARMACEUTICAL

One of the most difficult problems is to select the right antigen for raising the monoclonal antibody for later use. The antigen can be selected from surface or part of a single cell - benign or malign. Having raised the antibody one must use labelling methods without destroying the molecule and thereby the immunoreactivity of the molecule. Today most people use labelling with I-131 by Iodogen which is an exchange reaction, but other methods with chelating agents are in progress.

After labelling the radiopharmaceutical must be tested for immunoreactivity before use. All labelling work has to be done under aseptic conditions like other radiopharmaceutical preparations and this should include the primary preparation of the monoclonal antibody. It must be secured that the preparation before labelling is free from bacteriae, vira, and pyrogenes. Stability of the final product must be known before use - some labelled products are unstable and must be used within hours while others can be used later. The amount of free radionuclide must be known since it can affect the in vivo results.

Several isotopes can be selected for labelling. At present, most work have been done with isotopes of "medium" half-life because it gives one the opportunity to measure the time for optimal detection of tumor uptake.

However, more and more work are being done with Tc-99m because the time for maximum uptake for most antibodies seems to be within a limited time after injection in vivo. A different approach must be used when selecting a radionuclide for therapy. The most used isotopes here are beta-emmision isotopes. Different types of labelling must be used and the high irradiation dose to the molecule by selfirradiation must be taken into account. It would be optimal to use the same method for labelling a product both to diagnosis and therapy because it allows one to draw conclusions between biodistribution of the product and thus get more exact information about the final goal - the therapeutic dose to a given tumor.

3. SAFETY TEST

When starting a study with monoclonal antibodies for diagnosis or therapy, one must be sure that there are no side effects of the used antibody. The most common method used for this is a simple subcutaneous test - injection of 10 - 20 microliter antibody solution under the skin to examing whether there is any reaction. It is important to do this both with murine and human antibodies because they are gamma G-components and therefore may cause allergic reactions. In most studies today this is the only test being performed routinely but it may be followed by a number of sophisticated tests on blood samples.

The subcutaneous test should be sufficient to allow you to start an examination. Only a few percentage of reactions have been seen even when using murine antibodies.

Another and more difficult problem araise when the same antibody is used several times for scintigraphic and therapeutic studies in the same patient. It has been shown that a single dose of antigen may lead to formation of antibodies against the injected product and investigations may have to be stopped.

4. IN VIVO HUMAN STUDIES

Having started the injection of a given antibody for a given tumour type in a patient with a well known localisation of the tumour, the investigation can be divided in two parts:

1) investigation of the bio-distribution
2) investigation of localisation by scintigraphy.

4.1 Biodistribution

The bio-distribution can be measured by taking blood samples at different time intervals. The removal of the radiopharmaceutical from the blood stream can be determined. At the same time one may use column chromatography or HPLC to detect the stability of the monoclonal antibody in vivo. It is important to detect the amount of free radionuclide and if possible the amounts of free compared with conjungated antibody.

The importance of knowing the biodistribution of a given monoclonal antibody is that it is often very different from antibody to antibody; even for the same antibody labelled with different radionuclides and using the same labelling method. This may leed to different results both with respect to the results of the scintigraphic studies but may also have implications for the estimation in a therapeutic situation. It is also important to know the biodistribution in connection with the estimate of the tumour/no tumour ratio. This may help to estimate the background dose to the patient in a given therapeutic situation.

4.2 Scintigraphy

Instrumentation used for localisation of a radioactive monoclonal antibody used for in vivo studies are and will in the future be the computer connected gamma-camera given the opportunity to do data manipulation with all the information from the camera. Most work must be done with a rotating gamma-camera.

5. CONCLUSION

It is possible that the right antigen used to produce a monoclonal antibody, when radioactive after labelled can give you an exact diagnoses when used with an optimal detection system.

The starting point must always be a patient with known disease (primary tumour and/or metastasis) so one can differ between true positive and false positive results. When this have been done there may be prospects for daily clinical use and possibly therapy.

REFERENCES
1. Glennie MJ, Wyeth P. Radiolabelled antibody imaging and therapy: Theoretical considerations. In: Clinics in oncology 1986; 5:51-78.
2. Begent RHJ. Radiolabelled antibody imaging-clinical results. In: Clinics in oncology 1986; 5:79-91.
3. Pawlikowska TRB, Hooker G, Myers M, Epenetos AA. Treatment of tumours with radiolabelled antobodies. In: Clinics in oncology 1986; 5:93-108.
4. Marks MA, Adelstein SJ. Radiation doses from radionuclides administered for therapy. In: Clinics in oncology 1986; 5:109-124.
5. Strand SE, Norrgren K, Ingvar C, Brodin T, Hallstadius L, Ljungberg M. Parameters required in a dose planning model for radioimmunotherapy. In: Radionuclides for therapy 1986:75-90.
6. Blaser K. Immunological aspects of hybridoma technique and application of monoclonal antibodies. In: Radionuclides for therapy 1986:137-147.
7. Delaloye B, Bischof-Delaloye A, Buchegger F, Mach JP. Fundamental biokinetic measurements with respect to radioimmunotherapy. In: Radionuclides for therapy 1986:149-159.

PART 2

RADIOPHARMACY / RADIATION HYGIENE

Introduction

Radiopharmacy and Radiation Hygiene may interact in many ways. Handling of radioactivity in the daily practice of radiopharmacy may have an effect on the radiation dose received by the personel. It is therefore of great importance that the radiopharmacy staff have a thorougly understanding of radiation protection problems in order to keep such doses as low as possible. The use of radiopharmaceuticals for therapy and particularly the use of labelled antibodies, that may have to be radioactive labelled just before administration to the patient, stresses this problem. The way radioactivity is handled and disposed of may have implications for the environment. Waste disposal routine must therefore be well organised. The radiopharmacy should take the responsibility to make sure that up to date disposal technique is used. A theorethical problem is the Tc99 that nuclear medicine is spreading to the environment.

The correct "dose" to the patient is another important subject of interest to nuclear medicine and radiation hygiene. An amount of radioactivity that is sufficient to give good results but not higher than necessary is of equal importance. The validation of the system used for dispensing and controlling the "dose" given to the patient must therefore be considered in order to keep radiation doses as low as possible but also to make sure that optimal results are obtained. Too low a "dose" to give good results are absolutely inadmisable.

14. "DOSE" VALIDATION - HOW DO WE GUARANTEE THAT THE PATIENT IS GIVEN THE PRESCRIBED ACTIVITY?

S. MATTSSON

1. INTRODUCTION

As radiopharmacy is a multidisciplinary field encompassing both pharmacy and radiation physics, the popularization of the term "dose" is unfortunate. The term dose has one meaning when applied to radiation (i.e. absorbed dose) and another when used in the pharmacological sense (i.e. the prescribed amount of the radiopharmaceutical). Sometimes the amount of the radioactive element or the activity in a radiopharmaceutical is also called the "dose". The proper name for this quantity, which will be discussed in this paper, is, however, activity.

The identity and activity of the radionuclide must be known prior to administration to the patient. It is also necessary to consider the presence of the radioactive impurities, especially the level of "break-through" of the parent radionuclide in generator-produced radionuclides. Impurities may deteriorate the quality of the clinical result of the investigation and add to the absorbed dose to the patient. Appropriate checks of the chemical and physical form of the radiopharmaceutical as well as of its pharmaceutical properties are also necessary. These important problems are discussed elsewhere at this symposium.

Radiopharmaceuticals are used both for diagnosis and treatment. In Denmark and Sweden about 15.000 diagnostic nuclear medicine investigations are carried out each year, per million inhibitants; in the U.S.A. about twice that number. Therapeutic use of radiopharmaceuticals is less frequent, in Sweden about 500 treatments per year, per million inhibitants; in Denmark about 200.

2. RADIONUCLIDES FOR DIAGNOSIS

In diagnostic applications the administration of the wrong radiopharmaceutical might seriously effect the investigation; it will delay correct diagnosis and subsequently delay the treatment of the patient. Administration of too low activity will reduce the diagnostic value of the investigation and too high activity leads to an unnecessarily high absorbed dose to the patient. The activity needed depends on the characteristics of the patient and on the quality of the nuclear medicine instrumentation and the time available for the investigation.

The necessary precision and overall accuracy for activity measurements in connection with diagnostic applications in vivo have not been given much attention. This is because, in many cases, the examination involves the study of images which are relatively independent of the various precise activity administered, or because quantitative results are derived from the ratio between count rates from different samples in the same test. From the radiation protection point of view, ICRP (1) recommends that adequate accuracy (within ± 25%) should be maintained as part of a proper working technique.

The accuracy limit required in the United States is more rigorous; a maximum deviation of ± 10% from the prescribed activity is accepted. If the administered activity differs by more than 50% from the prescribed activity it is defined as a diagnostic misadministration (2). In most other countries there are no well defined limits on accuracy of the administered activity in in vivo diagnosis. It is, however, generally accepted that the activity should be checked prior to administration and that the remaining activity in the empty syringe etc. should also be measured. This is, however, not possible when ultra-short-lived, generator-produced radionuclides are used.

Administration of the wrong radiopharmaceutical or the "wrong" activity seems to be a rare occurrence in nuclear medicine. In a recent study in the U.S.A. (3) the risk was found to be around 1 per 10.000. In 74% of the reported misadministration the wrong radiopharmaceutical was given, in 22% the radiopharmaceutical was given to the wrong patient and in 4% the activity was reported to be incorrect. Even if the risk is low it is necessary to develop improved procedures to prevent such errors.

The various Pharmacopoeias (Ph Eur 2nd Ed II-3 and II-7, Ph Nord 63 Add) also give some guidance on accuracy needed when measuring activity. The maximal deviation accepted from the activity stated on the label is for a number of specified radiopharmaceuticals containing:

Tc-99m, I-131, H-3, F-18, Na-24, P-32, K-42, Cr-51,
Co-58, Fe-59, Se-75, Br-82 or Au-198   +/- 10%

I-125, Co-57 or Hg-197   +/- 15%

Xe- 133 or Kr-85   +30%/-20%

3. RADIONUCLIDES FOR THERAPY

The necessity for correct quantification is higher when radiopharmaceuticals are used for therapy than when they are used for diagnostic applications.

For <u>external</u> radiotherapy using accelerators or ^{60}Co-sources it is generally accepted that the overall uncertainty in absorbed dose to the tumour volume have to be within $\pm$ 5% (4,5).

It is possible to attain this accuracy using photon beams, if multiple and irregular fields can be avoided. With electron beams the $\pm$ 5% accuracy requirement is sometimes difficult to attain, especially in volumes with tissue inhomogeneities, e.g. bone and soft tissue.

In <u>Brachytherapy</u>, the absorbed dose rate from a multi-source configuration may typically vary by $\pm$ 10-15% at a point on the surface of the target volume.

There is no reason why an accuracy of $\pm$ 5% should not also be the goal when tumours are treated with radiopharmaceuticals (<u>internal radiotherapy</u>). This goal is, however, not easily achieved. In internal therapy, the absorbed dose is not only determined by the administered activity and the radiation parameters of the radionuclide but also by the biokinetics of the radiopharmaceutical. The uptake and retention of the radionuclide in the target tissue relative to other tissues is of special importance for the therapy. The main types of internal radiotherapy include treatment of both benign and malignant diseases:

I-131 iodide for thyreotoxicosis
Au-198 colloid and Y-90 silicate for intraarticular treatment
I-131 iodide for thyroid cancer
P-32 phosphate for polycytaemia vera and other diseases
Sr-89 chloride for bone metastases
I-131 MIBG for malignant phaeocromocytoma and neuroblastoma.

In the future there will hopefully be an increasing use of radionuclide-labelled monoclonal antibodies for the treatment of various tumours.

When planning the treatment of malignant tumours as well as of benign diseases, such as thyreotoxicosis, it is important to make individual uptake and retention measurements before treatment, so as to be able to estimate the optimal administered activity more accurately (6). Even if measurements using a "test" activity are carried out, there will still be a considerable uncertainty in the estimated mean absorbed dose both to the target and to other organs, mainly because of difficulties in determining their volumes.

It is, of course, desirable to be able to estimate the activity required for successful therapy as accurately as possible, but one has to remember that there are other parameters like uncertainty in volume estimation, which also influence the total accuracy of the estimate of the absorbed dose.

The definition of a therapeutic misadministration therefore varies between countries; one legal criterion for misadministration defined by the United States Nuclear Regulatory Commission is the administration of an amount of activity that differs from the prescribed amount by more than 10% (2). Misadministration of course also includes the erroneous administration of a therapeutic amount of a radionuclide to a patient not requiring treatment at all.

4. DETERMINATION OF RADIONUCLIDE INDENTITY, ACTIVITY AND PURITY

4.1. Gamma-emitting radionuclides

Determination of the identity, activity and purity of gamma-emitting radionuclides can be performed using several types of instruments (7):

1) A Ge detector used in conjunction with a multichannel analyser
2) A NaI(T1) detector used together with a single channel analyser (or a multichannel analyser)
3) An ionization chamber. By measuring the absorption of the photon fluence with different absorbers surrounding the radionuclide, the identity and gross contamination can be assessed.

4.1.1. Gamma-spectrometry using Ge detectors. Any laboratory, which routinely performs analyses on gamma-emitting radionuclides should have access to a high-resolution Ge spectrometer system. Determination of the impurities present in the Tc-99m eluates from Mo-99 generators provides an excellent example of the advantages of using a Ge spectrometer system (8). The detection effiency of a Ge spectrometer, as well as of a NaI(T1) spectrometer, must be determined as a function of photon energy for various source-detector distances and source configurations. Such calibrations are based on the full-energy-peak efficiency, and provide the basis for one method of determining the activity of gamma-emitting radiopharmaceuticals for which calibration standards of known activity are unavailable.

4.1.2. Measurements using NaI(T1) detectors. The use of NaI(T1) detectors for the assay of gamma-emitting radionuclides in clinical laboratories is well established. NaI(T1) detectors are normally used for routine quantitative measurements on radionuclidically pure samples. The system can be used to perform a rough pulse-height analysis by adding a single-channel or a multichannel analyser. In this way the detector can be used for radionuclide identification, purity control and activity determination.

4.1.3. Ionization chambers as activity meters. Once the identity of the main radionuclide has been confirmed and the purity checked, the activity of the radiopharmaceutical (in the absence of significant radiocontaminants) can be measured using calibrated ionization chambers. Ionization chambers from which the activity can be directly read off have thus become the most common type of instrument in quantitative preadministration assays of radiopharmaceuticals. As follows from the discussion in the introduction of this paper, these instruments should not be called "dose calibrators".

Most of the activity meters available today are variations on the basic design, type 1383A beta-gamma ionization chamber, developed for the National Physical Laboratory in the UK (9,10). The instrument is designed so that the sample is almost completely surrounded by the sensitive volume of the ionization chamber. This arrangement provides high geometrical efficiency which minimizes the effects of small variations in sample position and volume. Many manufacturers today use chambers filled with argon up to a pressure of 20 atmospheres, giving 20 times higher sensitivity with only a doubling of the background, compared with an air-filled chamber at atmospheric pressure.

Although ionization chambers cannot distinguish between photons of different energies, rough purity and identification checks can be made either by measurements of the half-life of the sample or by surrounding the sample with absorbers so that low-energy photons are absorbed to a considerable degree. The ratio between the signals with and without the absorber gives an indication of the identity of the radionuclide. If the ratio is higher than normal, this can also be an indication of the presence of an impurity emitting higher-energy gamma rays than those of the principal radionuclide, e.g. Mo-99 in Tc-99m.

However, because of the lack of energy selectivity, these devices should only be used to measure the activity of sources known to be pure.

4.2. Pure beta-emitting radionuclides

Methods commonly used to obtain the activity of pure beta-emitting radionuclides (H-3, C-14, P-32, S-35, Y-90 etc.) are gas proportional counting and liquid scintillation counting.

The latter technique is normally available at most hospitals and radiopharmaceutical laboratories.

Another method which is commonly used, for radionuclides e-mitting beta-particles of higher energy (P-32, Y-90) is based on the measurement of the bremsstrahlung radiation produced by the deceleration of the particles in the solution and source container. The bremsstrahlung can be measured in an activity meter. Measurements have shown that accurate assays can be made if careful consideration is given to the material and geometry of the source container, and if an accurate calibration procedure is followed. Recent reports indicate that it is possible to measure the activity of P-32 with an accuracy of better than $\pm$ 5% using an ionization chamber activity meter (11).

4.3. Ultra-short-lived radionuclides

When Ultra-short-lived generator-produced radionuclides such as Au-195m, Ir-191m and Kr-81m are used, there is not sufficient time to measure the activity before administration. The only way to estimate the administered activity is to carry out test elutions before administation to the patient and to make sure that the elution yield is reproducible.

5. QUALITY CONTROL AND INTERCOMPARISON PROCEDURES

When using an ordinary activity meter the response for a particular radionuclide is a function of many variables (sample position, container material and shape, radionuclide volume, density, activity etc.) each of which may introduce significant errors. The different variables have been identified, and thoroughly discussed by Woods (12). Activity meter manufacturers normally claim that the accuracy in measuring the activity is in the region of $\pm$ 2-5% in a broad energy (20 Kev - 3 Mev) - and activity (4 kBq - 70 GBq) range. A number of intercomparisons (12,13,14,15) have, however, shown that there are significant problems involved in obtaining accurate values of radionuclide activity in clinical practice. It is clear from a UK intercomparison (15) that almost 50% of the results reported for measurements on Co-57 deviated more than 5% from the true value. When measuring I-125 activity the corresponding figure was 90%, sometimes the measured value deviated from the true by a factor of 3 or more (12,15). Other studies show much better results both for Co-57 and I-125 (16,17).

Under all circumstances there is a need for quality control procedures, which will eliminate the errors or allow appropriate corrections to be made.

Regular checks according to internationally adopted protocols (18,19,20), recalibration or participation in intercomparison measurements are all suitable means of maintaining instruments performance according to requirements. Several countries now perform regular intercomparisons by distributing blind samples to hospitals from a central laboratory.

There is also increasing pressure to ensure traceability of almost any measurement to the relevant national standard. Traceability of activity measurements can be obtained in two ways:

1) using "absolute" standards from a national laboratory, for each and every radionuclide for which the instrument will be used, or

2) using an instrument (21,22,23) which is of well defined type, and which has been calibrated at a national standards laboratory, combined with the use of a calibrated check source.

"Absolute" standards are solutions of radionuclides in which the activity has been accurately determined utilizing special methods such as 4 Pii beta-gamma coincidence counting and other methods (7). Such absolute standards are available for most radionuclides from several laboratories around the world. They are furnished with a certificate giving the activity concentration at the reference time, method of standardization, precision of the measurement (24), the decay scheme, best estimate of physical half-life and other information such as impurities and their concentration. The overall uncerntainty of the activity normally lies within 0.7-4.5%.

Control sources which are normally used to check activity meters today are cheaper "reference solutions", standardized using stable ionization chambers calibrated by means of absolu-

tely standardized solutions. Such "reference solutions" are a-
vailable from several laboratories in a range of activities of
the most used radionuclides. The overall uncertainty of the activity quoted lies normally within $\pm$ 2-10%.

6. RECOMMENDATIONS

1) Prevent misadministration of radiopharmaceuticals by continous improvement of control procedures.

2) Continuous quality control of activity meters according to internationally adopted protocols must be performed.

3) Standards, for the most commonly used radionuclides should be distributed annually, by national authorities (possibly as blind tests). In the future all measurements of activity - not only in the radiopharmaceutical field - should be traceable back to a national standards laboratory for activity.

REFERENCES
1.   ICRP (International Commission on Radiological Protecti-
     on): The handling, storage, use and disposal of unsealed
     radionuclides in hospitals and medical research establish-
     ments. ICRP Publication 25. Oxford: Pergamon Press, 1977.
2.   NCRP (National Council on Radiation Protection and Measu-
     rements); Nuclear medicine - Factors influencing the
     choice and use of radionuclides in diagnosis and therapy.
     NCRP Report No. 70. Bethesda: NCRP, 1982.
3.   McElroy NL: NCR Reports on Misadministrations and Announ-
     ced Safety Inspections. J Nucl Med 1986; 27: 1102.
4.   ICRU (International Commission on Radiation Units and Mea-
     surements): Determination of absorbed dose in a patient
     irradiated by beams of X or gamma rays in radiotherapy
     procedures. ICRU Report 24. Washington: ICRU, 1976.
5.   Brahme A: Dosimetric Precision Requirements in Radiation
     Therapy. Acta Radiol Oncol 1984; 23: 379.
6.   ICRP: Protection of the patient in nuclear medicine. ICRP
     Publication xx. Oxford: Pergamon Press, 1987. (In press).
7.   NCRP (National Council on Radiation Protection and Measu-
     rements): A handbook of radiactivity measurements procedu-
     res, Second edition, NCRP Report No. 58. Bethesda: NCRP,
     1985.
8.   Finck R and Mattsson S: Int J Nucl Med Biol 1961; 3: 89.
9.   Dale JWG, Perry WE and Pulfer RF: Int J Appl Radiat Isot
     1961, 10: 65.
10. Dale JWG: Int J Appl Radiat Isot 1961; 10: 72.
11. Woods MJ: A feasibility study of the use of radionuclide
     calibrators for the assay of pure beta-emitters. NPL Re-
     port RS(INT)85, October 1986.
12. Woods MJ: Quality control of radionuclide calibrators. In:
     Quality control of nuclear medicine instrumentation, Ed.

by Mould RF, London: The Hospital Physicists' Association, 1983.

13. Lundéhn I: Testing of isotope calibrators. Report SSI: 1973-22. Stockholm: Statens strålskyddsinstitut, 1973. (In Swedish).

14. Naversten Y: 1973 Personal communication.

15. Woods MJ: Intercomparison of Radionuclide Calibrators in U.K. Hospitals. Int J Nucl Med Biol 1983; 10: 103.

16. Jensen M, Ennow K, Samuelsson G and Lindborg L: Results of measurements on samples of known activity using activity meters at some Swedish hospitals in October 1977. Report SSI: 1978-012. Stockholm: Statens strålskyddsinstitut, 1978. (In Swedish)

17. Jönsson B-A and Ydström K: Quality control of activity meters using accurately determined activity standards (1984) Report RADFYS 85:13, Malmö: Dept of Radiation Physics, Malmö General Hospital, 1985. (In Swedish).

18. Cradduck TD, Busemann-Sokole E and Roedler HD(eds): Review of quality control in nuclear medicine. München: MMV Medizin Verlag (bga Schriften 8/86), 1986.

19. IAEA (International Atomic Energy Agency): Quality control of nuclear medicine instruments. Vienna: IAEA (IAEA-TEC-DOC-317), 1984: 17-34.

20 American College of Nuclear Physicians: Initial testing and quality control for radionuclide dose calibrators. Rochester, N.Y., 1984.

21. Woods MJ, Callow WJ and Christmas P: The NPL Radionuclide Calibrator - Type 271. Int J Nucl Med Biol 1983; 10: 127.

22. Woods MJ: Design considerations for the UK secondary standard radionuclide calibrator - type 271 + 671. Presented at the meeting of the American Nuclear Society, Washington, November 1986.

23. Woods MJ: Personal communication, 1987.

24. ICRU (International Commission on Radiation Units and Measurements): Certification of standardized radioactive sources. ICRU Report 12, Washington: ICRU, 1968.

15. GOOD RADIOPHARMACY PRACTICE. DAILY PRACTICE WITH SPECIAL REFERENCE TO THERAPY

C.R. LAZARUS

1. INTRODUCTION

In order to achieve a therapeutic effect a radiopharmaceutical must be delivered to, and concentrate in, the target organ or lesion for a few days or weeks. The time and concentration should be sufficient to deliver a radiation absorbed dose which will produce the desired therapeutic effect. The radiation absorbed dose will depend on the type of radiation emitted by the radionuclide. Radiations which produce few ionisations per unit path length, eg, x- and gamma rays are not suitable for this type of therapy, whereas radiations which are locally absorbed, eg, alpha, beta, internal conversion and Auger electrons, can produce the necessary irradiation. Beta-emitting radionuclides are usually used in therapy.

Some of the earliest uses of radionuclides in medicine were for therapeutic purposes. After many years with little growth in the application of radionuclides, the last few years have seen a revival of interest. This is largely due to developments in diagnostic radiopharmaceuticals, which have shown potential for therapy when labelled with beta rather than gamma-emitting radionuclides. The number of radionuclides used as unsealed sources for therapy is rather limited, but includes iodine-131, phosphorous-32, yttrium-90.

Other radionuclides such as gold-198, rhenium-186, palladium-109 have also found applications.

The preparation and supply of radiopharmaceuticals for therapy will involve staff handling fairly large quantities of beta-emitting radionuclides.

However, this must be done in such a manner that the final product is sterile, free of pyrogens, and of a quality suitable for administration to patients.

This chapter will consider some of the hazards associated with this type of work, and the ways in which the hazards can be dealt with, and provide a radiopharmaceutical suitable for administration to patients.

2. RADIATION HAZARDS

A radiation hazard from an unsealed radioactive material can arise either from external irradiation of the body, or by entry into the body. The latter can occur by ingestion, inhalation or absorption through the skin.

2.1 External irradiation

The major hazard from external irradiation arises with gamma-emitters where the gamma ray has a long range in air. Beta particles in air have a range of about 3.65 metre per MeV, and the dose rate can be high at a considerable distance from an unshielded source. The wall of a container may not be sufficiently thick to absorb the beta radiation, and the surface dose rate should be taken into account. Bremsstrahlung radiation may be produced if the beta-energy is sufficiently high. Procedures and facilities for handling radioactive material must take account of these hazards, particularly when handling higher quantities of radioactivity used in therapy.

2.2 Internal irradiation

Entry of radioactivity into the body can occur when it is released into the environment by, eg, spillage, aerosol formation, or release of volatile radioactive material such as 131-I.

During preparation of a radiopharmaceutical, especially for therapy, radioactivity is usually used in a concentrated form in a small volume. Spillage of even a small volume can lead to a significant contamination hazard. The radiation dose from an unsealed source entering the body depends, not only on the radionuclide and its emissions, but also on its chemical and physical form, its mode of entry into the body, and its route of metabolism.

Again, facilities and procedures must be designed to cope with these hazards, and procedures developed in case of emergency.

3. LEGISLATION

National regulations for registration of premises, accumulation and disposal of radioactive waste (1), authorisation to administer radioactive materials (2), and record keeping should be followed where applicable.

A certificate of registration of premises will usually specify conditions concerning limits to the quantities of radioactive materials on the premises, the care and custody of the material, and the keeping of adequate records. National Health Service hospitals in the UK are issued with a notification instead of a certificate, and a copy of the notification must be displayed on the premises.

Authorisation must be obtained to accumulate and dispose of radioactive waste. Copies of the certificate of authorisation, showing the limit of the accumulation and disposal of radioactive waste, must be displayed.

Disposal of small quantities of radioactivity may be exempt from the regulations. Disposal of substantial quantities in the UK is usually via the public sewer, a specified tip or an incinerator.

In the UK the control of administration of radioactive materials to persons is under the Medicines (Administration of Radioactive Substances) Regulations (1978) (2). Prior authorisation is required for the administration of radioactive materials to persons in the form of a certificate. The certificate indicates the particular radiopharmaceuticals which may be administered by the holder, the route of administration. Valid scientific support and facilities must be declared on an application for a certificate.

The maintenance of records is usually a specified condition of the certificates. Checking of dispensed quantities of activity, before administration to patients, should be confirmed using an ionisation chamber.

Details of the type and activity of a radionuclide administered must be recorded. Stocks of radioactivity must also be controlled and recorded.

Enforcement of the above regulations in the UK is by the Radiochemical Inspectorate of the Department of the Environment.

Radiopharmaceuticals in UK are "drugs" under the meaning of the Medicines Act 1968 (3), and are under the controls of this act, as well as the controls on radioactive materials. The preparation of radiopharmaceuticals is now specifically covered in the Guide to Good Pharmaceutical Manufacturing Practice, GMP (4). Radiopharmaceuticals must be prepared and handled in such a way as not to prejudice the safety, quality and efficacy requirements of the Act.

4. FACILITIES AND EQUIPMENT

A laboratory for the preparation of radiopharmaceuticals for diagnostic and therapy use will need to be designed for pharmaceutical and radiochemical work. In addition space must be made for storage of radioisotopes, which may be in considerable quantities if used for therapy.

The type of facility required for handling unsealed radioactive materials is graded according to the quantity of radioactivity to be handled, and the radiotoxicity of the nuclides concerned (5). The maximum activities which can be handled in any type of laboratory may be altered depending on the nature of the work to be carried out. Generally the more complex and hazardous the procedure, the lower will be the maximum activity. Laboratories used for preparation of both diagnostic and therapeutic radiopharmaceuticals will need to be designated as Controlled Areas (6).

Areas in the laboratory, equipment and fittings, which are liable to become contaminated must be designed so as to minimise contamination, and allow easy decontamination. The flooring, walls, ceiling, benches and other surfaces should be smooth, impervious and easily cleaned. The flooring should be continuous vinyl and coated with a sealant which can be stripped off if necessary.

Plastic laminates or stainless steel are suitable for bench surfaces, and gloss paint provides a non-absorbent washable coating for walls. The benches should also be sufficiently strong to take the weight of lead shielding. The laboratory should be designed to minimise dust traps, especially ledges and inaccessible places. Only equipment which is essential to the work of the laboratory should be installed.

Wash hand basins, operated with foot, knee of elbow taps should be provided at the exit of the laboratory, near to the changing facilities. Protective clothing to be worn only in the laboratory, and removed before leaving, can be put on, taken off, and stored in an entry lobby to the laboratory. Suitable washing and changing facilities for controlled areas are required by the UK Approved Code of Practice (6).

Radioactive materials, when not in use, must be stored in a lockable, shielded safe, which is large enough to prevent accidental breakage or spillage due to overcrowding. Expired radiopharmaceuticals should be removed from the store.

Where there is a possibility of airborne contamination either by volatilisation of the radionuclide, or aerosol formation, during preparation, then the work should be carried out in a fume cupboard or workstation with total exhaust, and meeting current standards of performance (7). The operation of these pieces of equipment should prevent the spread of contamination from the working area into the laboratory. Recirculating types of workstation are unsuitable in this case due to entrapment of airborne radioactive material in the recirculating air.

In order to provide conditions suitable for the preparation of radiopharmaceuticals intended for parenteral administration, the facility must satisfy both radiation safety and pharmaceutical safety requirements. Both sets of requirements with respect to surfaces, and finishes of walls, floors and ceilings are similar. Other pharmaceutical requirements have been extensively discussed elsewhere (4, 5, 8-10).

5. WORKING PROCEDURES

Working procedures for the preparation of radiopharmaceuticals must be designed to prevent internal and external contamination. When handling therapeutic quantities of radioactivity the radiation protection requirements of the operator will assume a greater significance than the pharmaceutical requirements, although the latter must be included in the design of the working procedures.

5.1 Internal contamination

To prevent ingestion of radioactive materials pipetting should not be carried out by mouth, but using automatic dispensing aids. Other mouth operations such as eating, smoking and application of cosmetics are not permitted in laboratories where radioactivity is handled. Special clothing, including overshoes, should be worn in dispensing areas, and removed on leaving the laboratory. In aseptic areas sterile gowns, masks and hats will also need to be worn.

The purpose here is to prevent the spread of any released contamination to outside the laboratory, and to minimise the amount of airborne contamination taken into the aseptic area.

The absorption of radioactivity through the skin is a possible cause of internal contamination. Disposable gloves must always be worn when handling radioactive materials. Surgical rubber gloves must always be worn when handling radioactive materials. Surgical rubber gloves may decrease the beta dose to the hands more efficiently than examination grade gloves, by up to 30% (11). Gloves should also be impervious to radionuclides in order to protect the hands from contamination In radioiodination procedures it is particularly important to protect all skin surfaces, and gloves should, therefore, cover the wrists as well as the hands. It may be necessary to wear two pairs of gloves during this type of work. Gloves should be put on and removed without the hands touching the outside of the gloves. After use the gloves should be monitored for radioactivity before disposal, and the hands should be washed thoroughly.

Gloves should not be worn outside active areas, and if they become contaminated they must be changed immediately in order to prevent spread of contamination. Care should be taken not to touch equipment such as door handles, taps, switches etc with contaminated gloves.

For the preparation of radiopharmaceuticals intended for parenteral use, it is necessary to wear steriles gloves, or at least treat them with a suitable disinfectant after putting them on, but before commencing work.

Inhalation of radioactivity can be minimised by the prevention of airborne radioactivity, and by the containment and prevention of spreading of any radioactivity which may be released into the air. For this purpose a properly ventilated fume cupboard should be used.

Fume cupboards are suitable for the handling and preparation of oral doses of radioacitivity, eg, 131-I drinks, and for preparations which do not need to be sterile. Parenteral preparations will need to be handled under sterile conditions, and a unidirectional laminar flow workstation, providing a working atmosphere with air filtered to BS 5925 Class I becomes necessary (12). These workstations must totally exhaust air to outside the laboratory if the hazard of release of volatile radioactivity exists. Shielded glove box type of workstations, such as microbiological safety cabinets Class III, and conforming to BS 5726 (13) are suitable for this type of work.

Radioactive liquid handling should be carried out in trays, preferably lined with absorbent paper where possible, to confine any spilled radioactivity. The use of non-sterile paper in aseptic areas is precluded, and any spills should be immediately taken up with sterile absorbent material, eg, gauze squares. Dispensing areas should be monitored for radioactivity at the end of procedures to check for spillage.

5.2 External irradiation

External irradiation can be reduced using a combination of distance, time and shielding.

5.2.1 Distance. Radioactive sources should never be handled directly with the fingers, but using remote techniques including tongs and forceps. With gamma ray sources the variation of dose rate with distance follows the inverse-square law, and significant reductions in radiation exposure can be achieved by keeping as far from the radiation source as possible, and handling sources at arms length.

Beta-emitting radionuclides have a maximum and average range in absorbing materials such as tissue and air. These emissions may be totally absorbed by the walls of the container, although Bremmstrahlung radiation can be produced with high energy emitters. The range of these particles in air should be borne in mind when open procedures are used to prepare high activity radiopharmaceuticals for therapy.

5.2.2 Time. The time taken to carry out any radiolabelling procedure should be kept to a minimum. It is advisable to rehearse the procedure beforehand with inactive materials. The introduction of the radionuclide should be left as late as possible in the radiolabelling procedure, so that the number of steps involving handling of radioactivity is kept to a minimum.

5.2.3 Shielding. All radioactive material should be kept well shielded, either in lead pots or behind lead walls. Glass sheets incorporating lead provide useful screens to protect operators from work areas, but still allow the work to be clearly viewed. Vials can be shielded in lead or tungsten pots, but these should be of sufficient thickness to provide the required attenuation. Syringe shields, again of lead or tungsten, should be used during dispensing to reduce the radiation dose to the fingers.

The handling of large quantities of radioactivity required for therapy may require a greater amount of shielding. However, this can be minimised by placing the shielding close to the source.

Lead shielding should be kept painted and clean in sterile areas.

5.3 Practical considerations

To reduce the radiation dose to operators, both from internal and external hazards, and at the same time maintain the sterile integrity of the preparation, it is desirable to carry out the radiolabelling procedure quickly and in a closed system. This becomes particularly important in the handling of the larger quantities of radioactivity used for therapy.

Ferens et al (14) described a remote iodination apparatus for the radiolabelling of murine monoclonal antibody fragments with up to 11,000 MBq of 131-I. Their technique produced a radiopharmaceutical of quality suitable for use in humans.

The radiation dose to the chemist performing the radiolabelling handling 155 GBq 131-I over the course of one year was low using their labelling apparatus. The doses compared favourably with a technician doing open chloramine-T labelling in a fume cupboard with low activities of 125-I. Haisma et al (15) have also described the radioiodination of monoclonal antibodies for diagnosis and therapy using a one vial method.

Iodination and separation of bound and free iodide using an ion exchange resin are carried out in the vial. The procedure takes less than 15 minutes and produces a sterile, pyrogen-free product, suitable for human use, and safe for the operator.

6. MONITORING

Good radiopharmacy practice includes monitoring of the environment for radioactive contamination of surfaces and external radiation dose rate. It also involves monitoring the environment for contamination with microorganisms on surfaces, in the air, and in products (4). The assessment of radiation doses received by individuals either from external or internal irradiation must be undertaken by personnel monitoring.

Surface contamination with radioactivity may be assessed by wipe tests at the end of each radiolabelling procedure. Monitoring equipment, sensitive to the radionuclide used, should be available to check radiation dose rates from surfaces. Such equipment should be suitable for the purpose, tested before use, and periodically examined to ensure no damage, and calibrated at regular intervals. Suitable records should be maintained of all monitoring checks.

Monitoring of personnel for external irradiation is usually with a personal film badge or thermoluminescent dose meter (TLD). They provide a measure of the whole-body dose. Dosemeters can be worn on fingers or wrists. It is important to monitor internal contamination when handling large quantities of some radionuclides, eg, 131-I in therapeutic drinks and radiolabelling of antibodies.

Measurement can be made of the uptake of radioiodine in the thyroid gland with a suitable gamma ray detector. Beta and beta-gamma emitters can be monitored by assaying levels of the radionuclides in urine or blood. Verbruggen and DeRoo (16) have examined the packing material of sodium 131-I-iodide therapy capsules, and found all the packing inside the metal transport containers of some capsules, especially the filling material surrounding the lead container, to be contaminated with 131m-Xe, as well as 131-I. They recommend opening these containers in well-ventilated areas, such as fume cupboards.

It is good practice to survey the shipping containers of therapy radioiodine immediately on receipt for both external contamination and external radiation level. Miller et al (17) have described a detailed procedure of monitoring radioiodine containers and contents.

7. WASTE DISPOSAL

Radioactive waste disposal must be in accordance with national legislature, and records of all disposals must be made. Solid wastes such as empty source vials, contaminated syringes, gloves, etc can be disposed of by incineration or burial. It may be necessary to allow waste to decay before it is incinerated if the limits of this type of disposal are low. Liquid wastes, such as radiopharmaceutical residues, can be disposed of into the sewers via a suitable sink, sluice or toilet, with adequate flushing.

8. EMERGENCIES

Plans must be made to deal with emergencies which may arise when handling unsealed radioactive sources. Radioactive spills should be dealt with immediately, but decontamination of personnel should take priority.

Contaminated clothing should be removed and the skin decontaminated where necessary. Records of the incident should be maintained.

REFERENCES
1. Radioactive Substances Act, HMSO, London, 1960.
2. The Medicines, (Administration of Radioactive Substances) Regulations HMSO, London, 1978.
3. Medicines Act, HMSO, London, 1968.
4. Guide to Good Pharmaceutical Manufacturing Practice, Department of Health and Social Security, HMSO, London, 1983.
5. Kristensen K. Preparation and Control of Radiopharmaceuticals in Hospitals. Technical Reports Series No 194, IAEA, Vienna, 1979: 12-16.
6. The Ionising Radiations Regulations. Approved Code of Practice. HMSO, London, 1985.
7. Hughes D. The Design and Installation of Efficient Fume Cupboards. Special Report No 8, Br J Radiol 1974; 47: 888-892.
8. The Hospital Preparation of Radiopharmaceuticals. HPA Report No 16, Hospital Physicists' Association, 1977.
9. Guidelines for the Preparation of Radiopharmaceuticals in Hospitals. BIR Special Report No 11, British Institute of Radiology, London, 1975 (Revised 1979).
10. Facilities for the Hospital Preparation of Radiopharmaceuticals. Nucl Med Com 1980; 1: 54-57.
11. National Council on Radiation Protection and Measurements: Report No 37: Precautions in the Management of Patients Who Have Received Therapeutic Amounts of Radionuclides. Washington DC, NRCP, 1970.
12. British Standards Institution. Environmental Cleanliness in Enclosed Spaces. Part 1. Specification for Controlled Environment Clean Rooms, Work Stations and Clean Air Devices, BS5295, Part 1, 1976.
13. British Standards Institution. Specifications for Microbiological Safety Cabinets, BS 5726, 1979.

248

14. Ferens JM et al. High-Level Iodination of Monoclonal Antibody Fragments for Radiotherapy. J Nucl Med 1984; 25: 367-370.
15. Haisma HJ et al. Iodination of Monoslonal Antibodies for Diagnosis and Radiotherapy Using a Convenient One Vial Method. J Nucl Med 1986; 27: 1890-1895.
16. Verbruggen AM, and DeRoo M. Contamination of the Packing Material of Sodium Iodide (131I) Therapy Capsules with and Unexpected Radionuclide. Eur J Nucl Med 1983; 8: 406-407.
17. Miller KL et al. Review of Contamination and Exposure Hazards Associated with Therapeutic Uses of Radioiodine. J Nucl Med Technol 1977; 7: 163-166.

Other reading

1. The Institut of Physical Sciences in Medicine. Report No 46. Radiation Protection in Radiotherapy. Eds McKenzie Al, Shaw JE, Stephenson SK and Turner PCR. IPSM Publications, London, 1986.
2. International Commission on Radiological Protection. The Handling, Storage, Use and Disposal of Unsealed Radio-nuclides in Hospitals and Mecical Research Establishments. ICRP 12, 1977.
3. International Commission on Radiological Protection. Recommendations of the international Commission on Radio-logical Protection, ICRP Publication 26, ICRP 13, 1977.

16. WASTE DISPOSAL

KLAUS ENNOW

1. INTRODUCTION

Radioactive waste is looked upon as an inevitable or natural consequence of the uses of radioactive materials in various parts of the society, including nuclear medicine and biomedical research. This is right, but must never be an excuse for being more relaxed in waste disposal principles than in other areas of radiation protection. On the other hand too strict limits for disposal of radioactive waste will make daily work in radiopharmacy and nuclear medicine too difficult and therefore it is very important in this field to find the right balance between the need to maintain the standard of medical service and the need to keep the irradiation of personnel and population "as low as reasonably achievable".

Many years of public concern over the risk for future generations caused by the disposal of "high-level" nuclear waste, has forced the national and international agencies to review the radiation protection criteria for waste disposal. Although the agencies now do agree on how to apply the principles of radiation protection on waste disposal (1), there still exists a public opinion which has great influence on the national legislation. Dispersal of radioactivity and contamination of foodstuffs due to accidents in nuclear reactors has also heightened the level of public fear of all releases of radioactivity into the environment.

To illustrate this two "case stories" (from the time after april 1986) are given here: Recently it happened for two university departments that they were refused entrance to the major incineration plant where animal carcasses containing radioactivity have been incinerated for many years. Following danish legislation the institutes tried to get rid of the animals to the national disposal service for radioactive waste, but were refused again because of low concentration of radioactivity, although of nuclides of relatively long half-life. One of the institutes involved the municipal authority (for chemical waste) but this was mostly interested in burrial of animals in the past at the premises of the institute. The real problem was the private delivery of radioactive waste to the incineration plant and a possible solution would be to let this be untertaken by a professional contractor which can handle the waste safely and is trusted by the workers at the plant.

The second story: A company tracing the movement of groundwater around an old sanitary landfill by measuring the concentration of tritium, one day found a very high tritium activity in the first sample from a drilling in the middle of the dump. The high value could have been due to gaseous decay products (like methane) but the reason was never found as neither the company nor the authorities were able to reproduce the high level in subsequent measurements. A newspaper brought a picture showing empty packing materials with clearly visible "Radioactivity" labels and the public fear of contamination of the groundwater with radioactivity caused much more concern in the municipal council than other contaminants in the leacheate. Burrial in a municipal tip is not always a controlled disposal and incineration should be preferred.

There are probably many other "case stories" demonstrating the public alertness to any kind of releases of radioactivity, emphasizing the need to take public acceptance into consideration when giving guidelines for disposal of radioactive waste from hospitals and biomedical research institutes. One solution would be to make "collection and storage" the method of choice in any case, but this is not necessary to fulfill the requirement of keeping all radiation doses as low as reasonably achievable. It is costly and it is almost impossible to employ in daily work.

2. PRINCIPLES OF DISPOSAL

The general principles of disposal of this kind of radioactive waste have remained almost unchanged for some decades as can be seen by comparing the recommendations given in an "old" ICRP publication (no. 5 1964), in a later ICRP publication (no. 25, 1976), in NRPB Draft Guidelines 1983 (2) and in IAEA safety series no. 70 1985 (3).

Two principal ways to deal with radioactive waste are recognized: (i): the waste can be stored under controlled conditions either permanently, e.g. in a centralized treatment plant, or temporarily until the radionuclides have decayed to a low level, or (ii): the waste can be diluted and dispersed into the environment.

Although the general principles have remained unchanged the practical guidelines for disposal of liquid and solid waste have of course been altered. Small amounts of solid waste is still believed to be best disposed of by the method used for ordinary refuse (local authority refuse service (2)) but for higher activities of solid waste the alternative disposal has changed from "burrial and incineration" to transfer to a special (commercial) disposal service which will be available in many countries having nuclear research and nuclear power production.

3. CLASSIFICATION OF RADIOACTIVE WASTE

Radioactive waste is extremely heterogeneous and could be defined and classified in many ways: what is dealt with here is only "non-nuclear" waste: low-level radioactive waste (LLRW), produced in hospitals and biomedical research institutes.

In order to be able to manage the disposal of LLRW in a practical way and to follow the line of development mentioned above the following classification of "non-nuclear" waste is suggested:

class-1: LLRW which can be disposed of by the methods used for most non-radioactive waste,

class-2: LLRW which cannot be handled in agreement with condition (1) and therefore must be disposed of in the same way as the corresponding (low level) nuclear waste, (i.e. centralized collection and storage).

4. LIMITS FOR LOW LEVEL RADIOACTIVE WASTE

The limits for disposal of LLRW of class-1 will depend on the type of waste: solid, liquid, organic liquid or gas and on the existence of local and public waste treatment systems for disposal of different types of non-radioactive waste.

Following the general principles of "dilution", "concentration" and "delay for decay" the method for disposal of class-1 and class-2 LLRW will be:

class 1: a: incineration: diluted in (i) normal refuse or in (ii) hospital-risk-waste for both solid and liquid LLRW.

b: public sewer for aqueous liquid LLRW, including urine. (incineration or collection of organic liquid waste.)

c: release to atmosphere of gaseous LLRW

class-2: collection for concentration and storage in an authorized facility (e.g. used for storage of nuclear-LLRW)

LLRW of class-2 can be converted into class-1 by decay during storage in the institution or by dilution.

Limits for the activity, concentration and external dose-rate for class-1 to be disposed of as normal waste need to be fixed. This is necessary for the protection of personnel, e.g. during collection and transport, and the protection of the public, but is also needed to make the daily separation of class-1 and class-2 waste possible.

The exposure of man from the final dispersion of class-1 LLRW in air and water in the environment needs to be evaluated. Models or such evaluations (mostly designed for disposal of nuclear waste) are described in publications from ICRP (4) and IAEA (5) and will not be dealt with here.

The control of disposal must follow the basic principles of the ICRP dose limitation system and must be optimized, i.e. the resulting doses must be "as low as reasonably achievable".

The result of such model evaluations will show that the most of the nuclides, which are used in medicine and biomedical research in limited amounts, can reasonably be released to the atmosphere by incineration with neglible or small effect on the environment. This will certainly be the case for H-3 and C-14 and even for I-125 (as solid LLRW from RIA work) when combusted in a greater institutional or urban incineration plant.

In some models the purpose of the calculations is to set limits for "exempt" or "de minimis" quantities (in the nordic countries known as "inactive refuse") which can be disposed of with no radiation protection problems. The calculations are based on a recommended "de minimis" risk level (10^{-7} per year) and "de minimis" quantities must be derived from "generic models" (6).

Class-1 LLRW should not be identified by "de minimis" waste. This would inevitably leads to great problems in getting enough places for storage in centralized or commercial disposal services, as has recently been discussed in the USA (7). The cost of such storage of small activities in great volumens of LLRW as special disposal sites including additional external exposure of personnel, would far exceed the momentary value of the reduction of radiation doses and would therefore not be warranted from a socio-economic point of view.

As all waste contain some radioactivity of either natural radionuclides or fall-out nuclides it is reasonable to define a class "zero" waste but this should be considered as non-radioactive to disposed of as any other ordinary laboratory refuse. The activity limit for "inactive" refuse must be so low, that handling does not involve any problem from a radiation protection point of view and the expected effect on the environment must be negligible. An example of this type of waste is empty packing material and other material used in the laboratory in situations where the probability of contamination is low. All

kind of "Radioactivity" labels must be removed before disposal
as this waste is non-radioactive (cfr. the case story above).
In Denmark, as an example, the limit for "inactive" refuse of
sealed and un-sealed radioactive sources is 0.1 MBq per kg waste.

5. PRACTICAL GUIDELINES

Recommended limits for class-1 LLRW have recently been published by the Radiation Protection Institutes in the Nordic
Countries (8). Details can be found in the publication and will
not be repeated here. The limits for class-1 are given in terms
of ALI. This has been adopted in Swedish regulations (see Annex
II in IAEA safety series no. 70 (3) and partly in Danish regulations. For solid LLRW (class-1) the difference between Danish
and Swedish regulations could illustrate different approaches
to the interpretation of the principles behind the limits. It
is assumed that solid waste is disposed of in good-quality
packages, e.g. strong plastic bags or boxes, each containing an
activity less than the limits. The surface dose rate for each
package must be below 5 microSv/h (0.5 mrem/h). In addition, a
limit could be given (like in Sweden) for the total activity to
be disposed of per month from each workplace or, as an alternative (like in Denmark), disposal should only be permitted if
the incineration plant is able to treat class-1 LLRW containing
all activity which can be purchased under the licence issued.
An example is given in the table:

```
Radionuclide  Dose rate      DK               S (a)
-----------------------------------------------------------------
S-35          5 microSv/h  50 MBq/bag  80 MBq/bag   800 MBq/month
I-125,I-131   5 microSv/h   5 MBq/bag   1 MBq/bag    10 MBq/month
-----------------------------------------------------------------
        (a) certain limits for mixtures
```

The limits given in Danish regulations were originally given
for LLRW produced daily in hospital laboratories, e.g. RIA
counting vials, gloves, paper tissue etc. The risk of internal
exposure due to leakage and spill from this kind of waste during storage in the institution, e.g. to the air, is higher

than the risk of exposure to population and environment when diluted by combustion in an incineration plant having an extensive and constant production of gaseous effluent and ashes.

The most important feature in the regulations for the disposal of this kind of class-1 LLRW is the protection of the staff during storage and transport. The surface dose rate limit has been adopted from the international regulations for the safe transport of "execpted package" to allow transport from institution to municipal refuse disposal plant. It is required to examine carefully the complete system used to collect and transfer the refuse. If the system is not found satisfactory, it is recommended to use an existing disposal system for speci al waste, e.g. special-risk-hospital waste or to use a private contractor to enxure proper handling by personnel who could be informed about safe handling and transport of radioactive material.

It is important that LLRW is segregated prior to disposal and that the segregation is carried out during work: different waste bins and containers for solid and liquid LLRW should be available. The routes of segregation are illustrated in Figure 1.

The principle of limitting the surface dose rate could also be used in practice as a method for sorting the waste containing radionuclides with half-lives below one month. For most nuclides emitting gammarays or high-energy betarays the surface dose rate will be the limiting factor (assuming no lead shielding) - even for I-125: a waste bin containing a uniform distribution of RIA counting vials will give a surface dose rate in excess of 5 microSv/h at a total activity of 4-5 MBq. Therefore in many situations it could be decided from measurements of dose rate using a suitable monitor if the waste belongs to class-1, should be stored for decay or treated as class-2 LLRW.

6. DISPOSAL OF LIQUID LOW LEVEL RADIOACTIVE WASTE

Liquid LLRW of small volume, e.g. in bottles or syringes, could be collected in plastic containers together with solid waste if a suitable absorbing material is added. Aqueous LLRW

256

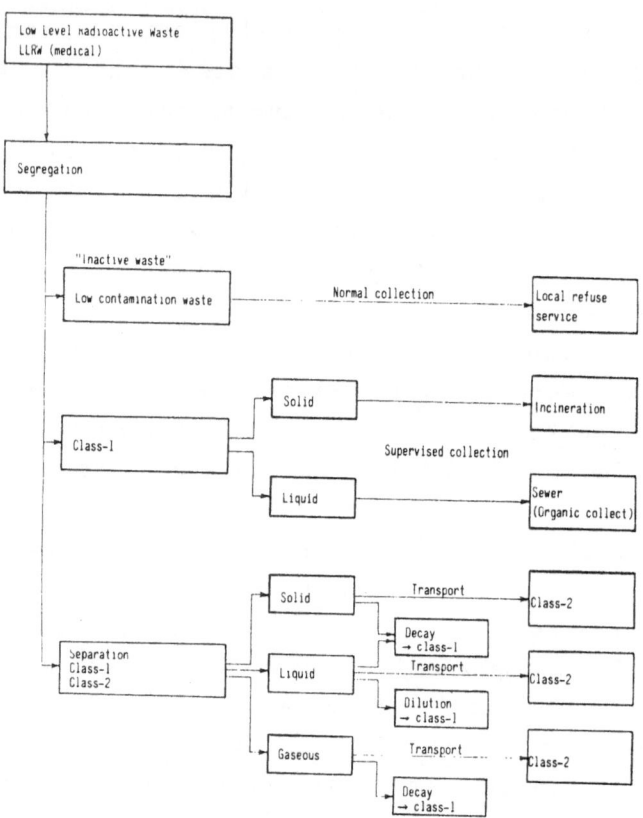

FIGURE 1. Segregation of Low Level Radioactive Waste from hospitals and biomedical institutions.

should only be poured into the sewer on purpose if the volume of the recipient in the environment (sea, lake, river etc.) is great enough to ensure dilution far below concentration recommended for drinking water and if the disposal is otherwise acceptable as evaluated from models of the pathways from water to humans or if the disposal is in accordance with transboundary agreements.

If the recipient is the sea and never used for drinking water liquid LLRW must only be poured into the sewer if the drains has been constructed to enxure dilution to the concentration required for "inactive" waste before discharge to the public sewerage system. In Denmark this limit has been set at 0.1 MBq per litre for protection of the plumbers and sewage plant workers in case of an accidental intake of sewage water (9). One possibility would be to dilute this concentration before disposal which would be almost impossible in many cases (for dilution of 1 ALI of tritium a volume of 30,000 litre would be needed).

The consumption of tapwater in hospitals and biomedical institutes and hence the discharge to the sewer is so enourmous during day time that dilution of liquid LLRW is hardly ever a problem during normal working hours, when disposed of through approved drains. Only that kind of liquid LLRW which will be disposed of during night and weekends, when the water flow is low, could cause troubles. Patients given radiopharmaceuticals for diagnostic or therapeutic purposes necessarily have to use the toilets on every hour and therefore urine and faces from these patients is a special type of LLRW.

The problems involved in the discharge of urine from patients treated with high activities of P-32 and I-131, e.g. for cancer therapy, has been dealt with for more than 35 years (10) and many other methods of disposal are applied in different countries. The growing interest in using new radiopharmaceuticals for radiation therapy still calls for regulations and recommendations for this problem.

If the dispersal of I-131 into the environment is found reasonable, then the major objective would be the protection in the hospital from external radiation from urine stored in the department or in tanks or cesspools and the protection of the technical staff of the hospital servicing these pools and toilets and drain.

7. SUMMARY

In daily work as much as possible of the radioactive waste should be collected as "solid waste". By measurement of the external surface dose rate it is possible to separate the waste containers to be stored for decay or to be send for treatment in a centralized (commercial) disposal service. Liquid class-1 LLRW should only be disposed of through the sewer if the LLRW is mixed with other types of waste which is otherwise impractical to handle: if the concentration is low (e.g. below 0.1 MBq/litre) or if the LLRW is contained in urine and faeces.

REFERENCES
1. Webb GAM: Radiological criteria for the disposal of solid radioactive wastes. Phil Trans R Soc London 1986; A319: 17.
2. National Radiological Protection Board: Draft guidance notes for the protection of persons against ionising radiations arising from medical and dental use. Consultative Document. London: Her Majesty's Stationary Office, 1983.
3. International Atomic Energy Agency: Management of Radioactive Wastes Produced by Users of Radioactive Materials, Safety series no. 70, IAEA, Vienna 1985.
4. International Commission on Radiological Protection, Publication 46, Annals of the ICRP 1985; 15: no. 4.
5. International Atomic Energy Agency: Safety series no. 57, IAEA, Vienna 1982.
    International Atomic Energy Agency: Safety series no. 64, IAEA, Vienna 1984.
6. International Atomic Energy Agency: De minimis concept in radioactive waste disposal, IAEA-TECDOC-282, Vienna 1983.
7. See SNM Newsline in The Journal of Nuclear Medicine, January 1985 and April 1986.
8. The Radiation Protection Institutes in Denmark, Finland, Iceland, Norway and Sweden: Application in the Nordic countries of international radioactive waste recommendations, Helsinki 1986.
9. Ennow K: Derived limits for I-131 in waste water, poster presented at Third European Symposium on Radiopharmaceuticals, Elsinore 1.-4. May 1987.
10. U.S. Department of Commerce: Recommendations for Waste

Disposal of Phosphorus-32 and Iodine-131 for Medical U-
sers, NBS Handbook 49, Washington D.C., 1951.

17. TC-99 - A WASTE PROBLEM?

ASKER AARKROG

1. INTRODUCTION

Technetium-99, the only radiologically important environmental technetium isotope, decays by beta emission with a maximum energy of 0.292 MeV and a specific activity of 0.63 TBq kg^{-1} (TBq = 10^{12} Bq). The maximum yield from thermal neutron fission of U-235 is 6.06%. Several mechanisms exist for producing Tc-99 apart from direct fission. Of these, the (n,gamma) reaction with Mo-98, is shown below:

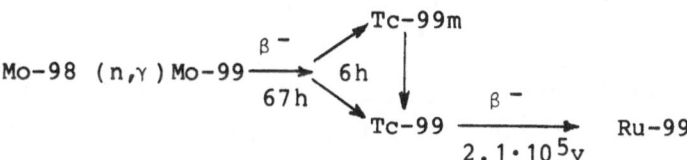

Whether Tc-99 is a waste problem depends on:
- The quantities in which the radionuclide is produced.
- The amounts released to the environment.
- The environmental behaviour, i.e. how easy is Tc transferred to man.
- The dose factor: Sievert pr Bq ingested or inhaled by man.

This paper discusses these items and furthermore briefly describes how Tc-99 can be used in environmental studies.

2. SOURCE TERMS

Technetium-99 is produced and released from the nuclear fuel cycle, from atmospheric nuclear explosions and from technetium used in medicine.

2.1 The nuclear fuel cycle

By 1983 the global electricity production by nuclear reactors was 762 GW(e)y (1) or 2500 GW(th)y. At a production rate of 6 TBq Tc-99 pr GW(th)y (2) the corresponding total amount of Tc-99 generated would be 15 PBq (PBq = 10^{15} Bq). Luykx (3) has estimated that of this about 1 PBq Tc-99 has been discharged to the environment, mostly from liquid discharges to the sea from the two European nuclear reprocessing plants: Sellafield in the UK and Cap de la Hague in France. Sellafield alone in discharging to the Irish Sea accounts for 60% of the total (4,5). Atmospheric discharges of Tc-99 from the nuclear fuel cycle is at least 2 orders of magnitude less than those to the aquatic environment (2). In the USA the most important source of Tc-99 is discharged from gaseous diffusion enrichment of uranium. The discharges from such plants (Oak Ridge, Paducah & Portsmouth) in 1977 were 2 TBq to the water and 0.17 TBq to air (2).

2.2 Atmospheric nuclear tests

From the fission yield ratio Tc-99/Cs-137 = $1.44.10^{-4}$ in detonated nuclear devices (6) and from the production of Cs-137 by nuclear test explosions (7) it is estimated that the global inventory from this source is 0.14 PBq Tc-99. Most of this will be in the ocean.

2.3 Medicine

Ennow (8) has estimated the annual production of Tc-99m to be of the order 20-30 PBq. As the halflife of Tc-99 is $3\cdot10^{8}$ times longer than that of Tc-99m, 20-30 PBq Tc-99m decay into 0.1 GBq Tc-99 (1 GBq = 10^{9} Bq). Up to now (1987) the total production of Tc-99 from the use of technetium in medicine may be an order of magnitude higher, i.e. approximately 1 GBq Tc-99.

2.4 Summary of source terms

The nuclear fuel cycle is the most important source of Tc-99, contributing a total discharge of 1 PBq. Fallout from all atmospheric nuclear tests comes next with a contribution of 0.14 PBq. Compared with these two sources, the 1 GBq produced from technetium used in medicine is insignificant.

3. RADIOECOLOGY

Radioecology describes the relationships between radioactive substances or radiation and the environment. Thus this science includes the movement of radionuclides within ecological systems and their accumulation within specific ecosystem components such as air, water, soil and living organisms.

Under aerobic conditions the most soluble chemical species of Tc in water is the pertechnetate ion (TcO_4^-), which is highly stable over broad pH ranges. Thus, technetium shows in general a low sorption in soils as well as in marine sediments.

3.1 Terrestrial radioecology of Technetium

In 1974, data became available from potted-plant experiments (9) that indicated that the concentration of Tc in the plants was 50 times that in the soil. Later experiments under field conditions have shown that the concentration ratio of vegetation to soil for Tc is between 1 and 20.

The rate of soil to plant transfer of Tc, when applied as TcO_4^- to a soil, often decreases over time. This is partly due to changes in chemical form from the highly soluble readily available TcO_4^- to less available insoluble forms such as TcO_2 and various organic complexes (10). However the migration of Tc out of the rootzone is also important. The transfer of Tc to milk and meat from vegetation seems to be low. The concentration ratios milk/pasture vegetation and meat/pasture vegetation are only of the order of 10^{-3} (11). The concentration ratio eggs/dry food is in the order of 0.2 (12). Hence vegetable food is the most important pathway of Tc to man.

3.2 Aquatic radioecology of Technetium

Most of the Tc-99 in the environment is in the oceans, present as TcO_4^- in the form of a solute following the water masses. Fish accumulate Tc from the seawater. The concentration ratio (CR) Bq kg^{-1} fish/Bq kg^{-1} water is 30 and shellfish show a CR of 10^3 (13). Certain brown algae (e.g. Fucus vesiculosus) show a CR of 10^5 on a dry weight basis (5), whereas green and red algae show considerably lower values. When Tc is discharged to a river an important pathway arises from crop irrigation (14). In this case drinking water is another possible pathway but it is usually less important than irrigation.

3.3 Summary of technetium radioecology

Technetium is in general highly mobile in the environment as the anion TcO_4^-. It is taken up by the roots of terrestrial plants, but the high mobility will, on the other hand, remove it from the root zone relatively fast. If it is reduced it may stay in the root zone, but in that case it usually becomes less available to the plants. Vegetable food is the main pathway in the terrestrial environment.

In the marine environment Tc will remain in the water column and in the long rung will be evenly distributed in the oceans. The main pathway will be from fish and shellfish comsumption.

4. DOSES

The effective dose equivalent commitment from consumption of 1 Bq Tc-99 is $3.4 \cdot 10^{-10}$ Sv and 1 Bq Tc-99 inhaled gives a dose of $2 \cdot 10^{-9}$ Sv (15). The annual dose from background radiation (exclusive contribution from radon) is $1 \cdot 10^{-3}$ Sv, and the collective dose to the world population ($5 \cdot 10^9$ persons) from one years background radiation is $5 \cdot 10^6$ person Sv.

4.1 Doses from unit releases of Tc-99

Hoffmann et al., (16) have calculated the effective dose equivalent from an annual release of 1 TBq Tc-99 to the atmosphere to the critical population groups living in the vicinity of the source.
The combined terrestrial pathways gave $2.4 \cdot 10^{-5}$ Sv y^{-1}, of which $1.9 \cdot 10^{-5}$ Sv y^{-1} came from vegetable food. The dose from inhalation was in significant.

According to Quinault & Grauby (14), 1 TBq Tc-99 released annually to a river would give $6.8 \cdot 10^{-5}$ Sv pr year.

If we assume that 1 TBq Tc-99 is released annually to the North Sea (70 000 km^3), the effective dose equivalent to a person consuming 100 kg fish and 20 kg shellfish pr year would be $3.4 \cdot 10^{-10}$ Sv y^{-1}

$$\frac{3 \cdot 10^{12}(30 \cdot 100 + 10^3 \cdot 20) \; 3.4 \cdot 10^{-10}}{70,000 \cdot 10^{12}}$$

(The value 3 above is the mean residence time in years in the North Sea).

The collective effective dose equivalent commitment (CEDEC) from 1 TBq Tc-99 discharged annually to the world's oceans ($1.5 \cdot 10^{18}$ m^3) would result into a mean concentration of

$$\frac{1 \cdot 10^{12} \cdot 2.1 \cdot 10^5}{1.5 \cdot 10^{18} \cdot \ln 2} \quad \text{Bq m}^{-3} = 0.20 \text{ Bq m}^{-3}$$

The annual amounts of fish and shellfish consumed globally is $17 \cdot 10^6$ and $3 \cdot 10^6$ tons, respectively. The total annual intake of Tc-99 from seafood becomes:
$$(17 \cdot 10^6 \cdot 30 \cdot 0.20 + 3 \cdot 10^6 \cdot 10^3 \cdot 0.20) \text{ Bq} = 0.71 \cdot 10^9 \text{ Bq}$$
corresponding to a collective effective dose equivalent of 0.24 person Sv pr year to the global population. We may also say that the discharge of 1 TBq Tc-99 to the world's oceans result in a CEDEC of 0.24 person Sv. As the ocean is the ultimate sink for atmospheric as well as liquid discharges of Tc-99 we may consider the above calculation as an estimate of CEDEC for any unit release (1 TBq) of Tc-99 to the environment.

4.2 Actual doses from present releases of Tc-99

In the chapter on source terms it was concluded that about 1 PBq Tc-99 had been released to the environment from the use of nuclear energy in power production.
Most of this has passed the North Sea, as it comes from the two European reprocessing plants, in the U.K. and France.

The effective dose equivalent commitment to a member of the critical group becomes: $3.4 \cdot 10^{-10} \cdot 10^3 = 3.4 \cdot 10^{-7}$ Sv or 0.34

o/oo of one year's background radiation. To an average person eating 10 kg fish and 1 kg shellfish pr year the effective dose equivalent commitment becomes $1.9 \cdot 10^{-8}$ Sv.

The CEDEC from 1 PBq Tc-99 becomes: $10^3 \cdot 0.24 = 240$ person Sv or 0.05 o/oo of one years background dose to the world population.

The Tc-99 doses from nuclear weapons testing and medicine are trivial.

5. CONCLUSION

Technetium-99 does not constitute a waste problem at present and even a substantial expansion of nuclear power production which is the main source of Tc-99 will not change this conclusion.

6. TRACER STUDIES

In recent years the development of a convenient analytical method for determining Tc-99 in environmental samples has led to the addition of Tc-99 to the list of useful tracers in marine research.

6.1 Radiochemical determination of Tc-99.

The analytical method used for determining Tc-99 in environmental samples was that developed by Holm et al. (17). Technetium was extracted from sulphuric acid solution with tributyl phosphate and back-extracted with sodium hydroxide solution. Tc-99m was used as a radiochemical-yield determinant. Prior to the measurement on an anticoincidence, shielded GM gas-flow counter, the Tc was electroplated onto stainless-steel discs.

6.2 Tracer studies in the North Atlantic Ocean

Since 1970 Tc-99 has been discharged to the Irish Sea from Sellafield in the U.K. The annual mean discharges in the seventies were around 50 TBq. By sampling brown algae (Fucus vesiculosus, which concentrates Tc-99 from the seawater) along the coasts of the Irish Sea, the North Sea, Norway, Spitzbergen and Greenland, it has been possible to trace the sea currents in the northern North Atlantic over a distance of nearly 10,000 kilometers.

It has been shown that it takes approximately eight years for a pollutant to diffuse from the Irish Sea to Baffin Bay between Greenland and Canada. A pollutant coming from the North Sea is diluted by a factor of 100 when it appears in the coastal waters of Greenland.

REFERENCES
1. IAEA. Reference Data Series No. 2. Nuclear Power Reactors in the World. International Atomic Energy Agency, Vienna. 1984.
2. Till J E. Source terms for technetium-99 from nuclear fuel cycle facilities. In: Technetium in the Environment, Elsevier Applied Science Publishers, London & New York, 1984: 1-20.
3. Luykx F. Technetium Discharges into Environment. In: Technetium in the Environment, Elsevier Applied Science Publishers, London & New York, 1984: 21-27.
4. BNFL 1978-85. Annual Report on Radioactive Discharges and Monitoring of Environment. British Nuclear Fuels Ltd, Risley Warrington, Cheshire, U.K.
5. Aarkrog A, Boelskifte S, Dahlgaard H, Duniec S, Hallstadius L, Holm E, Smith J N. Technetium-99 and cesium-134 as long distance tracers in Arctic waters. Estuarine, Coastal and Shelf Science (In press) 1987.
6. Harley J H. (Ed.). HASL procedures manual, HASL-300, Environmental Measurements Laboratory, U.S. Department of Energy, New York, 1987: 602.
7. UNSCEAR: Ionizing Radiation: Sources and Biological Effects. United Nations Scientific Committee on the Effects of Atomic Radiation 1982 Report to the General Assembly. New York 1982: 773.
8. Ennow, K. Personal communication. 1987.
9. Wildung R E, Garland T R, Cataldo D A. Preliminary studies on the uptake of technetium by soybeans. In: Pacific Northwest Laboratory Annual Report for 1974 to the USAEC Division of Biomedical and Environmental Research, Part 2, Ecological Sciences, Batelle-Northwest Laboratory, BNWL-1950 PT2. 1974.
10. Hoffman F O, Garten C T, Lucas D M, Huckabee J W. Environmental behaviour of technetium in soil and vegetation, implications for radiological assessments. Envir Sci Technol 1982; 16: 214-217.
11. Till J E, Shor R E, Hoffman F O. Environmental Effects of the Uranium Fuel Cycle - A Review of Data for Technetium. NUREG/CR-3738, Oak Ridge, Tennessee, Oak Ridge National Laboratory. 1985.
12. Thomas J M, Cadwell L L, Cataldo D A, Garland T R. Distribution of orally administered and chronically fed Tc-95m in Japanese quail tissues and eggs. In: Technetium

268

in the Environment, Elsevier Applied Science Publishers, London & New York, 1984: 349-357.

13. IAEA. Sediment Kd's and concentration factors for radio-nuclides in the marine environment. Techn. Rep. Ser. No.247, International Atomic Energy Agency, Vienna, 1984: 73.

14. Quinault J, Grauby A. Estimations des Risques Radiologiques Liés à un Rejet Concerté de Technetium dans l'Environment. In: Technetium in the Environment, Elsevier Applied Science Publishers, London & New York, 1984: 377-383.

15. ICRP. Limits for intakes of radionuclides by workers. ICRP Publication 30. Pergamon Press, Oxford. 1979.

16. Hoffman F O, Gardner R H, Bartell S M. The Significance of environmental exposure pathways for technetium. In: Technetium in the Environment, Elsevier Applied Science Publishers, London & New York. 1984: 359-376.

17. Holm E, Rioseco J, Garcia-Leon M. Determination of Tc-99 in environmental samples. Nuclear Instrumentation and Methods in Physics Research 1984; 223: 204-207.

PART 3

LEGAL ASPECTS OF THE INTRODUCTION OF NEW
RADIOPHARMACEUTICALS

Introduction

At the first European symposium on Radiopharmacy and Radiopharmaceuticals in 1983 some of the key questions discussed were as
follows:
"A very general problem were approached from many sides: How
can we best reach a sensible level for the requirements for
safety and efficacy. At what level do we set our standards? How
much money is the society prepared to spend on extra safety?
Who will take the responsibility? This problem is of course in
nature a political one but at its basis it requires scientific
information, on which risk estimates may be based".
   During the four years since this first symposium industri,
hospitals and competent authorities have taken a great interest
in the subject of securing the safety and efficacy of new
radiopharmaceuticals. Both national and international organisations are preparing legislation or guidelines. 1987 will
probably see guidelines on the registration of radiopharmaceuticals from Nordic Councils committee on drugs and guidelines
or directives from the European Economic Community. The World
Health Organisation has also included the subject in its
Nuclear Medicine Quality assurance programme as can be seen
from chapter 18 where a summary report from a WHO meeting is
given.
   Radiopharmaceuticals must in principle fulfil the same
reguirements with regard to safety and efficacy as other drugs.
There are however special problems to consider. The way they
are used (few administrations, small amount of chemical substance, part of a diagnostic system) may along with the very
limited market allow some deviation in the balancing of cost-
effectiveness.
   Specifications must be set and relevant quality control
methods developed including raw materials and final labelled
product. The numbers of studies in animals is a question for

discussion along with questions such as mutagenecity and carcinogenicity testing. It is common practice in relation to approval of non radioactive drugs to consider rather narrow indications and to require that each indication must be documented by clinical trials.

For radiopharmaceuticals it has to be remembered that they generally are a small part of a diagnostic system. It may therefore not be useful to work with too narrow indications and it may not be relevant for the licensing authorities to embark themselves too deeply into approving diagnostic systems.

Instead the effort might be better used on securing a uniform quality of the product and a safety testing and description. Clinical efficacy may to a large extent depend on types of equipment and the evaluation methods used. Here of course there are considerable difference between radiopharmaceuticals used for diagnosis and therapy. The latter being much more comparable to non-radioactive drugs. A close cooperation between industry and hospitals to identify the usefulness and safety of new radiopharmaceuticals needs to be further developed both with regard to economics and liability.

18. REPORT ON THE WHO WORKSHOP FOR ADMINISTRATORS IN THE FIELD OF RADIOPHARMACEUTICALS

J. TURNER

1. INTRODUCTION

The workshop was organised by the World Health Organisation (WHO) in collaboration with the Isotope Pharmacy, National Board of Health, Denmark and held between 28-30 April 1987 at the WHO Regional Headquarters in Copenhagen. It was attended by 18 participants from developed and developing countries including members of regulatory and international authorities and scientific staff from the radiopharmaceutical industry.

2. OBJECTIVES

The principle goal of the workshop was to draft internationally acceptable recommendations on common regulatory aspects of radiopharmaceuticals and on appropriate training and development activities at national level.

3. BACKGROUND

The regulatory aspects of radiopharmaceuticals had previously been discussed at the 1973 IAEA/WHO Symposium on Radiopharmaceuticals and Labelled Compounds. In view of the new trends in nuclear medicine it was felt during the 1984 IAEA International Conference in Japan that it would be useful to hold an international workshop for administrators in the field of radiopharmaceuticals in order to consider basic requirements in this area.

The workshop noted that nuclear medicine services are currently vailable in approximately 50% of WHO member states, ranging from 100% of the European countries to about 11% of countries in the African Region. A survey (1) showed that 16 of the 38 countries which replied to a questionnaire had no regulatory control of radiopharmaceuticals. In Europe in 1983 out of 23 countries investigated 8 had no regulations relating to the licensing of radiopharmaceuticals, 6 had special regulations and in 9 countries they were covered by general pharmaceutical regulations (2).

4.PRELIMINARY DISCUSSIONS

The workshop considered presentations from a number of its members. T. Bringhammer spoke about the latest draft Nordic guidelines on the data necessary to support a licence application for a radiopharmaceutical. He emphasised the need for the same criteria of safety, quality and efficacy to be met as are required for conventional medicines. This would include mutagenic and carcinogenic potential, a subject about which considerable discussion arose later. Ligands could now be designed for their intended purpose, he said, due to developments in synthetic chemistry, monoclonal antibodies and proteins derivatives from recombinant DNA techniques rather than being discovered by empirical methods. This offered great potential for diagnostic agents but also raised new considerations for regulatory authorities.

H. Roedler discussed the balance of biological detriment to the patient from radiation and the expected benefit, after optimisation of the radiation dose. Some of the newer agents such as some monoclonal antibodies had reversed the trend towards use of lower radiation dosage, measured as effective dose equivalent, because of the radionuclides employed but further developments were allowing reduction of dosage again. He noted that dose studies performed in healthy animals can give misleading indications of action in diseased human organs.

Quality Assurance in this field, he said, involved considering the clinical need, alternative approaches, selecting the optimum agent and method of administration and ensuring the correct functioning of all equipment and procedures.

H. Dige-Petersen described nuclear medicine as presently exclusive, complicated and often expensive, a high-tec speciality with very limited application when considered within the total health-care system. Having said this she expressed the wish that it would become more available to aid general practitioners in local communities. She acknowledged that by public demand regulation was increasingly visible and wide-ranging. To achieve sensible use and appropriate control of radiopharmaceuticals requires communication to be effective between the innovators, the users, the regulators and the public. In this way antagonisms could be avoided. Developments in nuclear medicine were outlined and Dige-Petersen finally offered as a solution to current problems the development of "the art of using poor radiopharmaceuticals better".

5. PAPERS TABLED

The workshop also had written papers from members detailing the present arrangements for control of radiopharmaceuticals in their respective countries and giving some manufacturer's views on regulations. It was apparent that in North America and Europe at least there is much work in progress to decide what modifications should be made to the existing data requirements for standard pharmaceuticals before applying them to radiopharmaceuticals. Clearly radiation aspects need to be addressed but there was discussion on the extent to which other conventional studies, including toxicity and mutagenicity, were relevant.

The Nordic countries and the UK will this year produce guidance for applicants for new licences and Sweden has requested further data on all existing products. Proposals for regulations to remove the exemption of radiopharmaceuticals from the

EEC Directives on Medicinal Products are expected to be made early in 1988.

6. VISIT

As an integral part of the workshop, participants visited the Department of Nuclear Medicine at Herlev Hospital, Copenhagen, and the Isotope Pharmacy of the National Board of Health. The latter demonstrated how effectively a small, centralised and specialist unit can monitor and control the radiopharmaceuticals used throughout the country.

7. DRAFT RECOMMENDATIONS

The workshop divided into groups to draft recommendations on the various aspects of regulatory control and on training and development at a national level. The full report will be produced later this year by WHO. The key aspects identified and some of the proposals made are indicated briefly below.

7.1 Policy

Radiopharmaceuticals form a special group of drugs but the same regulations which are applied to other drugs are valid for them. In addition radiopharmaceutical and radiation hygiene aspects must be considered when the safety, quality and efficacy of the product is being evaluated. Radionuclide generators and non-radioactive preparations which are designed to be mixed with a radioactive solution before administration should be included within the control of radiopharmaceuticals. The medicinal use of radiopharmaceuticals should be subject to strict government control.

7.2 Registration of Products by Authorities.

All radiopharmaceuticals should be registered before marketing, with provision for registration of existing products with minimal data. Registration of new products might be granted either after receipt of proof of registration of the same product in another acceptable country or after assessment of the safety, quality and efficacy according to the national requirements. Detailed guidance was drafted on the data which might be required.

7.3 Industrial Production.

Radiopharmaceuticals should be manufactured in accordance with the requirements of Good Pharmaceutical manufacturing Practice which are applicable to all pharmaceuticals, as described in the WHO or relevant national publication. Any potential conflict between product protection and operator protection, as might arise for example during the production of sterile products requiring forced, filtered ventilation, must be resolved without jeopardising the quality of the product or the safety of the operator. Recommendations are given on this and other considerations of GMP peculiar to radiopharmaceuticals.

7.4 Hospital Production.

Adequate facilities are required including qualified responsible management, trained staff, dedicated premises, suitable equipment and defined written procedures for production and quality control. There should be competence in radiopharmacy, medical physics and nuclear medicine.

7.5 Radiation Hygiene.

The key elements to avoiding unnecessary radiation dose to the patient are to avoid clinically unproductive examinations and to optimise the agent, the procedure and the dose. These elements are discussed and the protection of operators and the general population is considered.

7.6 Therapy with Open Sources.

It was noted that the development of new ligands offers the possibility of more selective targetting and therefore of an increase in the therapeutic applications for radiopharmaceuticals. Product registration, production and post-marketing surveillance should be on the same lines as those recommended primarily for diagnostic radiopharmaceuticals but the high dose levels involved (3700-7400 MBq) necessitate special facilities for storage, dispensing, administration and nursing care.

7.7 Quality Control by the Distributor, User and Authorities.

Special storage and distribution arrangements are required for radiopharmaceuticals so these should be subject to control and approval by the authorities.

The user of the radiopharmaceuticals should have basic procedures for assuring the quality of the products used, including scrutiny of all written material and, as appropriate, simple tests such as for the correct operation of radionuclide generators and for radiochemical purity. Any adverse findings must be reported to the authorties.

It is not recommended that every authority need establish its own specialised test facilities for radiopharmaceuticals. An alternative approach would be to make whatever investigation is practicable of the controls operated by and applied locally to the manufacturer and to require reports from users and suppliers of any defects found.

PARTICIPANTS
T Bringhammer, Department of Social Affairs, Sweden
P Cox, Rotterdam Radio-Therapeutic Institute, Netherlands (chairman)
H Dige-Petersen, Glostrup Hospital, Denmark
K Kristensen, The Isotope Pharmacy, Denmark
M Merlin, Companie ORIS Industrie, France
Y Megahed, Middle Eastern Regional Radioistope Centre, Egypt
T Paal, National Institute of Pharmacy, Hungary
H Roedler, Institute of Radioation Hygiene, Fed. Rep. of Germany
G Souchkevitch, Radiation Medicine, WHO Geneva
F Stock, Mallinckrodt Diagnostica, Netherlands
S Sullman, Amersham International plc, UK
J Svihovec, State Institute for Drug Control, Czechoslovakia
G Toth, Hungarian Academy of Sciences, Hungary
R Turaev, Ministry of Health, USSR
J Turner, Dep. of Health and Social Security UK
N Vinberg, The Isotope Pharmacy, Denmark
E Westerlund, International Atomic Energy Agency

REFERENCES

1. Kristensen K. Regularory Aspetcs of Radiopharmaceuticals in Radiopharmaceuticals and labelled compounds. IAEA, Vienna 1984: 383-394.
2. Safety and Efficacy of Radiopharmaceuticals, ed K Kristensen and E Nørbygaard. Nijhoff. Hague 1984.

19. CURRENT TRENDS IN THE REQUIREMENTS FOR SAFETY AND EFFICACY OF NEW DRUGS

HARRIET DIGE-PETERSEN, PER JUUL

1. INTRODUCTION

The regulatory requirements concerning drugs involve quality, efficacy and safety. These matters are dealt with in national, international and supranational rules and regulations (e.g. 1).

Whereas quality often may be considered in absolute terms, efficacy and safety obviously are linked together in a relative manner, and in most countries even this relative efficacy/safety ratio is requested to be compared to existing alternatives.

By way of introduction it can be stated that the requirements concerning radiopharmaceuticals closely follow the requirements concerning "ordinary" drugs - apart from the specific problems involved in radiation exposure. The administrative channels of procedure are most often different from those involved with "ordinary" drugs, but the principles are identical.

At the symposium on "Safety and Efficacy of Radiopharmaceuticals" 1983 several papers dealt with the individual aspects of quality, efficacy and safety (2). The present paper deals with "current trends" in these respects four years later.

The development within radiopharmacology involves new techniques (e.g. positron emission tomography), new diagnostic procedures (e.g. 131-methyliodobenzylguanidine (MIBG) scintigraphy in neuroblastoma), new areas of possible therapeutic use (e.g. 131-I-MIBG in neuroblastoma and pheochromocytoma) and use of radioisotopes in "high-technology-drugs" (e.g. monoclonal antibodies in the diagnosis and treatment of malignant diseases).

From a regulatory point of view radiopharmaceuticals have been dealt with in recent directives, rules and guidelines, and some of these shall be dealt with in more detail (3, 4, 5, 6, 7).

Before embarking upon the various rules and guidelines it should be stressed that this national, international and supranational intervention is not established to put obstacles, obstruction and impediment to progress - an often expressed view by industry, scientists and clinicians. The requirements are based upon historical experience (the Nuremberg Code and subsequent ethical declarations), more recent drug disasters (thalidomide and thorotrast) as well as the very recent backgrounds for all the "Goods": Good Manufacturing Practice, Good Laboratory Practice, Good Clinical Practice, Good Radiopharmacy Practice et cetera. Both industry and academia may consider the role of society, its insight in, influence on, and even control of drug development as a threat to the freedom of thought, research and trade. Admittedly the bureaucratic paperwork and the unavoidable delays are irritating, but they are part of the attempts by "society" to protect human individuals (volunteers and patients) and to ensure the marketing and use of optimal drugs considering the individual patient as well as society - in competition with other resource demanding activities within the health sector.

"Clinical freedom died accidentally, crushed between the rising cost of new forms of investigation and treatment and the financial limits inevitable in an economy that cannot expand indefinitely. Clinical freedom should, however, have been strangled long ago, for at best it is a cloak for ignorance and at worst an excuse for quackery. Clinical freedom was a myth that prevented true advance"(8).

2. DRUG REGULATION PRIOR TO CLINICAL TRIALS
2.1. Quality

By "quality" is understood the physico-chemical, microbiological and pharmaceutical characteristics of the drug: route of synthesis, structure analysis, chemical and radionuclidic purity, impurities arising from synthesis and/or degradation, stability et cetera.

The problems concerning the quality of radiopharmaceuticals are dealt with elsewhere in this symposium. They comprise the industrial phase as well as the final preparation for use (e.g. 9). It should be emphasized that quality requirements in some areas may be regarded as perhaps even more important than biological requirements (e.g. concerning toxicology testing). When biotechnological compounds (e.g. derived from recombinantDNA-technology and monoclonal antibodies) are evaluated the problems arising from the active ingredient as well as from impurities resulting from the biological synthesis or degradation may be difficult or impossible to solve through animal and human experiments due to a.o. imperfect immunological techniques as discussed elsewhere in this symposium and in recent papers and guidelines (4,5,6,10). When a new chemical compound is considered as an investigational new drug (IND) and when notifications/applications of clinical trials are evaluated less detailed information of chemical and pharmaceutical data is normally required compared to the requirements concerning an application for marketing of a new drug (NDA).

Specific guidelines concerning preclinical quality requirements for radiopharmaceuticals do not exist, but in principle the Nordic guidelines concerning clinical trials of "ordinary" drugs should be followed (11) - bearing in mind the special problems arising from biotechnologically derived compounds.

2.2. Preclinical investigations

The animal toxicological investigations necessary to initiate studies in humans are described in (11). With regard to a carcinogenic potential short-term (in vitro) mutagenicity tests shall normally suffice when considering clinical trials.

3. CLINICAL TRIALS

The flow-sheet of the development of "ordinary" drugs should preferably be followed also concerning diagnostic and therapeutic radiopharmaceuticals. A coherent plan involving the various clinical phases should be followed, and particular attention should-be paid to the randomized clinical trial comparing the new drug or procedure to existing alternative(s) as described in (12). An extensive reference list concerning the conduct of clinical trials is published in (7).

There seems to be an increasing international harmonization concerning the principles and practice of clinical trials as well as the regulatory requirements involved. The individual trials protocol should be evaluated by institutional review boards, research ethics committees and/or regulatory authorities. Apart from the scientific/ technical matters (purpose, justification, design, effect variables, statistical estimation of the necessary number of research subjects et cetera) the protocol should contain information of informed consent, responsibility, liability, insurance and economics involved. If the trial is to be performed in another country than that of origin of the drug, this should be justified. Many of these points are discussed in (7) and (13).

4. REGISTRATION REQUIREMENTS

The requirements are presented in numerous national, international and supranational rules and guidelines. The national requirements unfortunately differ to a certain extent, and particular conditions imposed by the Canadian, Japanese and U.S. regulatory authorities should be taken into consideration if applications for marketing are intended in these countries. Harmonization shall definitely occur - but at a very slow rate (14). In the EEC and Nordic countries very similar requirements exist (15,16, numerous guidelines on specific therapeutic groups).

4.1. Quality

Requirements are presented in the above mentioned references (4,5,6,15,16).

4.2. Efficacy

By "efficacy" is understood the diagnostic or therapeutic efficiency of the compound in absolute terms or in relation to

existing alternatives. The requirements obviously differ according to the product in question, e.g. diagnostic/therapeutic
drug. However, the basic principles of the randomized clinical
trial in most cases form the background for the evaluation. A-
mong the "current trends" (developing through the last 20
years) three points should be mentioned: dose-response relationship, comparison to existing optimal alternative(s) and
studies of interindividual variation. Relevant monographs concerning these points are given in (7). The "alternatives"
should be viewed in a broad context depending on the compound
in question, e.g. a reference drug, other diagnostic procedures
involving radiopharmaceuticals, clinical chemical methods, X-
ray et cetera.

4.3. Safety

The evaluation of "safety" of the compound/procedure builds
on preclinical animal studies and experience from clinical
trials resulting in a rough estimate of risk, which should be
evaluated in context with the expected diagnostic/therapeutic
benefit. Also in this respect radiopharmaceuticals are dealt
with in parallel with "ordinary" drugs. With regard to the preclinical (animal toxicity) studies the usual problems: chronic
toxicity, teratogenicity and carcinogenicity studies are particularly difficult to solve when concerning biotechnological
products.

5. TECHNOLOGY ASSESSMENT, DRUG UTILIZATION

Drugs are most often marketed based upon a limited clinical
experience. Phase 4 studies, i.e. large scale evaluation under
practical clinical conditions - often uncontrolled - are often
extremely difficult to perform and evaluate. Apart from the general problems involved the evaluation of diagnostic procedures
involving radiopharmaceuticals pose particular problems concerning the diagnostic strategies, different techniques and different equipment, whose quality may be difficult to standardize.
These studies have always been important, but their importance
increases due to the relative lack of resources necessitating
to put the possibilities in order of priority - even with re-

gard to the individual patient, the ultimate process of decision ("One man's provision another mans deprivation").

Drug utilization is defined as the marketing, distribution,
prescription and use of drugs in a society, with special emphasis on resulting medical, social and economic consequences.
Drug utilization is thus an important part of medical technology assessment. The radiopharmaceuticals as such in this respect may not represent a major problem, but the total technique involved may well do so (e.g. positron emission tomography).

In many countries the marketed drugs are reevaluated every 5
years, but the rules concerning this evaluation for continued
marketing are vague. The two major reasons for withdrawal of
drugs from the market are the occurrence of unacceptable adverse reactions or commercial reasons. A thorough reevaluation
comparing the drug/procedure to existing alternative(s) according to the state of the art is rarely undertaken. It may be
expected that this reevaluation shall play a major role in the
determination of the fate of the drugs on the market and their
use (including radiopharmaceuticals).

6. ETHICS
Ethical considerations form an integral part of drug development, evaluation and regulation. Also in this respect radiopharmaceuticals are treated as "ordinary" drugs. Particularly
concerning research involving human subjects international and
supranational rules and declarations have been issued. A recent
monograph excellently describes these ethical problems (17).
Several problems of ethics are mentioned in the EEC document
(7) and have been dealt with in (13).

The discussion of ethics is closely linked to "risk". The
risk involved in the research involving human subjects and in
the diagnostic and therapeutic use of drugs is indeed very
small. However, it is often difficult or impossible to state
even a rough estimate of the size of the risk, and even when
this is possible, the estimate may not be understandable to the
public, which furthermore may have "unscientific" interpreta-

tions of the figures. This is sometimes of a particular concern when working with radiopharmaceuticals. A recent report from a meeting dealing with benefit/risk decisions gives an excellent introduction to this important area (18).

7. PROMOTION AND RESEARCH

Only 10-12 out of 20,000 new chemical entities (NCE) reach the stage of clinical trials, and only 1-2 out of these reach marketing. The total time of development of a new drug may be 15 years and the total cost may amount to 150 million US $. The economical risk to the individual drug company is therefore great and the existing patent protection systems may be inadequate. As a result the EEC has implemented new measures (1987) concerning "high-technology products" including those derived from biotechnology (3). According to this "high-tech directive" drugs developed by means of biotechnological processes (e.g. rDNA technology and monoclonal antibodies) and "other" high technology medicinal products must be dealt with in a common EEC-procedure, i.e. considered by the Committee for Proprietary Medicinal Products (CPMP). The applications must be dealt with according to a rapid multistate time schedule ("the 120 days procedure"). If a marketing authorization is granted, the high-tech product shall be "protected" from generic equivalents for a period of 10 years from the time of marketing. Among candidates for the high-tech procedure apart from those derived from biotechnology are mentioned new drug delivery systems, new indications, medicinal products based on radioisotopes et cetera, provided that the products can be considered of "significant therapeutic interest."

Thus society may actively promote the development of certain drugs/procedures. On the other hand the initiative almost exclusively lies with the industry, and so far the Western societies have not exerted any influence on this process.

8. DISCUSSION

Radiopharmaceuticals in the legal and administrative sense are drugs, and their development, evaluation and use shall follow established rules and guidelines with regard to quality, efficacy and safety. The development of "high-tech" medicinal products (including "bio-tech" drugs) puts particular emphasis on quality aspects and gives rise to special problems with regard to preclinical (animal toxicity) studies. Considering the clinical phases of drug development particular emphasis shall be -put on randomized clinical trials comparing the new drug/ procedure to existing, optimal alternatives.

New EEC directives and rules may encourage the development of high-tech drugs through the establishment of a rapid registration procedure and a prolonged "patent protection."

REFERENCES
1. The rules governing medicaments for human use in the European Community. III/182/87. February 1987.
2. Kristensen K, Nørbygaard E (eds.). Safety and efficacy of radiopharmaceuticals. Martinus Nijhoff Publ. 1984.
3. EEC Council Directive 87/22/EEC of 22.12.86 relating to the placing on the market of high technology medicinal products particularly those derived from biotechnology.
4. EEC Notes to applicants for marketing authorizations on requirements for the production and quality control of medicinal products derived by recombinant DNA technology. Draft, January 1987.
5. EEC Notes to applicants for marketing authorizations on the requirements for the preclinical biological safety testing of medicinal products derived from biotechnology. Draft, March 1987.
6. Radiopharmaceuticals. Drug Applications. Nordic guidelines. Draft, Nordic Council on Medicines, January 1987.
7. EEC Recommended basis for the conduct of clinical trials of medicinal products in the European Community. Draft, March 1987.
8. Hampton JR. The end of clinical freedom. Brit med J 1983; 287: 1237-1238.
9. Hammermaier A, Reich., Bögl W. Qualitätskontrolle von in-vivo Radiopharmaka. Institut für Strahlenhygiene, Bundesgesundheitsamt, 1986.
10. Lasagna L. Clinical testing of products prepared by biotechnology. Regulatory Tox Pharmacol 1986; 6: 385-390.
11. Clinical Trials of Drugs. Nordic guidelines. Nordic Council on Medicines Publication no. 11, 1983.
12. Juul P. Clinical trials of radiopharmaceuticals. In Kristensen K, Nørbygaard E (eds.): Safety and efficacy of radiopharmaceuticals. Martinus Nijhoff Publ. 1984: 179-190.
13. Towards an international ethic for research involving human subjects. Report of the summit bioethics conference, Ottawa, 1987 (in press).
14. Lasagna L. On reducing waste in foreign clinical trials and postregulation experience. Clin pharmacol Ther 1986;

          40: 269-372.
15.   Drug Applications. Nordic guidelines. Nordic Council on
      Medicines Publication no. 12, 1983.
16.   Notice to applicants for marketing authorizations for
      proprietary medicinal products in the member states of the
      European Community. III/158/54. (Revision 1987).
17.   Levine RJ. Ethics and regulation of clinical research.
      Urban & Schwarzenberg 1986 (2. ed.)
18.   Walker SR & Asscher AW (eds.). Medicines and risk/benefit
      decisions. MTP Press Ltd. 1987.

20. RELATIONSHIPS BETWEEN INDUSTRY, HOSPITALS AND AUTHORITIES

R. D. NEIRINCKX

1. INTRODUCTION

The common denominator between the commercial companies, wanting to optimise profits from existing and novel pharmaceuticals, and the national regulatory licensing authorities, is that both want to make safe, new drugs available to the patient population. For example, the EEC Rules which govern medicaments (1) state that the primary purpose of the comunity rules relating to the medicinal products is to safeguard public health whilst at the same time ensuring that the development of the pharmaceutical industry and trade in medicinal products will not be hindered.

This could be accomplished on a worldwide basis if the following conditions were met:

1. Uniform regulations
2. Unequivocal standards of acceptability
3. Unequivocal proof of safety and efficacy for any new drug
4. Realistic balance between risk and benefit
5. Timely response to submissions

These ideal circumstances do not exist because of:

1. Nationalistic pride
2. Rapid growth in scientific knowledge, which continuously expands our capability for novel and/or more accurate analysis of pharmacological effects.
3. Unexpected technological developments in drug design and production techniques which create new concerns
4. Finite resources of the pharmaceutical company

5. Lack of resources at regulatory agencies

This results in:

1. Contradicting requirements from different national authorities

2. Uncertainty in both producers and regulatory authorities about what represents sufficient information

3. Delays in licensing and improved diagnosis and treatment

2.SPECIAL SITUATION OF RADIOPHARMACEUTICAL DRUGS

Historically, new in-vivo radiopharmaceuticals have been introduced by academic researchers and clinicians who discovered, produced and applied these relatively simple radiopharmaceuticals in their patient population. They subsequently published their data in the open literature. These published references which relate to pharmacology, toxicology and clinical results may be used in the regulatory submissions (2) as long as the products have an established use and known effects - including side effects - on human beings. This was confirmed by the US Department of Health and Human Services' Guidelines (3). This simplified the licensing of the early radiopharmaceuticals by commercial manufacturers such that is could be accomplished after a relatively short and low cost licensing effort, which made the commercial availability of these products possible. Extensive time delays and resource expenditure on these low-volume and low-price products would throttle any further developments in nuclear medicine. Recently, however, radiopharmaceutical agents have become much more complex molecules, whose development mirrors that of conventional pharmaceutical drugs. The identification and development of novel chemical entities now require the co-ordinated effort of relatively large research and development teams. Consequently it is industry rather than academia which has come to the forefront of new development in in-vivo diagnostic agents. This also means, however, that at the time of commercial involvement there is no established use of the new drugs yet and the manufacturer is responsible for satisfying all the regulatory requirements applicable to the new drug.

In-vivo diagnostic agents are unlikely to be used more than once in each patient so they are much safer than standard drugs, but it also means that their market is orders of magnitude smaller than that for standard therapeutic drugs. Despite this the diagnoses made with radiopharmaceuticals may be unique and be a determining factor in the current follow-up treatment of a patient. Hence, the benefit-over-risk ratio can be very high for radiopharmaceuticals and hence their existence should be protected. This will not happen if the same restrictions are applied to radiopharmaceuticals as are being applied to the other pharmaceuticals because the low sales of a typical radiopharmaceutical can never warrant the amount of support work needed.

3. RADIOPHARMACEUTICAL LICENSING REQUIREMENTS
3.1 Conditions for marketing drug

The Council Directives (2,4,5,6) lay down the conditions for marketing authorisation of drugs. This includes the requirements for tests and trials to be carried out and the rules controlling manufacture and control of these products. Ihe Directive 65/65/EEC (2) describes in its Article 4 what the content should be of an application aimed at bringing a proprietary medicinal product to the market. In summary such an application should mention the name or the corporate name of the person responsible for the product the name of the proprietary product, the qualitative and quantitative particulars of all the constituents of the product, a brief description of the method of preparation, the therapeutic indications, contrary indications and side effects, pathology, pharmaceutical form and the route of administration, the controlled methods used by the manufacturer, the results of physico-chemical, biological and microbiological tests, the results of pharmacological and toxicological tests and the results of the clinical trials.

The EEC Directives (2,4,5,6) specify that the following toxicological and pharmacological tests should be carried out for pharmaceuticals: toxicity, foetal toxicity, reproductive function examination, carcinogenicity, pharmacodynamics and pharmacokinetics. In toxicity testing one must differentiate between the single dose toxicity and the repeated dose toxicity or sub-acute toxicity.

3.2 Unique characteristics of radiopharmacuticals

Radiopharmaceuticals have unique characteristics which ought to be considered before the same requirements imposed on therapeutic drugs are imposed upon them. First, in-vivo diagnostic agents are not intended to have pharmacological effects (7) and they are normally only administered once to a patient. Hence toxicity is much less of concern than with a daily administered therapeutic drug. The toxicity is typically not that of the active ingredient (7). In a typical radiopharmaceutical the active ingredient is a radioactive no-carrier-added product which is present in vanishingly-small quantities. Pharmacokinetics of these compounds are very easily determinded and are indeed necessary as requested by the EEC Directives (3). The real safety issue is the radiation of the pharmaceutical and hence the radiation dosimetry calculations are very important. In many radiopharmaceuticals like the cyclotron isotopes no other incipient but this no-carrier-added isotope is present. For the kit-formulated Tc-99m agents, however, the complexing agents which are being used to synthesise the desired Tc-99m complexes are present in a vast excess in comparison with a no-carrier-added material, but in reality the quantities injected in the patient are very small, in the order of milligrams. Toxicology of these agents is being carried out although they are only injected once in the patient.

3.3 Required safety tests for radiopharmaceuticals

All radiopharmaceuticals, must undergo the single dose toxicity or acute dose toxicity. The EEC directives for drugs stipulate that a relatively short sub-acute test (2-4 weeks) should suffice for all single administration drugs. This was confirmed by the FDA guidelines for radiopharmaceuticals (7). Foetal toxicity can be ignored on condition that appropriate warning is given against use in pregnant or lactating women. Examination of the reproductive functions should only be carried out if previous animal tests have revealed anything suggesting harmful effects on progeny. Carcinogenicity should only be carried out in substances which are administered regularly over a long period of a patient's life or if the compound is structurally related to a known carcinogen (2,8). Pharmacodynamics should evaluate the variations which are caused by the new substance in the normal physiology. For diagnostic agents - with no known therapeutic effect - they should not be applicable. Pharmacokinetics must be carried out for all in-vivo diagnostic agents.

It would help the industry to know whether these interpretations of the directives are the correct ones for radiopharmaceuticals. This has already been accomplished in the USA through the FDA guidelines (3) which give a clear overview of the types of studies which will need to be carried out for a radiopharmaceutical. Since all radiopharmaceuticals are invariably administered in a hospital under medical supervision the regulatory authorities should consider whether the requirements for safety testing of radiopharmaceuticals should not be relaxed. Inherently it is very difficult, if not impossible, to determine the safety of the therapeutic agent itself. Tc-99m agents for example are only present in very small quantities and the production of the equivalent Tc-99 compounds give rise to products or in-vivo decomposition products which are different from the products encountered when no-carrier-added materials are being used. Under these circumstances it is doubtful whether data collected with Tc-99 compounds allow valid conclusions about equivalent Tc-99m compounds.

Saturation of metabolic processes for example can alter the fate of compounds, which becomes relevant when one considers the metabolic fate of radiopharmaceuticals in-vivo. Since the drug can only be followed through its emitted radiation, it is impossible to tell the chemical form in which the drug is present. Whereas HPLC analysis of body fluids might allow an estimate of certain physicochemical parameters of the excreted products it is very difficult to carry out the same analysis in the other organs of the human body. Because no chemical methods can be brought to bear on the no-carrier-added products it is impossible to prove through analysis of the body fluids the structure of the excreted products. The use of carrier material like technetium-99m compounds often leads to different species in-vivo. Thus evaluation of the in-vivo fate of radiopharmaceuticals must be based on circumstantial evidence and deduction rather than on chemical analysis of reaction products.

3.4 Differing Requirements

Apart from the necessity to have to face a wide range of scientific problems the R and D departments have to deal with different guidelines from national regulatory bodies. These guidelines contain very little information about the nature and extent of the scientific data required. The Food and Drug Administration guidelines for example deal mainly with the documentation aspects of the submission although indications are given of the kind and extent of desirable safety data (3). Although the EEC Directives summarise the nature of the scientific data that need to be provided in a drug application there are no such directives for radiopharmaceuticals. It is therefore up to the radiopharmaceutical research and development departments to decide on the deployment of their scarce resources, such that more limited data on their inherently safer drugs will still satisfy the regulatory requirements.

The differences in the requirements between the various regulatory authorities sometimes also complicates the decision on which data should be gathered. The insistence of the Food and Drug Administration on submission of all available data leads to the submission of data which have been gathered to satisfy other authorities, whether these are relevant or not. For example, for Tc99m labelled compounds compatibility studies are carried out with a number of different pertechnetate generators in order to provide marketing support for the ultimate product. However, this is essentially irrelevant to the quality of the technetium complex itself and complicates the more important licensing issues. Nevertheless, since those data are available they are required by the FDA.

4. COST VERSUS BENEFIT

Satisfaction of the regulatory requirements requires the collection of a very large amount of data, which span a wide spectrum of scientific expertise including physiology, pharmacology, analytical chemistry, physical chemistry, microbiology, toxicology and clinical evaluation of the drug. Ultimately all the data must be provided by the research and development department of the radiopharmaceutical drug manufacturers. Only a limited amount of research and development can be supported by an industry which services a relatively small market.

In the absence of well-defind guidelines for radiopharmacauticals the research and development departments of radiopharmaceutical companies depend heavily on the in-house regulatory departments to judge on the kind and extent of testing data which will be needed by various regulatory authorities. Once this decision is made the development programme - and to a certain extent the research programme - can be tailored to meet these requirements. The development networks for new radiopharmaceutical drugs must now not only incorporate the development of the drug from an interesting entity to a marketable product, but also, the basic research effort required to answer safety and pharmacodynamic questions about the new product.

Since the outcome of net-present-value calculations for new products is very dependent on the time delay between the discovery of a new agent and the achievement of market saturation it is very important to limit the delay between licence submission and approval to the shortest possible time. Hence the decision to omit additional data and of spending less time and resources on collecting these data must be made against the possibility that these omissions can result in deficiencies which would severely delay the ultimate granting of a licence. It would be very helpful if a mechanism existed whereby the Regulatory Authorities could advise on the shortcomings of existing data before the time of the Drug Application. For example, early feedback on the content of the Production and Control Sections of drug applications would allow a company to address any insufficiencies while clinical trials are ongoing and before these sections are finalised and added to the final application.

5.CONCLUSION

For most pharmaceuticals the expenditure involved in satisfying all of the requirements for the regulatory authorities runs in millions of dollars. However, most therapeutic drugs address very common disease states and thus very large potential markets. Under those circumstances the real cost of the regulatory process lies not in the gathering of the data but in lost sales due to extensive delays in the sale of the products. Preferential treatment for a drug may be obtained if it represents a major advance in treatment. Such a sense of priority is hard to obtain for any diagnostic agent since inherently it does not represent a long-awaited solution to a severe problem. Hence, licensing processes for new diagnostic agents, even if they represent major diagnostic advances, tend to have a lower priority and receive less attention.

It is obvious that the subjection of new radiopharmaceutical drugs to the full extent of testing, which is carried out for other drugs would quickly bankrupt the radiopharmaceutical industries.

A thorough understanding by the regulatory authorities of the special character of radiopharmaceuticals will be needd to allow a sensible limitation of the testing imposed on these agents. This can best be accomplished by interaction between the authorities and academic as well as industrial experts on the subject of nuclear medicine.

REFERENCES
1.   The Rules Governing the Medicaments in the European Community Commission of the European Communities, July 1984
2.   Council Directive 65/65/EEC. Official Journal of the European Communities, No 22, 9.2.1965: 369 - 365
3.   Guidelines for the Clinical Evaluation of Radiopharmaceutical Drugs. HHS (FDA) 81-320: 2.

4. Council Directive 75/318/EEC. Official Journal of the European
    Communities, No L147, 9.6.1975: 1.
5. Council Directive 75/319/EEC, No L147/1, 9.6.1975
6. Council Directive 83/570/EEC No L332/1, 26.10.1983
7. Guidelines for the Clinical Evaluation of Radiopharmaceutical
    Drugs. HHS (FDA) 81-320: 3.
8. Guidelines for the Clinical Evaluation of Radiopharmaceutical
    Drugs. HHS (FDA) 81-320: 4.

STUART R. HESSLEWOOD

1. INTRODUCTION

In all cases where radiopharmaceuticals are used in clinical practice, consideration of patient safety is of paramount importance and everybody has a contribution to make in achieving this aim. This requires close co-operation between hospitals, manufacturers and authorities to ensure that all materials used are safe, are of suitable quality and are efficacious.

The need for scientific information to form the basis of the standards set has long been recognized, but the answers to questions such as how much money is society prepared to expend to improve safety standards and who ultimately accepts responsibility for any damage to patients are still debated. Awareness of such factors will be enhanced by the eventual implementation of EEC directive 85/374 on Strict Product Liability. Under this directive the patient would have to prove that damage resulted from the product, but is not required to demonstrate that either the product was defective or that the producer had been negligent.

Administration of radiopharmaceuticals to patients takes place in hospitals and it is there that any adverse affects of the administration will be first detected. Harmful affects may be due either to radiation emitted or the chemical constituents of the radiopharmaceutical. The majority of radiopharmaceuticals are administered for diagnostic purposes using small quantities of chemicals which often have no demonstrable pharmacological activity, and the most recently published surveys indicate that the number of reported adverse reactions to radiopharmaceuticals has remained low (1,2). At a recent symposium on Radiopharmaceutical Dosimetry, it was suggested that it was rare for radiopharmaceuticals to exhibit any toxicity other than that due to radiation hazards (3).

What steps should hospitals therefore adopt to maximise safety of patients in their care? The first obvious answer is to use products which have been granted product licences by appropriate authorities, since the granting of such licences is dependent upon the submission of review of data demonstrating the safety, quality and efficacy of the product.

However, the granting of a product licence cannot guarantee that an adverse reaction or patient damage will not occur and conversely the fact that a product does not have a licence does not necessarily mean that it is unsafe. It would seem prudent to use materials which have been granted product licences, since in the event of an adverse reaction occuring with an unlicensed material, the prescriber may have to justify his choice of radiopharmaceutical.

Inevitably, economic factors have to be considered, particularly at times of financial stringency. Where nuclear medicine is competing with other specialities for limited resources, it is important that cost of materials does not rise excessively. The development of a monopoly situation in supply of radiopharmaceuticals could defeat this objective since competition between manufacturers ensures costs are kept under careful review. It is therefore in the hospital's interest to see as many products as possible licensed such that a wide range of both diagnostic and therapeutic agents is available, and they should therefore co-operate with manufacturers and encourage them to seek licences for their products. Part of the cost of radiopharmaceuticals accrues from testing procedures carried out to demonstrate suitability for a product licence. It is again in the hospital's interest to ensure any irrelevant tests which do not contribute to the safety, quality and efficacy of the radiopharmaceutical are avoided since it is inevitable that there will be the temptation to use unlicensed materials if they are cheaper than licensed alternatives.

It is also recognized that the size of the whole radiopharmaceutical market worldwide is small compared with other medicinal products. In view of the comparatively limited use of some radiopharmaceuticals and therefore their financial return, manufacturers may decide not to proceed with product licensing if the cost of obtaining the data required by the licensing authority appears disproportionate. More importantly, the prospect of a lengthy, expensive procedure may deter companies from developing new radiopharmaceuticals.

Hospitals should therefore co-operate to ensure that standards are adopted which are relevant to situations on which radiopharmaceuticals are used. Further, the co-operation between national authorities to develop a unified approach to licensing, not only within Europe, but also worldwide should be encouraged. Within the United Kingdom, is it sensible that American manufacturer's of radiopharmaceuticals who have licensed their products through the FDA system do not have, and in some cases do not intend to seek U.K. product licences? There are also European manufacturers who sell products within the United Kingdom which do not possess appropriate licences.

The United Kingdom has a comprehensive licensing system for all medicinal products under the Medicines Act 1968. Extensive Guidance Notes on applications for product licences and also clinical trials have been published (4,5). However, these notes deal with all medicinal products and are not specific to radiopharmaceuticals. It is therefore important to highlight sections that are relevant to radiopharmaceuticals and provide the necessary data. In addition it is equally important to identify areas that are not relevant such that unnecessary expenditure can be avoided. It is encouraging that there are indications within the guidance notes that this situation is recognized. Even so, perhaps it is worth debating whether there should be a completely separate mechanism to handle radiopharmaceuticals since it is also necessary to consider certain parameters, e.g.

radiation dosimetry, which are not applicable to other medicinal products.

2. PRODUCT LICENCE REQUIREMENTS

Data required in product licence applications can be divided into three broad headings,

   i)   Chemical and pharmaceutical

   ii)   Toxicological and pharmacological

   iii)   Clinical

The chemical and pharmaceutical data will be obtained in the laboratory and the initial toxicological and pharmacological data, if present, is normally determined in animals.

The clinical data necessary will be obtained in humans and it is therefore important that properly controlled clinical trials are initiated as soon as possible, since the first two items are expensive to perform and they may not guarantee a safe, efficacious radiopharmaceutical. This can be exemplified by the experiences of one American Company in developing technetium labelled myocardial agents. Dimethyl phosphenoethane looked promising in animal studies. After spending approximately two million dollars in development, the first trials in humans showed that the radiopharmaceutical localized predominantly in the liver (6). This is one example of the well known difficulty in extrapolating data from one species to another and the ability to perform prompt clinical trials is therefore important. Mechanisms which promote this are to be encouraged. Within the United Kingdom, it is possible to apply for a Clinical Trials Certificate or alternatively a Clinical Trial Exemption.

The advantages of the latter are that

   i) Only summaries of data are required and it is suggested that this should not exceed 50-60 pages.

   ii) Exemption is granted automatioally <u>unless</u> the licensing authority raises objections within 35 days. Once granted an exemption is valid for 3 years.

Great care is necessary in the design of clinical trials to ensure that maximum information is gained for them. Effort ex-

pended in the design and evaluation of trials is normally re-
warded (7). With the information gained, the company should
then be able to decide whether or not it is worth proceeding to
full product licensing.

It is impracticable to discuss in detail all the specific
requirements outlined in the Guidance Notes. The hospital is,
anyway, not in a position to make a contribution towards the
data required for the application. Comments will therefore be
restricted to the consideration of specific topics which are
relevant to radiopharmaceutical products.

3. CHEMISTRY OF DRUG SUBSTANCE

There is a requirement to provide comprehensive data on the
chemical structure of the material, including the complete formula of the finished product. For the majority of radiopharmaceuticals administered to patients, the structure of the labelled molecule is unknown. As an example, phosphonates have been
widely used for bone imaging. The structure of the unlabelled
molecule is known, but the exact nature of the complex formed
with technetium is uncertain. There is evidence that more than
one complex may be formed (8). The fact that the precise structure is unknown should not, per se, inhibit the use of the radiopharmaceutical. Indeed technetium phosphonates for bone
imaging have been one of the most successful and widely used
radiopharmaceuticals over the last decade. In this particular
case and with other diagnostic radiopharmaceuticals which do
not exert any pharmacological activity, the efficacy of the radiopharmaceutical is largely dependent on its biodistribution.
Provided that the purity of unlabelled starting materials is
controlled and preparation technique is constant, significant
batch to batch variation can be avoided and hence a reproducible biodistribution can be obtained. Similar arguments could
also be applied to new radiopharmaceutioals, for example,
HMPAO, which has recently been introduced for cerebral blood
flow measurements. A structural formula for the technetium complex has been published (9), but again there is evidence that
there is not a unique product. However, studies in many centres

have suggested that this agent may be one of the most successful radiopharmaceuticals of the next decade even without the
knowledge of its precise structure.

Studies on the evaluation of structures of radiopharmaceuticals are nevertheless valuable despite the inherent difficulties they present. They may promote greater efficacy of the
agent if mechanisms can be found to remove components of the
radiopharmaceutical which do not contribute to the usefulness
of the study e.g. technetium phosphonate complexes that do not
accumulate significantly in bone lesions.

4. PHARMACOLOGY

In view of the small quantities of chemicals present in
radiopharmaceuticals, it is uncommon for them to possess any
pharmacological activity. In the case of radiopharmaceuticals
used for therapy, the pharmacological activity is usually due
to radiation emitted rather than the chemical composition. For
example, the chemical quantities of Sodium Iodide(I-131) administered for treatment of thyrotoxicosis or ablation of thyroid
carcinoma (Table 1) are much below the levels at which pharmacological activity of iodide can be expected.

Table 1 - Quantities of Sodium Iodide (I-131) Administered

Specific Activity 220 - 70 MBq / microgram

Treatment	Dose (MBq)	Quantity (micrograms)
Thyrotoxicosis	200	< 1
Ablation	4000	< 20

However, with the development of radiopharmaceuticals which
bind to specific receptors, pharmacological activity may exist.
Similarly pharmacological activity may be encountered with the
development of completely novel chemical entities for which it
may not be possible to predict potential effects. In such ca-

ses, it is necessary to investigate these possibilities, although the difficulty of extrapolating data between different
species would again indicate that human data is the most reliable.

A recent example of such an investigation is the search for
untoward pharmacological events following administration of therapeutic doses of Iodine 131 meta-iodobenzylguanidine (MIBG)
(10). This acts as an analogue of noradrenaline and hence concentrates in adrenergic nerve endings and could produce a hyper-
tensive crisis following intravenous administration by displa-
cing stored noradrenaline. Five patients receiving a total of
14 doses of up to 7.3 GBq containing as much as 7 mg of I-131
MIBG were investigated. The radiopharmaceutical was infused
over a ninety minute period and heart rate, blood pressure and
ECG showed no change during infusion or for 18-24 hours after-
wards. There was also no deterioration in 5 tests of autonomic
nerve function after therapy. In order to obtain this data,
patient co-operation was necessary which again highlights some
of the limitations of animal experiments. This agent has only
been therapeutically used on a limited number of patients thus
far, and even though diagnostic doses of this agent contain
less than 1 mg of MIBG it is prudent to continue monitoring patients carefully during administration in order that information on potential pharmacological actions can be gained.

5. TOXICITY TESTING

It has previously been suggested that there is a strong case
for special regulations to be applied to toxicity testing of
radiopharmaceuticals rather than using requirements for other
drugs (11), since the chemical quantities administered to patients are generally minute and the most likely cause of damage
will be due to the radiation emitted. This is exemplified by
thallium 201, which is administered as thallous chloride for
myocardial studies and localisation of parathyroid adenomas,
even though thallium is known to be an extremely toxic metal.
The radiopharmaceutical can be prepared at a specific activity
of greater than 3.7 GBq per microgram. Thus a dose of 100 MBq

administered to the patient would contain approximately 27 nano-
grams of thallium. When compared with the estimated dietary intake of thallium of 2 micrograms per day (12), it is obvious
that there is unlikely to be problems due to chemical toxicity.
However in an incident where 74 MBq of thallous chloride was
inadvertently injected subcutaneously, the patient developed
skin ulceration two years later which required skin grafting.
The damage was probably due to local radiation damage, estimated to be a maximum of 200 Gy at the injection site.

Acute toxicity tests are important when new chemical entities are being developed. However, classic LD 50 tests are not
applicable since it may be necessary to administer such large
doses of the radiopharmaceutioal that they present a significant radiation hazard to personnel performing the test. Testing the unlabelled material is therefore an alternative approach, but this has limited applications where the biodistribution is altered as a result of labelling, e.g. technetium
labelling of iminodiacetic acid derivatives.

There has been repeated comment on the application of prolonged toxicity testing, since the number of doses of a particular radiopharmaceutical administered to a patient is usually
small. Where repeated administrations do occur they may be
separated by several weeks or months and cumulative toxicity,
other than that due to the radiation, is doubtful. Published
data on the pattern and frequency of radiopharmaceutical administration is sparse and hence a survey was performed of all
patients referred to the Nuclear Medicine Department at Dudley
Road Hospital, Birmingham, during the years 1982 - 1986.

Dudley Road Hospital is a large District General Hospital
possessing three gamma cameras and offering a wide ranging Nuclear Medicine Service comprising approximately 4000 investigations per year. It is felt that the patient referral pattern
is likely to be representative of, though not identical to,
those encountered in many hospitals. Table 2 shows the frequency of administration of a radiopharmaceutical to a particular
patient.

Table 2 - Radiopharmaceutical Administration

Dudley Road Hospital 1982 - 1986

Frequency of Administration	Number of Patients	% of Total Patients
Once	15098	88.5
Twice	1422	8.3
x 3	350	2.1
x 4	104	0.6
More than x4	88	0.5

It can be seen that only 0.5 % of patients receive the same radiopharmaceutical on more than four occasions. Closer examination of the data revealed that the radiopharmaceutical which was most commonly used for repeated administration was technetium labelled medronate for bone imaging (Table 3).

Table 3 - Medronate Administration

Frequency	x1	x2	x3	x4	x5	x6	x7	x8	x9	x12
Number	3058	498	198	69	38	23	4	1	1	1
% of Total	78.6	12.8	5.0	1.7	1.0	0.6	0.1	0.02	0.02	0.02

In this case, less than 2 of patients received in excess of four administrations, the extreme being one patient who received twelve doses of technetium medronate. Analysis of this patient's administration record revealed that the twelve doses had been given over a period of 8.9 years with a minimum gap of 5 months between individual doses. It could therefore be argued that because of the long interval between doses, each could be regarded as a single administration and hence the relevance of prolonged toxicity testing brought into question. The radiation burden to the patient is cumulative and must also be considered. The Effective Dose Equivalent (E.D.E.) of a bone scan has been estimated to be 4mSv. Concurrent with the medronate, this patient had also received three doses of technetium labelled colloid for liver imaging (E.D.E. 1mSv) which further increased the radiation dose. The patient had therefore received 51mSv from radiopharmaceutical administration over a period of 8.9 years. There are currently no recommended limits for the radiation doses which patients can receive but this figure can be placed in context by comparing it with the annual limits of 5mSv for a member of the general public and 50mSv for a radiation worker in the United Kingdom.

6. POST MARKETING SURVEILLANCE

Clinical trials of radiopharmaceuticals necessarily involve small numbers of patients and hence the probability of encountering adverse effects during them is small 13). This makes post marketing surveillance an important aspect of the overall process of demonstrating drug safety and efficacy. It is a standard provision for product licences within the United Kingdom that the licence holder maintains a record of adverse effects of which he is aware occuring with the product. This is an area in which hospitals have an obvious role to play, not only by informing the manufacturer of the radiopharmaceutical, but also by reporting the event to a suitable centre for collation. The number of reported adverse reactions is small, but it has been suggested that not all reactions are reported (1). Reasons for this may be a lack of awareness of the importance of reporting reactions, the minor nature of the reaction or the difficulty in ascribing the reaction to the radiopharmaceutical.

The reporting of all reactions, even if trivial or unlikely to be due to radiopharmaceutical administration is important and every hospital should therefore co-operate in a scheme such as that organized by the European Joint Committee on Radiopharmaceuticals. A greater awareness of the reporting scheme and a willingness to contribute to it will enhance the confidence in the safety of radiopharmaceutical products.

REFERENCES
1. Keeling D.H. & Sampson C.B. Adverse Reactions to Radio-pharmaceuticals. United Kingdom 1977-1983. British Journal of Radiology 1984; 57: 1091-1096.
2. Atkins H.L. Reported Adverse Reactions to Radiopharmaceuticals remain low in 1984. Journal of Nuclear Medicine 1986; 27: 327.
3. Ketchum L.E. Radiopharmaceutical Dosimetry Symposium explores new estimates. Journal of Nuclear Medicine 1986; 27: 163-165.
4. Medicines Act 1968. Guidance Notes on Applications for Product Licences (MAL 2) 1986 HMSO London.
5. Medicines Act 1968. Guidance Notes on Application for Clinical Trials Certificates and Clinical Trial Exemptions 1984 HMSO London.
6. Gerson M.C., Deutsch E.A., Nishiyama H. et al. Myocardial Perfusion Imaging with 99mTc DMPE in Man European Journal of Nuclear Medicine 1983; 8: 371-374.
7. Dige-Petersen H. Evaluation of Clinical Information. In: Safety & Efficacy of Radiopharmaceuticals Ed. Kristensen K. & Nørbygaard E. Martinus Nijhoff, Boston 1984: 191-202.
8. Tanabe S., Zodda J.P., Libson K., Deutsch E. & Heinemann W.R. The Biological distributions of some Technetium - MDP components isolated by Anion Exchange High Performance Liquid Chromotography. Int. J. Appl. Radiat. Isotopes 1983; 34: 1585-1592.
9. Nowotnik D.P., Canning L.R., Cumming S.A. et al. Development of a 99Tcm labelled radiopharmaceutical for cerebral blood Flow imaging. Nuclear Medicine Communications 1985; 6: 499-506.
10. Sisson J.C., Shapiro B., Beierwaltes W.H. et al. Radiopharmaceutical Treatment of Malignant Phaeochromocytoma. Journal of Nuclear Medicine 1984; 25: 197-206.
11. Cox P.H. Preclinical Studies - Radiopharmacology & Toxicology. In: Safety & Efficacy of Radiopharmaceuticals Ed. Kristensen K. & Nørbygaard E. Martinus Nijhoff, Boston 1984: 117-129.
12. Kazantzis G. Thallium In: Handbook of toxicology of metals. Ed. Friberg L., Nordberg G.F. & Vouk V.B. Elsevier Amsterdam 1986; II: 549-567.
13. Juul P. Clinical Trials of Radiopharmaceuticals. In: Safety & Efficacy of Radiopharmaceuticals Ed. Kristensen K. & Nørbygaard E. Martinus Nijhoff, Boston 1984: 179-190.

22. RELATIONSHIP BETWEEN INDUSTRY, HOSPITALS AND <u>AUTHORITIES</u>

TRYGVE BRINGHAMMAR

1. INTRODUCTION

The use of a new radiopharmaceutical formerly often started in a hospital department where radiochemicals after some experimental work were used as radiopharmaceuticals.

Before being used in routine practice the efficacy and safety of the radiopharmaceutical were simply demonstrated by producing an image of an organ and estimation of absorbed dose.

Today when quite new radionuclide generators, substances and "carriers" (e.g. liposomes, autologous blood cells and monoclonal antibodies) are investigated, where the risks for and behavior in the human is little known, the evaluation of the place of a radiopharmaceutical in medical treatment must be based on detailed information about the drug.

To achieve this several countries have set up requirements for radiopharmaceuticals so that they will be as effective and safe as "ordinary" drugs.

2. APPLICATION FOR APPROVAL

Those products intended to be marketed must be approved by the regulatory authorities and a manufacturer has to file applications covering documentation proving that the product will comply with the following aim:

A radioparmaceutical shall be of satisfactory quality and suitable for its purpose. It must not, under normal use, cause adverse effects which are disproportionate to the value of the drug.

Guidelines for such applications should be set up by the authorities giving detailed information about which documentation must be presented. To make it easier for the applicant to file an application it would be of great value if guidelines from different countries could be harmonized.

The documentation should cover:
* Chemical and pharmaceutical documentation
* Toxicological and pharmacological documentation
* Clinical documentation
* Information on absorbed dose

2.1 Chemical and pharmaceutical documentation
The chemical and pharmaceutical documentation submitted must:
- clearly state the product's qualitative and quantitative composition,
- show that the manufacture takes place under conditions such that different batches do not differ from specifications stated,
- prove that the stability of the product meets stated specifications throughout the period of validity. As for semi-manufactured products stability has to be investigated before as well as after radiolabelling.

2.2 Toxicological and pharmacological documentation
The product must be investigated to such an extent that no unexpected effects of toxicologic, mutagenic or carcinogenic nature are likely to occur.

2.3 Clinical documentation
The clinical documentation must give evidence on the products value in medical treatment. Those indications applied for must be confirmed by well planned and performed clinical trials.

2.4 Information on absorbed dose
The estimation of absorbed dose must make it possible to evaluate the risk for unwanted radiation injury.

The requirements set up by different licensing authorities

have been accepted by most manufacturers and in recent years
the quality of the applications has been improved.

3. CLINICAL TRIAL

In principle, the documentation needed for an application
for a clinical trial is the same as for an application for approval. The information may, however, be preliminary and less
detailed.

An application for a clinical trial should include
* Trial protocol
* Documentation
  - chemical and pharmaceutical
  - animal-pharmacological and toxicological
  - human pharmacological or clinical (if there is any)
  - information on absorbed dose
These requirements have been accepted by the manufacturers.

Those who actually use the product for diagnostic or therapeutic purposes do not always follow generally accepted guidelines for the conduct of clinical trials. Deviations from trial protocols, laid down, are not rare and sometimes the physi-
cian uses the drug under trial in routine practice before it is
approved without ending the trial.

It is very important that the authorities and the manufacturers ensure that trials are well-designed and carefully planned.

The number of patients studied is far less important than
the adequacy of the design of the study.

4. WHAT CAN BE DONE?

What can be done to speed up the introduction of new radiopharmaceuticals without disregarding safety and efficacy?

I think the requirements set up have to be carefully discussed and evaluated. Those for "ordinary drugs" are sometimes too
extensive but sometimes not sufficient.

Furthermore I think it would be of great value if people involved in the process of bringing a new product into routine

practice could meet to increase the understanding of the work carried out by the manufacturer, hospital and regulatory agency. The meetings should not only be between the head officers but also between those who do the actual work.

PART 4

SELECTED ASPECTS OF GOOD RADIOPHARMACY PRACTICE

Introduction

Good Radiopharmacy Practice is the basis for all handling of radiopharmaceuticals in hospitals. It is based on general pharmaceutical good manufacturing practice and developments in this area should be transferred.

The emphasis on process validation should in particular be considered. It is an obvious duty for radiopharmacy to have available all information on production, quality control, safety and efficacy of relevant radiopharmaceuticals. It is of particular importance to help encourage clinicians to use the most effective and safe radiopharmaceuticals. Collection of information on adverse reactions and drug defect therefore become indispensible.

In order to be able to fulfil his job the radiopharmacist needs training in many fields allthough he of course cannot have specialist knowledge in all fields that may be necessary. He should, however, be able to identify the problems and to localize this specialist information.

Many radiopharmacies perform centralized preparation and dispensing followed by distribution to a number of nuclear medicine centers. In such cases they must take further responsibility for the quality of the product in comparison with a clinic using preparation kits and generators just in accordance with the manufactors instruction. Stability after distribution, dispensing and transport must be specially considered. A radiopharmacy developing its own formulation of a radiopharmaceutical must in principle be able to document safety and efficacy of this product. A production and quality assurance system based on good practice in the manufacturing of drugs should be established.

23. DESIGN OF A HOSPITAL SYSTEM FOR PRODUCTION OF RADIOPHARMA- CEUTICALS (QUALITY ASSURANCE PROGRAMME FOR A LABELLED BIO- LOGICAL PRODUCT)

C.R. LAZARUS

1. INTRODUCTION

The purpose of Quality Assurance is to ensure that a product is of the quality required for its intended use. This can only be achieved when all the activities involved in producing the product are taken into consideration. These considered activities must then be organised into a programme which enables the aim to be realised.

The design of a hospital quality assurance programme for the production of a radiopharmaceutical involves a description of the aims and problems associated with its production, and includes the raw materials, premises, facilities and equipment, preparation procedures, product controls, documentation, personnel and training.

The importance of a properly designed quality assurance programme cannot be underestimated. The short physical half-life of many radionuclides used in nuclear medicine requires that radiolabelling be performed in the hospital near to the site of use of the product. Few radiopharmaceuticals, compared to the total number used, are delivered from a commercial manufacturer in a form ready for direct administration to a patient. With those products which are ready for use the onus is on the manufacturer to provide a product of the required quality supplied according to his quality assurance programme.

In the case of hospital-produced radiopharmaceuticals, which include many biological products, the onus is on the hospital radiopharmacy to produce an adequate quality assurance programme.

It is advisable for a radiopharmacy to prepare a manual describing the quality assurance programme for the production of radiopharmaceuticals. This chapter will describe some of the important considerations when designing a programme, with the main emphasis on biological products. A programme for these products will be broadly similar for all radiopharmaceuticals prepared in the hospital, but further consideration should be given to raw materials, procedures and facilities, and personnel training, due to extra hazards attending the use and handling of biological materials.

2. AIMS AND PROBLEMS

The primary aims in producing any radiopharmaceutical are that it should be safe to administer to a patient, and be efficacious in supplying the data required, or the therapeutic effect intended. But, the processes leading to this goal should cause the minimum harm to personnel, including the operators engaged in supplying the radiopharmaceutical.

Protection of the patient is achieved when all the product ingredients are handled and processed in such a way that they are protected from microbial contamination from the environment, the operator and other products. Personnel must be protected from radiation hazards, and from biological hazards, such as pathogenic organisms, where these may be involved, eg, in the handling of autologous blood and blood components. The provision of adequate protection requires a careful consideration of all the risk involved and a course of action chosen to minimise the risks, or eliminate them as far as possible, to patients and personnel.

3. QUALITY ASSURANCE PROGRAMME

The writing of a programme is left to individual institutions, but the following factors should be included.

3.1 Raw materials

An increasing use of radionuclides with short physical

half-lives for radiolabelling biological products and other materials is now established, eg, Tc-99m (6 hours); I-123 (13.3 hours; In-113m (100 minutes); In-111 (67.4 hours). Other radionuclides with longer half-lives are, however, widely used, eg, Cr-51 (27.7 days); I-131 (8.04 days). The short physical half-life of some radionuclides often means that a full testing of a commercially obtained radionuclide is not possible before administration to a patient. Radionuclides should be purchased from a named and reputable supplier, whose record for providing material of the required quality is well-established. This may require a knowledge of his methods of radionuclide production, controls and tests used. A visit to the manufacturing facility, and observation of procedures, tests and documentation is advised. Radionuclides from generators should undergo the usual tests for radionuclidic purity, concentration, chemical purity, pH, sterility, freedom from particles and pyrogens.

Non-radioactive ingredients to be used in labelling by open procedures should be carefully considered for quality. These and cold kits should only be purchased from reputable manufacturers, and their quality demonstrated to be suitable, before their use in patients. With kits and preparations of human serum albumin, the albumin must be shown to be non-reactive when tested for hepatitis B antigen (HB_SAg). Chemicals of the highest grade, eg, "Analar", should be used to avoid the possibility of radiolabelling impurities present in the chemical.

The radiolabelling of monoclonal antibodies is now extremely popular. Very few are available commercially in a form suitable for radiolabelling for imaging or therapy.

Many institutions raise their own antibodies for a particular imaging or therapy purpose, but the production of these antibodies should only be undertaken by specialists in an appropriate department with suitable facilities and equipment. The person intending to use the antibody clinically must first, however, satisfy himself of several factors. The total process of antibody production must be documented and made available to the user, eg, the history of the production and characterisation of the hybridoma cell line, including such factors as the source of the parent myeloma line, fusion and efficiency of cloning procedures. Details of animals used including species, age, breeding conditions, etc, should be available. The possibility of viral contamination should be considered together with methods of purification of the antibody. The stability of the final product should be established, as well as sterility and freedom from pyrogens. A description of the appearance and other physical properties should be available. The control requirements for antibodies and conjugates has been considered by a working party of a joint committee of the Cancer Research Campaign of the National Institute for Biological Standards and Control (1).

Autologous blood components such as red cells, white cells and platelets are commonly labelled in many nuclear medicine centres. A definite possibility exists that a patient's blood is contaminated with bacteria or viruses, eg, hepatitis (HB_SAg). The presence of this type of contamination should, hopefully, be established before the radiolabelling process is considered. A decision whether to proceed with the process can then be taken. However, the operator must be protected from hazards associated with unscreened blood samples, or those which have slipped through any screening process. These hazards can occur with patients in renal units, those suffering from infective liver disease, defective or altered immunological competence, and drug addicts.

Measures to counter these hazards and protect operators should be agreed upon, and carefully described in the quality assurance programme. A quality assurance programme should be devised describing procedures for the ordering, receipt, storage and release of raw materials and blood samples. Detailed considerations for raw materials are given in various national Guides to Good Pharmaceutical Manufacturing Practices (2), and can be adapted for the preparation of radiopharmaceuticals.

3.2 Premises, facilities and equipment

An essential function of any quality assurance programme is

to describe the premises, facilities and equipment necessary for the preparation of a radiopharmaceutical. Recommendations for facilities have been discussed on many occasions, and are now well established (3-7). Additional guidance can be obtained from the GMP (2).

To minimise the possibility of product contamination, and radiation hazards to the operator, the use of closed procedures for radiolabelling should be adopted whenever possible. Whereas it is possible to radiolabel many biological products by closed procedure methods (and these should be encouraged) many are processed using open procedures. The problems associated with open procedures include the possibility of ingress of microorganisms into the preparation threatening its sterility, and the increased risk of release of radioactivity by spillage, aerosol formation, and loss of volatile radionuclides such as radioiodine. The handling of blood by open procedures is associated with the possible release of any microorganisms present in the blood sample.

Centrifugation is a procedure often used in separating blood components prior to their radiolabelling. Aerosols of blood can be formed during this process. Sealed centrifuge buckets, or the use of a windshield, should be used to prevent the spread of these aerosols.

Open procedures often require a sterilisation procedure, which introduces additional hazards involved in filtering or autoclaving radioactive materials. Monoclonal antibodies are often passed through a chromatography column to separate and remove unbound radioactivity. These examples of procedures involving handling radioactive materials by open procedures will introduce increased risks to the product and personnel.

Any departmental programme devised for the preparation of the above types of radiopharmaceutical must recognise the risks involved, and describe steps to cater for them.

In general the requirements necessary to achieve hygienic conditions and radiation protection in radiopharmacies are similar, eg, finishes of walls, surfaces etc. Radiopharmaceuti-

cals which are not terminally heat sterilised, and this includes biological products, can be prepared by aseptic techniques
in a unidirectional downdraught workstation situated within a
Controlled Area (BS 5295, Part 1) (8). The workstation must,
however, provide a BS 5295 Class I environment, and the controlled area must be finished to the required radiation standard.

Biological products using open procedures should be radiolabelled in a unidirectional downdraught workstation in a room
supplied with filtered air (BS 5295. Class I). When radiolabelling blood components a suitable separate area, preferably a
separate room, is advised (7). BS 5295 Class I air should be
provided in the work area, but in addition the workstation
should conform with the requirements of a Class II or Class III
microbiological safety cabinet, BS 5726, 1979 (9). Class II
cabinets provide a greater degree of protection to the operator
than other downdraught workstations, as well as protection to
the product, and are suitable for the handling and labelling of
blood components. Radioiodination procedures involve the additional hazard of volatile radioactive iodine. The recirculating type of cabinets are not suitable, but a cabinet with a
total exhaust facility may be used.

However, a Class III (BS 5726) cabinet, which is a totally
enclosed exhaust protective cabinet providing a gas-tight containment area, and fitted with glove ports, may be used. Air is
filtered to BS 5295 Class I before passing through the area,
and the exhausted air is passed through a HEPA filter, or exhausted remotely from the cabinet outside the building. Advice
on the use, maintenance and disinfection of these safety cabinets is available (10).

A range of high integrity containment cabinets is now becoming commercially available. These are designed to protect
the operator from the product, and to protect the product from
the operator and environment. They are designed on the glove
box principle, and offer a BS 5295 Class I environment or better. The cabinets can be modified by the manufacturer for their

intended purpose, eg, generator storage and elution, radioiodination, blood labelling with an integral centrifuge, and
other radiolabelling procedures. Lead protection can be built
into the design of the cabinet.

Quality assurance programmes must define the facilities and
equipment to be used for a particular radiolabelling purpose.
The maintenance, proper use of equipment, disinfection procedures, in addition to the laboratory clothing, cleanliness and
hygiene, must all be described in the programme.

3.3 Procedures

Procedures for radiolabelling materials should be described
in order to ensure that the product is of the required quality
for its intended purpose. With the added difficulties and hazards associated with the radiolabelling of biological materials, procedures must be well-defined to cope with the risks.
It is good radiochemical practice to run through labelling procedures "cold", ie, without the radionuclide, in order to anti-
cipate and solve problems prior to the introduction of the additional radiation hazard.

It is important that all procedures have been demonstrated to
produce the product of the required safety, but with an acceptable hazard to the operator. The latter may require monitoring
tests of the operator, eg, measurement of radioactivity in the
thyroid gland if radioiodinations are performed. Any significant changes in procedure, equipment or materials should be
validated before being brought into routine use.

A quality assurance programme should also include steps to
be taken if an untoward event occurs, eg, the procedures to be
adopted in case of a spillage or accidental puncture of the
skin with a needle during a blood labelling procedure.

A master formula describing all starting materials, procedures, labels, containers and processing controls and records
should be prepared, and form a major part of the quality assurance programme.

3.4 Documentation

Satisfactory documentation is a vital and indispensable part of a quality assurance programme. Its purpose is to define the system of control, to reduce the risk of error which verbal communication can introduce, to instruct personnel, and to trace defective products back through their various processing stages.

Documentation should be updated, clear, precise and contain all necessary, but no superfluous data. Amendments as a result of error, review or revision should be authorised, and alterations should be clear and signed.

3.4.1 <u>Specifications</u>. Specifications should include raw materials, packaging and the finished product. The specification should accurately describe the material so that there can be no ambiguity, enabling the same material to be purchased on each occasion. The name, identification code, supplier, physcial form and appearance, tests and limits for purity and identity, concentration, storage conditions and expiry date, and any necessary safety precautions, are some of the inclusions of a specification for raw materials and packaging.

For each radiolabelled product the following should be specified; name and batch number; description of physical appearance; control test methods; limits for identity, purity and assay; storage conditions and expiry; and any safety requirements to be observed.

3.4.2 <u>Master formula and method</u>. The master formula should describe all the starting materials, procedures, labels, containers, processing controls and storage conditions for each product and batch size.

3.4.3 <u>Batch manufacturing records</u>. A batch manufacturing record should show all the details associated with the preparation procedure, and include; batch numbers of raw materials; names and radioactive concentration of radio-nuclides and other materials; details of ingredients; results of yield measurements; the final yield and number of containers; in-process test results, and date and signature of operator and person authorising release of product if appropriate.

3.4.4 <u>Raw materials record</u>. Records should be made of all radioactive and non-radioactive starting materials. The record should describe the material received, its batch number, and the signed release by quality control where appropriate.

3.4.5 <u>Other documents</u>. These may include cleaning and maintenance of facilities and equipment; procedures and records of monitoring for particulate, microbial and radiochemical contamination; training of personnel: waste disposal; instructions for use of specialised equipment: records of instrument calibration; instructions for decontamination procedures; and records of servicing of equipment.

3.5 <u>Analytical testing</u>

An accepted problem with the supply of radiopharmaceuticals is the difficulty in completing tests on finished products before administration to patients. However, testing of quality for a product is an integral part of its supply, and full testing is important, even if it is retrospective, as it provides a check on the adequacy of facilities, procedures and materials. A quality assurance programme should be written for each radiopharmaceutical, and include a description of the tests to be performed on the final product, and those tests during the processing of the product. The latter are particularly important where certain final tests may prove difficult before administration of the final product to the patient.

Analytical testing should also be performed, where appropriate, on raw materials, containers and packaging.

3.5.1 <u>Sampling</u>. A batch size of a radiopharmaceutical is usually one vial, and normal pharmaceutical principles of sampling cannot be applied. When preparing a radiopharmaceutical, including a biological product, it is advisable to produce a sufficient surplus quantity of the product to provide the patient dose and material for the necessary testing.

3.5.2 <u>Frequency of testing</u>. It is probably sufficient with some radiopharmaceuticals, eg, those produced from commercial kits, to test a sample of a manufacturers lot, and not to test each

vial made from that lot. The frequency of testing of other products depends upon factors such as the source of the materials,
and the confidence in the quality of a manufacturer's products,
materials and processes. Radiopharmaceuticals prepared from raw
materials should be thoroughly and adequately tested, on each
occasion that a dose is prepared. The frequency of testing
should be stated in the quality assurance programme.

3.5.3 <u>Analytical tests</u>. Certain tests such as radionuclidic
identity, radioactive concentration, appearance, and freedom
from gross particulate contamination are simple to perform, and
can be tested on each product prior to patient administration.

Radionuclidic purity should be checked regularly, eg, generator eluates. Similarly particle size of particulate preparations should be regularly measured. Radiochemical purity tests
need only be checked regularly in the majority of cases, eg,
those produced from commercial kits.

However, the efficiency of labelling of biological products, especially blood components and monoclonal antibodies,
should be checked with each preparation, and prior to patient
administration. The variability in quality of the raw material,
ie, the patient's blood, can interfere with radiolabelling.
This can be due to the nature of the cells themselves, the patients physiology or medication. It is convenient and useful to
include a test for labelling efficiency in the radiolabelling
procedure, and then to perform a radiochemical purity check on
the finished product. When radiolabelling antibodies an in-
process control is possible by measuring the radioactivity in
the fractions as they are eluted from the chromatography column
used to purify the radiolabelled mixture. A final test for unbound radioactivity should also be performed prior to patient
administration.

Whilst a precise pH for most radiopharmaceuticals is not
crucial, it does become important for some, eg, the radiolabelling of monoclonal antibodies with In-111. However, even in
these cases, it is usually sufficient to use wide-range or mul-
ti-indicator pH strip papers, for both in-process and finished

product testing. Many biological products, eg, platelets are very sensitive to the procedures used in radiolabelling, and can suffer mechanical, chemical or radiation damage. The behaviour of the cells, both in vitro and in vivo may vary before and after radiolabelling. An alteration in the biodistribution of such a radiolabelled preparation may render it unsuitable for its intended purpose, and even undesirable in that an unintended radiation dose may be given to those body organs in which the final product localises. It is essential, therefore, with biological products, that tests of function before and after radiolabelling be performed and the results compared, before patient administration. Such tests include the ability of radiolabelled platelets to aggregate; white cells to maintain their function: and monoclonal antibodies to retain their activity.

Tests for sterility and freedom from pyrogens cannot be performed by official methods prior to patient administration. However, testing is still important, not so much as a control of the final product, but more as a control on facilities, equipment, procedures and technique.

3.6 Personnel and testing

There should be sufficient personnel qualified with the ability, training and experience appropriate to their tasks. The duties, responsibilities and training for each member of radiopharmacy personnel should be clearly described in writing in the quality assurance programme, and clearly explained to the member of staff.

Training for radiopharmacy staff should include the principles of good manufacturing practice (2) and good radiopharmacy practice (12), as well as theoretical and practical experience in the techniques they will use, eg, microbiology, chemistry and radiochemistry, radiation protection and radiopharmacy. Training should be to a level appropriate to the tasks to be performed, and the ability to perform to the required standard should be tested and reviewed at regular periods.

It is particularly important with biological products that

the associated hazards are made known to personnel. The need to protect the product from the environment and the operator, and the potential hazard of contaminated blood and its containment to protect the operator, should be very clearly explained. The causes of loss of viability and function of white cells, red cells and platelets during radiolabelling should be explained, and the techniques developed to prevent this should be described and demonstrated.

Training programmes should be reviewed regularly, and any special requirements, such as those associated with biological products, should be carefully considered, and written into the training schedule of the quality assurance programme.

3.7 Waste disposal

The disposal of radioactive waste should be in accordance with national regulations and national Codes of Practice. Radiolabelled biological waste presents additional hazards, other than those due to the radioactivity. Blood products and other biological waste materials should not be brought back into the radiopharmacy, where they can form substrates for microbiological growth. Procedures for the handling, storage and disposal of waste should be agreed upon and included in the quality assurance programme for the various products.

Products labelled with short-lived radionuclides can be stored for a few days, and then disposed of as inactive waste, providing there are no other hazards. With longer half-lives it may be necessary to store for longer periods. It is advisable, however, to dispose of biological waste materials as soon as possible after use. Usually small quantities of radioactivity are involved, and immediate disposal may be allowed within the regulations.

Special care must be exercised with radiolabelled cells which may carry an infective microorganism. In this case it is best to store the waste material in a secure container until radioactivity has decayed to the required level, and then it should be autoclaved prior to incineration. National guidance for the disposal of infected waste should be followed (10).

3.8 Standards for labelled products

Standards for some radiopharmaceuticals are available in pharmacopoeias, although generally there is a lack of official guidance, particularly for radiolabelled biological products. This is due in part to the variability of the raw materials used as biological products, and to the continous introduction into nuclear medicine of new agents. The onus for setting a standard, where one is not officially available, must fall on the institution preparing the product. With radiolabelled biological materials, the crucial test must be that the material is of a quality suitable for its purpose.

In which case the standard must be agreed upon between the user of the product as well as those formulating and preparing the product. It is possible that a variation in the standard of a product can be tolerated depending on its use. Thus a lower level of unbound Tc-99m pertechnetate in a labelled red cell preparation may be required when looking for the site of a gastrointestinal bleed, than when performing a cardiac blood pool study.

Standards should be decided upon and written into the quality assurance programme.

3.9 Environmental monitoring

A quality assurance programme should describe procedures and equipment for monitoring the environment for microbial and radiation contamination. Recognised methods using settle plates in the radiopharmacy and workstations should be performed at prescribed and regular intervals. Air sampling in rooms and workstations using centrifugal or slit samplers, and air velocity measurements in workstations should be carried out at prescribed intervals. Air particle counts in rooms and workstations need not be performed so frequently.

Microbiological safety cabinets should be serviced regularly to check their conformation with BS 5726. However, before testing, and especially if filters are to be changed, contamination of the cabinet and filters with radioactivity should be checked.

Similarly steps should be taken to ensure the protection of maintenance and service personnel if it is suspected that cabinets and filters are contaminated following radiolabelling of infected blood.

Radiation monitoring of rooms, facilities and equipment should also be performed at predefined intervals according to methods described in national codes of practice (11). Monitoring should include wipe tests of benches and surfaces, levels of external radiation, and air radioactivity concentration where necessary.

Suitable records of the equipment used and results obtained should be maintained.

3.10 Radiation safety

Procedures for the preparation and supply of all radiopharmaceuticals should be designed so as to cause the minimum radiation exposure to personnel including patients and operators. Many radiolabelled biological products have long effective half-lives in the body, especially those labelled with I-131. Effective quality assurance programmes should ensure that the preparation and control of radiopharmaceuticals, including biological products, do not deliever an unnecessarily high radiation burden to patients. Radiation from internal and external sources should be kept well below permissible levels.

A major radiological problem in radiolabelling biological products is the use of iodine radioisotopes. The volatile nature of iodine makes it a potential airborne contamination risk. Work with volatile and gaseous radioisotopes should be carried out in well-ventilated areas, in non-recirculating workstations. The totally enclosed glove box cabinets, flushed with filtered air which is exhausted externally from the building, or trapped in a remote filter, are the most suitable. Monitoring of internal contamination of operators is important when handling iodine radioisotopes, particularly if open procedures are used. Thyroid gland uptake of radioactivity, and measurements in urine, should be assessed at frequent intervals, if this type of work is done regularly. Procedures for dealing with accidents should be clear and visually displayed in a prominent place.

4. <u>CONCLUSION</u>

An effective quality assurance programme for the production of radiopharmaceuticals, including radiolabelled biological products, involves many considerations. The most important of these have been raised in this chapter. Radiopharmacies must prepare their own programme, bearing the above points in mind, to suit their own practices, facilities and staff.

REFERENCES

1. Begent RHJ et al: Operation Manual for Control of Production, Preclinical Toxicology and Phase I Trials of Antitumour Antibodies and Drug Antibody Conjugates. Br J Cancer 1986; 54: 557-568.
2. Guide to Good Pharmaceutical Manufacturing Practice. Department of Health and Social Security, HMSO, London, 1983.
3. Bell N: Design Criteria in Relation to Protection of the Patient. In: Safety and Efficacy of Radiopharmaceuticals, Kristensen K, Nørbygaard E. Martinus Nijhoff Publishers, The Hague, 1984: 311-325.
4. Ennow K: Design Criteria in Relation to Protection of the Personnel and the Environment. In: Safety and Efficacy of Radiopharmaceuticals, Kristensen K, Nørbygaard E (eds). Martinus Nijhoff Publishers, The Hague, 1984: 326-332.
5. Lazarus C: Present status for the Design of Laboratory Facilities. In: Safety and Efficacy of radiopharmaceuticals, Kristensen. K, Nørbygaard E (eds). Martinus Nijhoff Publishers, The Hague, 1984: 333-348.
6. Facilities for the Hospital Preparation of Radiopharmaceuticals. Nucl Med Commun 1980; 1: 54-57.
7. Guidance Notes for Hospitals. Premises and Environment for the Preparation of Radiopharmaceuticals. Department of Health and Social Security, London, 1982.
8. British Standards Institution, Environmental Cleanliness in Enclosed Spaces, Part 1. Specification for Controlled Environment Clean Rooms, Workstations and Clean Air Devices, BS5295, Part 1, 1976.
9. British Standards Institution, 1979. Specifications for Microbiological Safety Cabinets. BS 5726, 1979.
10. Code of Practice for the Prevention of Infection in Clinical Laboratories and Post-mortem Rooms. Department of Health and Social Security, HMSO, London, 1978.
11. Approved Code of Practice. The Protection of Persons Against Ionising Radiation Arising from any Work Activity. HMSO, London, 1985.

12. Kristensen K: Preparation and Control of Radiopharmaceuticals in Hospitals. Technical Report Series No 194, IAEA, Vienna, 1979.

24. NEW DEVELOPMENTS: LABORATORY FACILITIES/PRODUCT QUALITY.

KNUD KRISTENSEN

1. INTRODUCTION

The quality of a radiopharmaceutical may be seriously influenced by the production environment. In order to prepare a product of a suitable quality, production must take places in a system based on a number barriers to separate the product and the environment from interchange. In the case of radiopharmaceutical these barriers have a double function of protecting the product as well as the staff and the environment. The questions to be answered are what kind of barriers are needed for different types of products, are they effective and are they cost-effective. Or in other words what is the minimum that will be sufficient. The parameters most influenced by environmental conditions will of course be the purity of the product but also the identity may be influenced by the risk of mix-up of different products in too narrow facilities. Bell, Ennow and Lazarus (1,2.3) described in 1983 comprehensively the situation at that time. This paper intend to review the developments since then.

2. GENERAL DEVELOPMENTS

The methods we have available to test the quality of product have their limitations. For economic reasons it would be impossible to fully test all products. Inspection control and simple tests at hospitals on receipt of radiopharmaceuticals forms along with the clinical experience on biodistribution, the basis for a drug defect registration (4). This methods does not, however, give us much information on the effect of the handling at the hospital. For specific tests it should be mentioned that sterility test has its statistical limitation in relation to the standards of "not more than one unsterile unit per 1 million units produced" (1). Validation of procedures therefore seems to be the most effective method to get an impression of the quality level obtainable for products produced in a given system. But also this method is of limited value if one wishes to establish any quantitative relationship between laboratory facilities and product quality. Member states of the Pharmaceutical Inspection convention (PIC) met in Oslo in 1985 to discuss Premises for Pharmaceutical Manufacture (5). There is not much to be found on the problem discussed here. Emphasis were placed on trends from fully air-controlled rooms to smaller enclosures and the importance of validation. The human factor was given a central position illustrated by the following statement by Falck (6): "planners should be equally concerned with the psychological and physical design when planning premises for pharmaceutical manufacture". Training programmes were also given great attention. There were now change in room classification. The highest standard required corresponds to class 100 in the US Standard. The proposed revised US Federal Standard (7) will introduce class 1 and 10. This is mainly inspired by the electronics industry and they are necessary for the radiopharmaceutical area.

3. THE DEVELOPMENT IN THE RADIOPHARMACEUTICAL AREA

3.1 Industry

The radiopharmaceutical industry has in recent years made quite large investments in new facilities. There are no publications on the design of such facilities, but from personal experience it is obvious that the standards of facilities for radiopharmaceutical production has been improved considerably at many producers during recent years.

3.2 Hospitals

Also a number of hospitals, particularly in United Kingdom, have invested in new facilities, probably very much influenced by the Notes for guidance from the DHSS in 1982(8). Aberdeen

(9) is one good example where a complete suite with separate rooms for different types of work has been built. Another approach is the use of sealed enclosures where one can lower the requirement to the air of the room (10). An assesment was made by a committee of the UK Radiopharmaceutical officers. One of the question discussed was the risk of leaks in gloves. Gloves considered the weakest part of the system. It was concluded that although a situation with leaks in the system could not be excluded it seems likely that this probability does not exceed the likelihood of "its occurence in a conventional clean-room installation where the difficulties of maintaining a Class I condition in the manned state are well known. "These units are well designed and provide an environment of high quality for pharmaceutical manipulations with excellent operator protection.

4. CONCLUSIONS

It was not possible by reviewing the literature to find new data on the quantitative relationship between product quality and laboratory facilities used for the preparation. So we are still left with the question: How much investment in such facilities is needed. We are in urgent need for research in this area. We need model studies but also full scale validation studies in the newer facilities will help further developments and may establish quantitative data.

REFERENCES
1. Bell N. Design Criteria in Relation to Protection of the Product in Kristensen K. Nørbygaard E. (eds) Safety & Efficacy of Radiopharmaceuticals Nijhoff, The Hague 1984: 311-325.
2. Ennow K R. Design Criteria in Relation to Protection of the Personel and the Environment in Kristensen K. Nørbygaard E. (eds) Safety & Efficacy of Radiopharmaceuticals Nijhoff, The Hague 1984: 326-332.
3. Lazarus Cr. Present Status of Recommendations for the Design of Laboratory Facilities in Kristensen K. Nørbygaard E. (eds) Safety & Efficacy of Radiopharmaceuticals Nijhoff, The Hague 1984: 333-348.
4. European Society of Nuclear Medicine Newsletter 8. Eur J Nucl Med 1984; 9: 388-389.

338

5.   Premises for Pharmaceutical Manufacture. EFTA secretariate Geneva 1985.
6.   Falck LP. Premises and the Human being in Kristensen K. Nørbygaard E. (eds) Safety & Efficacy of Radiopharmaceuticals Nijhoff, The Hague 1984: 209-216.
7.   King GJ, Mc Donongh J. Airbone Particulate Cleaness Classes for Clean Room and Clean Zones. Nord Tidskrift för Renlighets-Teknik 1986; 15: 20-24.
8.   Guidance Notes for Hospitals. Premises and Environment for the Preparation of Radiopharmaceuticals. Department of Health and Social Security, London. 1982.
9.   Tan KKC, Doherty J, Lyall D, Will IG. New Aberdeen radiopharmacy. The Pharmaceutical Journal 1986; Dec 13: 786-787.
10. Mather SJ (chairman) Working party report. An assesment of the "Amercare" Containment System. London May 1986.

25. PROCESS VALIDATION

E. BACHMANN

1. INTRODUCTION

Process validation is a requirement of the Current Good Manufacturing Practices Regulations for Finished Pharmaceuticals (United States) 21 CFR Parts 210 and 211, and of the Good Manufacturing Practice Regulations for Medical Devices, 21 CFR Part 820.

Assurance of product quality is derived from careful attention to a number of factors including selection of quality parts and materials, adequate product and process design, control of the process, and in-process and end product testing. Due to the complexity of today's medical products, routine end product testing alone usually is not sufficient to assure product quality for several reasons. Many end product tests have limited sensitivity. In some cases destructive testing would be required to show the manufacturing process was adequate and in other situations end product testing does not reveal all variations that may occur in the product that may impact on safety and effectiveness.

The basic principles of quality assurance have as their goal the production of articles that are fit for their intended use. These principles may be stated as follows:

a. quality, safety, and effectiveness must be designed and built into the product;

b. quality cannot be inspected or tested into the finished product;

c. each step of the manufacturing process must be controlled to maximize the probability that the finished product meets all quality and design specifications.

Process validation is a key element in assuring that these quality assurance goals are met. It is through careful design and validation of both the process and controls that a manufacturer can assure that there is a very high probability that all manufactured units from successive lots will be acceptable. Successfully validating a process reduces the dependence upon intensive inprocess and finished product testing. Process validation also lowers costs by reducing the proportion of defective finished products which must be scrapped or reworked.

The FDA offers the following as one definition of process validation:

> Process validation is a documented program which provides a high degree of assurance that a specific process will consistently produce a product meeting its pre-determined specifications and quality attributes (1).

2. GOOD MANUFACTURING PRACTICE AND VALIDATION

Good Validation practice forms an important part within the frame of the Good Manufacturing Practice regulations (FIP-GUIDE (2)) and is an essential element in ensuring evidence that, provided the production instructions are carried out and the prescribed operation conditions are followed, then the manufacturing process employed in the production of a pharmaceutical product can be relied upon to yield the specified end-product.

Validation of the manufacturing steps performed, the facilities employed and the equipment used is not new in principle. Data are available in each and every production unit. What is new, however, is the need for the systematic correlation and documentation of the designated essential operations.

Every pharmaceutical product and each group of products has its own special problems and is subject to its own particular difficulties in areas of development, manufacture and control.

No universally applicable procedure can be drawn up for Good Validation Practice. However, the crucial points to which attention must be paid in validation should be established, especially with respect to determining the critical manufacturing steps for which significant deviations from the operating directions may not be immediately evident from control checks of the end-products.

Good Validation Practice in the sense of these guidelines means establishing that every essential operation in the development and manufacture including the control of pharmaceutical products, is reliable and reproducible; and when following stipulated production instructions and control procedures is capable of providing the desired product quality (2).

3. THE IMPORTANCE OF VALIDATION

A reduction in batch rejections, reworks, and re-samples is a likely outcome for validated processes due to the establishment of proper process controls. This has been the case within numerous firms. Sterility retesting has been nearly eliminated over the last several years, partially as a result of sterilization validation.

A reduction in utility costs is frequently possible as a result of optimized processes using appropriate, not arbitrary, controls. Steam sterilizer validations studies have reduced cycle time by two-thirds, while still maintaining an overkill cycle.

Increased throughput often results from proper process validation which reduces unnescessary process time usually incorporated into un-validated systems as a safety factor. Reduction of processtime may also result in the avoidance of major capital expenditures when operating near full capacity. The need for a new steam sterilizer was avoided by reducing the cycle time on the existing unit.

The improved product quality attributed to process validation has resulted in fewer complaints about process related failures. The reduction in complaints is due to improved uniformity of the product made by a validated process.

The additional process knowledge gained from validation can result in reduced testing requirements at the inprocess and finished goods stages. This is a direct consequence of the reduced variation in process performance and the greater confidence afforded by the validation process. Employees develop a greater awareness of processes and the need for adherence to procedures through the attention given to process controls brought about by validation. Process managers and supervisors, quality control personell and production operators have all evidenced a greater awareness of the need for training, the requirements for accuracy in records, and adherence to procedures, as a consequence of validation efforts conducted in their areas.

Validation is good business practice. It is no longer a mere regulatory requirement, but a mechanism for better process control. The pressures to increase profitability, without compromise to product quality require enhanced methods for product preparation. This can be achieved today through the employment of a sound validation program (6).

4. VALIDATION IN PHARMACEUTICAL PRACTICE

4.1. What is validation

Validation is by no means an entirely new concept, but one which has long been inherent in any serious scientific or technological exercise. If validation is kept within bounds a useful purpose is served in focusing attention on the need to maintain a questioning attitude to the processes of manufacture and a penetrating, systematic approach to their evaluation (3).

To prove that a process works is, in a nutshell, what we mean by the verb "to validate" (4).

At an American Society of Quality Control (ASQC) conference on process validation it was recommended that manufacturers take a common sense approach to process validation and make sure that relevant practices are documented as such.

It was emphasized that process validation should be nothing much more than organized common sense - something many firms have been doing for years, with the probable exception that we have not been documenting it to the extent that we should (5).

4.2. Which process should be validated

It is generally accepted that processes requiring validation are, primarily, new processes, those used in steril manufacture and "problem" processes, for example, those expected to result in problems of content uniformity.

In the PIC guidelines (13) is written that "Critical steps during manufacture shall be validated". This does not refer only to the manufacture of sterile products.

4.3. How

It is impossible to give hard and fast rules on how to validate since the manufacture of pharmaceuticals involves such big variety of processes.

Some guidelines are established concerning objectives i.e. that one should aim to develop the best possible method of manufacture for a given product and that this should be documented.

Practical help can be obtained from e.g. FDA's guide.

A great deal of literature exists, especially in the area of sterile production. A few examples are given on the list of references (7-14).

4.4. When

When any new master formula and method is adopted, steps should be taken to demonstrate that it is suitable for routine production and that the defined process, using the materials and equipment specified, will consistently yield a product of the required quality.

Significant changes in processing methods, equipment or materials should be accompanied by further validation steps to ensure that the changed conditions continue to yield consistently a product of the required quality.

From time to time processes and procedures should undergo critical appraisal to ensure that they remain capable of achieving the intended results.

Validation studies should be conducted in accordance with previously defined procedures and a record made of the results. The extent and degree of the work will depend on the nature and complexity of the product and process (9).

4.5. Who

The manufacturer of pharmaceutical products is responsible

for validation with respect to Development, Production and Quality Control Activities. This responsibility comprises kind ranges, organisation and control of validation. The governmental regulation should be limited to fixing the manufacturer's responsibility for validation in the interest of drug safety. On this basis, it is the governmental inspector's task to verify whether the manufacturer carries out a validation and whether the methods chosen are appropriate and in keeping with the present state of science and technical knowledge (2).

REFERENCES

1. Guideline on general principles of process validation, march 1984 (FDA, USA).
2. "FIP-guidelines". Die Pharmaceutische Industrie 1980; 42 Nr. 10.
3. Sharp J.R. The Pharm Journal, Jan. 11, 1986.

4. Fry, E. Process validation policy" paper presented at Swedish Academy of Pharmaceutical Sciences seminar, April 11 to 13, 1984.
5. The Gold sheet, Jan. 86.
6. Agalloco, J.P. Journal of Parenteral Science and Technology 1986; 48: No. 6 nov/dec. 1986.
7. Loftus and Nash (eds), "Pharmaceutical process validation", New York: Dekker, 1984.
8. Fry, Ed., "Validation theory and concepts", in collected papers of seminar on Validation, Dublin, June 14-17, 1982, Pharmaceutical Inspection Convention. Geneva: European Free Trade Association, 1982.
9. Guide to Good Pharmaceutical Manufacturing Practice, 3rd edition, Department of Health, London: HM Stationary Office, 1983.
10. "Validation of steam sterilisation cycles", PDA Technical Monograph No. 1. Philidelphia, Pa: Parenteral Drug Association, 1978.
11. "Validation of aseptic filling for solution drug products", PDA Technical Monograph No 2, Philidelphia, Pa: Parenteral Drug Association, 1980.
12. "Validation of dry heat processes used for sterilisation and depyrogenisation". PDA Technical Report No 3, Philadelphia, Pa: Parenteral Drug Association, 1981.
13. "Validation". PIC seminar june 1982, EFTA secretariat, Geneva, 1982.
14. Sucker, M. Praxis der Valiedierung. APV seminar. Wissenschaftliche Verlagsgeselschaft GmbH, Stuttgart, 1982.

26. THE RADIOPHARMACY AS AN INFORMATION CENTRE

C.B. SAMPSON

1. INTRODUCTION

During the past decade the need for information on therapeutic pharmaceuticals has been evidenced by the rapid growth of drug information centres both locally and nationally. It is generally accepted that the provision of drug information services to the medical profession has improved the quality of patient care (1-3). Similarly in the field of nuclear medicine; as the variety and complexity of diagnostic procedures has increased over the years so has the need for information on radiopharmacy and radiopharmaceuticals become more apparent.

Traditional drug information centres are poorly equipped to deal with the information requirements of the nuclear medicine community and in many areas the local or regional radiopharmacy has assumed the role of the "radiopharmacy information centre". The functions of a radiopharmacy information centre can be conveniently categorised under the following headings:

The provision of information to nuclear medicine personnel both locally and nationally on:-

    adverse reactions and unusual biodistributions;

    specific pharmaceutical or pharmacokinetic properties of the radiopharmaceutical;

    formulation, preparation, stability and quality assurance;

    regulatory requirements associated with the use of the radiopharmaceutical;

    information on paediatric dosage;

    new techniques in radiopharmacy;

Monitoring of product literature
Monitoring of defects in the product or packaging
Data collection

The above list contains classes of information which could
and should be handled by most radiopharmacy information centres. However certain classes of information may be directed to
the radiopharmacy information centre but are sometimes handled
more appropriately by other departments such as medical physics. These include information on internal radiation dosimetry
and possible causes of technical artefacts, and will not be
discussed further. Consideration will be given to each of the
above groups and if important clinically, specific examples of
information will be discussed. It is emphasised however that in
a brief review of this nature it is only possible to give a
general overview. Fuller details may be obtained from the references listed in the bibliography.

2. PROVISION OF INFORMATION TO NUCLEAR MEDICINE PERSONNEL

2.1 Adverse reactions and unusual biodistributions

The importance of the radiopharmacy information centre in
dealing with adverse reactions is well illustrated by its role
in the monitoring of the changing pattern of adverse reactions
as new products become available and less effective products
become obsolete. For example, the original United Kingdom
survey on adverse reactions (4) showed that out of a total of
77 reports 58% were associated with the use of iron hydroxide
particulates for lung scanning. A later survey however (5)
which was for 1977 to mid 1986, showed that most adverse
reactions are now due to diphosphonates and colloids and
together total 54% out of a total of 102 reactions.

Observation and analysis of the characteristic symptoms
associated with a particular radiopharmaceutical is another
important function of the radiopharmacy information centre.
Thus a typical diphosphonate reaction presents a maculopapular
erythematous rash which usually appears several hours after
injection (6). Most diphosphonate reactions are accompanied by

pruritis. Instances of dermographism have also been reported as well as malaise, nausea and vertigo. Reactions associated with colloids are usually mild and transient, but the few which are more severe can be categorised as vasomotor or bronchial. In the first category there have been reports of pallor, flush, pulse changes and hypotension, and in the second category bronchospasm, wheezing and dyspnoea. Reactions associated with antimony sulphide colloid tend to be more severe than those with other colloids and reports have been received of severe headache, dyspnoea and tachycardia. Reactions from albumin particulates tend to be similar symptomatically to those of colloids and include dyspnoea, chest discomfort, hypotension, nausea and vomiting.

As regards the incidence of adverse reactions reliable figures are difficult to obtain. American sources quote an incidence of between 1-6 reactions per 100,000 injections (7) and Abra et al (8) quote an incidence of 3 reactions per 100,000 doses. It is apparant from these figures that there is almost a negligible likelihood of an adverse reaction occuring. Indeed literature surveys have shown that the hazards of radiopharmaceuticals are considerably less than those of all other injectable preparations (6).

The function of the radiopharmacy information centre in investigating the causes of abnormal or unexpected biodistribution is becoming increasingly important as it has been established that many factors can alter the biokinetics of the tracer. These may be related to the way in which the radiopharmaceutical is dispensed or administered, or to factors inherent in the patient such as interaction with the patient's medication. The most difficult part in dealing with examples or abnormal biodistribution is sifting through all the factors that may be responsible for the occurrence and then pin-pointing the one applicable in a particular case.

The radiopharmacy information centre is generally well adapted to fulfill this role by virtue of the fact that data collection particularly for instances of abnormal biodistributions is

a prime function of the centre. For example, it has been reported that contamination of a radiopharmaceutical can sometimes
give rise of abnormal biodistribution. Adams et al (9) showed
that hydrochloric acid could leak out from the aluminium crimp
of a sulphur colloid syringe and excess aluminium in the vial
of radiopharmaceutical was sufficient to flocculate the colloid
particles to a size of 150 microns and consequent entrapment in
the lungs. More recently it has been observed (10) that techne-
tium-99m tin colloid could leach out impurities from the rubber
plunger of a disposable syringe to form a compound which is renal-
ly active. Again it has been observed (personal observation)
that PIPIDA can react with the lubricant oil of some disposable
syringes to form a glue-like substance. Millar (11) has shown
that low labelling yields of Tc-99m pyrophosphate may be due to
interaction between stannous ions and materials leached from a
Teflon catheter.

As regards patient-related factors which can cause altered
biodistribution of tracer nearly 400 papers have been published
(for reviews, see 12 and 13) in which the patient's medication
has been implicated in causing markedly altered biodistribution.

The alteration in biokinetics was so marked in some instances that completely erroneous diagnoses were made. Examples of
drugs cited include corticosteroids which can affect tumour vi-
sualisation, cytotoxics which can cause unusual biodistribution
of 67-Gallium and antibiotics which can produce unusual renal
images. It is evident that a systematic approach is needed for
the collation and dissemination of information on drug interference and the local or regional radiopharmacy centre is generally regarded as the most appropriate centre to fulfill this
function.

2.2 Specific pharmaceutical or pharmacokinetic properties of the radiopharmaceutical

Information on specific chemical or pharmacokinetic properties may be appropriately handled by the radiopharmacy information centre and examples of the type of information under this

category whether the blood clearance of Tc-99m DMSA in a child is similar to that of an adult: or whether there is any significant difference in the pharmacokinetics of Sodium Iodide-131 in capsular form as compared to solution. Although it is usually appropriate for radiopharmacies to handle this class of information it is likely that in some institutions clinicians themselves may be better equipped to deal with such information by virtue of their easy access to text books of clinical nuclear medicine.

2.3 Formulation, preparation, stability and quality assurance

Information pertaining to preparation, formulation, stability and quality assurance is an ever-increasing field which requires continual up-dating and monitoring. For example there has been much recent interest in the use of Tc-99m DMSA(V) for imaging of medullary cancer of the thyroid. The material is available only in Japan (14) and the question arose of the availability of a similar preparation in the United Kingdom.

After exhaustive enquiries the material was found to be unavailable. However, it was possible to modify an existing standard British kit to achieve the Japanese formula (15) and to use the preparation successfully in a sizeable number of patients. The information was then dissipated to British and European institutions via the radiopharmacy information centre. The question then arose as to a satisfactory method of chromatographically analysing the radiopharmaceutical.
Recent work by Bharij and Theobald (16) provided this information so it is evident that within a short space of time an important new product together with its method of analysis had become available to other radiopharmacies and nuclear medicine departments.

2.4 Regulatory requirements associated with the use of the radiopharmaceutical

Radiopharmaceutical kits and generators can be purchased from a variety of suppliers throughout Europe, USA and Canada, and although licensed for use in the country of manufacture they may not necessarily be licensed for use in other countries. The question then arises as to whether the material should be used at all; whether alternative products should be sought, or whether the material is regarded as exempt from full licensing regulations according to the Medicines Act 1968. The radiopharmacy information centre has a vital role to fulfil in interpreting these questions and arguably the most important task is to ascertain the legal status of a particular radiopharmaceutical at a given time. The legal status of radiopharmaceuticals can be conveniently categorised as shown in Table 1, but it is emphasised that in a number of countries, e.g. Finland, Italy, Luxembourg and Portugal special licensing regulations for radiopharmaceuticals are not in operation and the comments above do not apply.

Table 1. legal status of radiopharmaceuticals

Names of products which are licensed in country of use

Names of products which have had licence applications submitted

Names of products which have licences in the process of preparation

Names of products which are not the subject of licences

Names of products which have been refused a licence

Names of products which are not licensed and for which there is no alternative

---

Other regulatory functions of the radiopharmacy information centre will sometimes include dealing with matters such as: the authorisation of nuclear medicine personnel to administer radioactive substances. In the United Kingdom the Regional Health Authority is generally responsible for certifying that a particular clinician is licensed to administer radiopharmaceutical injections. It is possible however, that in some institutions the radiopharmacist will assume this function.

2.5 Information on paediatric dosage

Information on paediatric dosage is generally handled within the radiopharmacy information centre and requests are associated with the need to obtain a desired diagnostic effect with the absolute minimal radiation dose to the patient. During 1960-1975 paediatric dosage was generally based on a simple weight proportion as compared with that of an adult. In 1976 however, the FDA conducted a survey of paediatric dosages and concluded that those based on adult body weight were too low. The liver of an infant is larger compared with its total body weight than that of an adult, and the correct dose should therefore be based on organ ratios rather than total weight ratios. A number of methods for determination of paediatric dosages have been proposed (17) and it is usual for the radiopharmacist in consultation with the clinician to decide on an appropriate method of calculation.

2.6 New Techniques in radiopharmacy

As with all medical sciences techniques and applications are changing continually, and for the radiopharmacy information centre to function effectively continual updating of information on new developments is essential. There has been an almost explosive increase in the use of radioactive aerosols (18) and labelled blood products (19). The most recently published techniques for technetium labelled leucocytes (20, 21) appear promising and it is likely that during the next few years much information will be published on these new techniques.

Exciting developments in the field of immunoscintigraphy (22) will add greatly to the mass of information that can be expected to be handled by information radiopharmacists. As regards positron emitters information input/output has not yet been clearly defined but it has been predicted that the global increase in the number of cyclotron units will greatly increase levels of information to be dealt with by the radiopharmacist.

3. MONITORING OF PRODUCT LITERATURE

Monitoring of product literature is a necessary function of

the radiopharmacy information centre to acquire information on dispensing techniques, recommended dosages, and possible adverse reactions. Knowledge of different manufacturers's dispensing techniques is of great significance because a technique which is for one brand of material will not necessarily be appropriate for another. For example, techniques to reconstitute albumin particulates vary. Some manufacturers will suggest ultrasonication or shaking whereas others will recommend simple mixing. It is known that deviation from the recommended technique can alter the particle size and a consequent alteration in biodistribution patterns.

Occasionally errors on product literature are noticed. A recent check through the literature for a brand of DTPA revealed that the manufacturer had claimed that there was no known adverse reaction to the material (personal observation). It is known from the latest survey on adverse reactions that the converse is true (5). Monitoring of manufacturers' vial labels by the radiopharmacist can sometimes lead to important additional information and this is exemplified by an instance where the manufacturer labelled the total activity of material in the vial but had omitted the actual volume. Representations by a number of radiopharmacists led to the omission being corrected.

4. MONITORING OF DEFECTS IN PRODUCT OR PACKAGING

Radiopharmaceuticals, as with therapeutic drugs are characterised by standards of integrity and purity and when these standards deviate from accepted specifications the product may be regarded as defective. The radiopharmacy information centre either local or national has an important role to fulfil in the collation and dissemination of information on such defects and the data obtained is relevant to both manufacturer and user. For the manufacturer the reporting of product defects acts as a post-market surveillance system and focusses attention on deviations from expected standards. For the clinician and pharmacist defective product reporting is neccessary to alert them to the fact that occasionally radiopharmaceuticals do not perform as expected and in the event of this occuring alternative products should be sought.

Examples of information on drug defects which had had impor- tant implications for nuclear medicine are afforded by the results of a recent United Kingdom survey (23).

Table 2. Reported defects in the UK, 1972-1984 (Sampson & Hessle- wood, 1986)

Free pertechnetate	153
Excessive lung uptake on liver scint.	80
Elution failure	20
Faulty elution vials	19
Needle problems	16
Excessive liver uptake on lung scint.	15
Faulty packaging	13
Leakage of vials	12
Increased background levels	12
Unusual levels of Tc-99m	11
Others	36
	387

From the results shown in Table 2, it can be seen that out of a total of 387 defective product reports during the period 1972-1984, 153 referred to products which were found to have excess levels of free pertechnetate after reconstitution. These facts were brought to the attention of the manufacturer and sub- sequent re-formulation of the offending product resulted in a dramatic decrease in the number of adverse reports. As regards the many reports received of excessive lung uptake with liver material, again the offending product was traced to a particu- lar manufacturer and re-formulation produced a greatly improved product.

The function of the radiopharmacy information centre acting as a post-market surveillance unit is furter illustrated by the results of the latest survey on generator malfunctions (Hesslewood, 1987, unpublished). As shown in Table 3, out of a total of 116 reports 82 referred to the products of one manufacturer and 34 reports to the other two manufacturers. Again representations to the manufacturer have produced improvements to the product.

Table 3. Generator defects, UK 1985/1986
          (Hesslewood, 1987 unpublished)

Generator faults (elution problems or volume discrepancies)	
	GENERATOR A 82
	GENERATOR B 32
	GENERATOR C 2
	116

---

5. DATA COLLECTION

The logical goal of the radiopharmacy information centre staff might be to set up a searchable on-line database that is specific for radiopharmacy or nuclear medicine. The feasibility of developing such a database depends largely on the size and workload of the staff involved and the number of outside reviewers that could contribute to the indexing of information contained in the database.

In the United Kingdom such a unit has recently been installed (Bristol General Hospital, Directors Mrs. A.M. Palmer) and at present the unit deals mainly with information on abnormal biodistribution as a result of drug interference. The Bristol scheme acts as a local rather than a national system and it is to be hoped that the system will become more nationally and the literature reference is inserted into the database file and retrieval of information on possible drug/ radiopharmaceutical effects is easily obtained.

At present databases specific to radiopharmacy or nuclear medicine have not yet been developed. However, MEDLINE (which indexes thirty journals pertaining to nuclear medicine) has been used with sucess in the United Kingdom, Europe, and the USA. Collection of data on adverse reactions, defective products, and abnormal biodistributions is generally accomplished throughout Europe and the USA by means of official reporting systems. In the United Kingdom the reporting system (Table 4) is required to submit details of the patient, the diagnostic

Table 4. Adverse Reaction Reporting Scheme, United Kingdom

CONFIDENTIAL
Results will not be made known to any person without the express permission of the person submitting this report but are 'banked' with the European Reporting Scheme, and the general DHSS Adverse Report Scheme.

REPORT OF AN ADVERSE REACTION ATTRIBUTED TO A RADIOPHARMACEUTICAL

1. Patient .... Initials .... Hospital No. ....
    Age ....   Sex ....
    Date of Test ....   Nature of Test ....
    Clinical Diagnosis ....

2. Radiopharmaceutical: Radionuclide .... Chemical Form ....
    Brief details of materials, source, method of preparation & storage - refs.if any
    ....
    ....
    ....
    Has a commerçial manufacturer, if involved, been informed? YES / NO

3. Nature of Reaction: Any clinical observations and treatment, if required ......
    ....
    ....
    ....
    Has the patient received this or a related radiopharmaceutical before?
    ....

4. Approximate number of times this preparation has been used uneventfully.
    ....
    Other drugs etc. currently being given: ....
    ....

5. Any other comments ....
    .... continue overleaf.

Signed ....   Name ....
Address ....

Return to: The Medical Assessor, Radiopharmaceutical Adverse Reaction Reports,
British Institute of Radiology, 36 Portland Place, London W1N 3DG marked CONFIDENTIAL

test performed, and the number of times the preparation has been used "uneventfully". This last detail is particularly relevant to ascertain the approximate incidence of reactions in a given number of uneventful injections. The completed questionnaire is then sent to the Medical Assessor British Institute of Radiology, then to the Department of Health and Social Security. Details are also sent to the European Reporting Scheme. Instances of abnormal biodistribution and defective products are treated separately and reports from regional radiopharmacy specialists are collated by a central unit (Regional Radiopharmacy, Birmingham, Director, Dr. S. Hesslewood) for onward transmission to the European Scheme.

The European Reporting Scheme is more exhaustive (Table 5) and includes details of any defect in packaging or contents. It is also required to categorise the probability that the adverse reaction is in fact due to the radiopharmaceutical. It is well known that a casual relationsip is sometimes difficult to establish, and the requirement to assess the probablity as "low", "medium", or "high" is useful so that a possible cause/effect relationship be evaluated statistically. The completed report is sent via national delegates to the European Joint Committee on Radiopharmaceuticals in Denmark.

Table 5. European Reporting Scheme

JOINT COMMITTEE ON RADIOPHARMACEUTICALS

EUROPEAN NUCLEAR MEDICINE SOCIETY   SOCIETY OF NUCLEAR MEDICINE – EUROPE

ADVERSE REACTION DRUG DEFECT REPORTING SYSTEM	SEND TO	National delegate or direct to addr	European Joint Committee on Radiopharmaceuticals THE ISOTOPE-PHARMACY 378 Frederikssundsvej, DK-2700 Brønshøj. Denmark

Radiopharmaceutical (name-code)	Manufacturer	Lot no

* If relevant: Radionuclide generator (code)	Manufacturer	Lot.no

Key index – Please mark | Date of Incident.

☐ ADVERSE REACTION:
   Type

Detailed description: (see also questions in the text)

☐ Allergic
☐ Pyrogenic
☐ Drug effect
☐ Other:

   Reaction
☐ Moderate
☐ Severe
☐ Fatal

   Probability of connection to
   R.Ph. Administration.
☐ Low
☐ Medium
☐ High

☐ RADIOPHARMACEUTICAL DEFECT:
☐ Transport damage
☐ Label
☐ Package insert
☐ Appearance
☐ Rad.surface contamination
☐ Radioactive concentration
☐ Total radioactivity
☐ Radiochemical purity
☐ Radionuclidic purity
☐ pH
☐ Elution efficiency
☐ Particulate contamination
☐ Biodistribution
☐ Sterility
☐ Pyrogens
☐ Other

Please continue if needed

Report sent by:

Name.
Occupation:
Institution:
Address.

Telephone

Date: Signature:

The recently revised American Reporting Scheme consists of two separate report forms (Tables 6, 7). The first of these is

Table 6. Defective Product Reporting Scheme, The United States Scheme

---

Approved OMB No. 0910-0012 Expiration date February 29, 1988

	DO NOT USE THIS SPACE
Drug Product Problem Reporting Program	DATE RECEIVED
	REFERENCE NO

NOTE: IF PROBLEM/DEFECT INVOLVES A RADIOPHARMACEUTICAL OR "COLD KIT," FURNISH THE ADDITIONAL INFORMATION AS INDICATED IN SHADED AREAS BELOW

1 PRODUCT NAME, DOSAGE FORM, STRENGTH, NDC NUMBER
(FOR RADIOPHARMACEUTICALS, ALSO INCLUDE RADIOACTIVITY CONCENTRATION AND ASSAY TIME)

2 LOT NUMBER(s) AND EXPIRATION DATE(s)	**RADIONUCLIDE**	**"COLD KIT"**
LOT NUMBER	LOT NUMBER	LOT NUMBER
	CALIBRATION DATE	EXPIRATION DATE
EXPIRATION DATE	EXPIRATION DATE	
	(ALSO INDICATE MANUFACTURER(S) IN 3. BELOW)	

3 NAME AND ADDRESS OF THE MANUFACTURER, PACKAGER AND OR DISTRIBUTOR ON THE LABEL

4 REPORTER'S NAME *(Please print or type)*

5 PRACTICE LOCATION
   a Name, Address and Zip Code

   b Telephone *(include Area Code)*

6 PROBLEMS NOTED OR SUSPECTED *(If more space is needed, please attach separate page)*

NOTE This is a voluntary reporting program authorized under Chapter V of the Federal Food Drug, and Cosmetic Act and your identity will be provided to the Food and Drug Administration You have the option of further restricting, or permitting the disclosure of your identity	PLEASE INDICATE	☐ NO OTHER DISCLOSURE ☐ DISCLOSURE TO MANUFACTURER OR DISTRIBUTOR ONLY ☐ DISCLOSURE TO MANUFACTURER OR DISTRIBUTOR AND TO OTHER PERSONS WHO REQUEST A COPY OF THE REPORT ☐ **DISCLOSURE TO THE SOCIETY OF NUCLEAR MEDICINE**
SIGNATURE OF REPORTER		DATE
RETURN TO	Project Director DRUG PRODUCT PROBLEM REPORTING PROGRAM c/o United States Pharmacopeial Convention Inc 12601 Twinbrook Parkway Rockville, Maryland 20852 OR	CALL TOLL FREE ANYTIME **800-638-6725*** IN THE CONTINENTAL UNITED STATES *In Maryland, call collect (301) 881-0256 **Monday through Friday**

---

known as the "DPPR" form and is used to report problems of quality of radiopharmaceuticals to the Drugs Product Problem Reporting Programme. The DPPR Programme is sponsored by the Society of Nuclear Medicine, the Food and Drugs Administration and the United States Pharmacopeial Convention, and a number of other pharmaceutically orientated organisations. Examples of problems will include labelling errors, container problem, foreign matter and unexpected biodistribution. An interesting

Table 7. Adverse Reaction Reporting Scheme, The United States Scheme

DEPARTMENT OF HEALTH AND HUMAN SERVICES PUBLIC HEALTH SERVICE FOOD AND DRUG ADMINISTRATION (HFN-730) ROCKVILLE, MD 20857 **ADVERSE REACTION REPORT** (Drugs and Biologics)	Form Approved OMB No 0910-0230
	FDA CONTROL NO
	ACCESSION NO

I. REACTION INFORMATION

1 PATIENT ID/INITIALS (In Confidence)	2 AGE YRS	3 SEX	4-6 REACTION ONSET			B-12 CHECK ALL APPROPRIATE:
			MO	DA	YR	

7 DESCRIBE REACTION(S)

☐ PATIENT DIED

☐ REACTION TREATED WITH Rx DRUG

☐ RESULTED IN, OR PROLONGED, INPATIENT HOSPITALIZATION

☐ RESULTED IN PERMANENT DISABILITY

13 RELEVANT TESTS/LABORATORY DATA

☐ NONE OF THE ABOVE

II. SUSPECT DRUG(S) INFORMATION

14 SUSPECT DRUG(S) (Give manufacturer and lot no for vaccines/biologics)

20 DID REACTION ABATE AFTER STOPPING DRUG?

15. DAILY DOSE	16 ROUTE OF ADMINISTRATION

☐ YES   ☐ NO   ☐ NA

17 INDICATION(S) FOR USE

21 DID REACTION REAPPEAR AFTER REINTRODUCTION?

18 DATES OF ADMINISTRATION (From/To)	19 DURATION OF ADMINISTRATION

☐ YES   ☐ NO   ☐ NA

III. CONCOMITANT DRUGS AND HISTORY

22 CONCOMITANT DRUGS AND DATES OF ADMINISTRATION (Exclude those used to treat reaction)

23 OTHER RELEVANT HISTORY (e g diagnoses, allergies, pregnancy with LMP, etc)

IV. ONLY FOR REPORTS SUBMITTED BY MANUFACTURER	V. INITIAL REPORTER (In confidence)
24 NAME AND ADDRESS OF MANUFACTURER (Include Zip Code)	26 -26a NAME AND ADDRESS OF REPORTER (Include Zip Code)

24a IND/NDA NO FOR SUSPECT DRUG	24b MFR CONTROL NO	26b TELEPHONE NO (Include area code)

24c DATE RECEIVED BY MANUFACTURER	24d REPORT SOURCE (Check all that apply) ☐ FOREIGN ☐ STUDY ☐ LITERATURE ☐ HEALTH PROFESSIONAL ☐ CONSUMER	26c HAVE YOU ALSO REPORTED THIS REACTION TO THE MANUFACTURER? ☐ YES ☐ NO	
25 '5 DAY REPORT? ☐ YES ☐ NO	25a REPORT TYPE ☐ INITIAL ☐ FOLLOWUP	26d ARE YOU A HEALTH PROFESSIONAL? ☐ YES ☐ NO	Submission of a report does not necessarily constitute an admission that the drug caused the adverse reaction

NOTE. Required of manufacturers by 21 CFR 314 80

difference in the new scheme is that the reporter has a choice of disclosure of his identity. Identity will be provided to the Food and Drugs Administration but the reporter can elect to have no other disclosure.

The Adverse Reaction Report is required to submit details concomitant drug therapy, relevant history (e.g. allergies, pregnancy, previous diagnoses) and full details of the duration of administration and route of administration. The completed form is sent directly to the FDA.

It is generally agreed that one of the problems associated with assessing the incidence and number of adverse reactions and abnormal biodistributions is that unusual occurrences are not always reported. It has been estimated (24) that less than 10% of adverse reactions ever get to be reported. It is thought by many that the reporting of adverse reactions and abnormal biodistributions is of no real significance in nuclear medicine but it is only by thorough and careful monitoring that a true picture can be obtained of such instances.

6. CONCLUSION

In conclusion it can be seen that the radiopharmacy information centre is an integral part of the nuclear medicine facility. It has been estimated (25) that 6,000 to 7,000 scientific articles are written daily; that the overall increase in scientific information is 13% per year; and that the base of information doubles every 5.5 years.

If these figures are extrapolated to radiopharmacy information it is evident that the next decade will bring a huge increase in information likely to be handled by the radiopharmacist. The use of new radiodiagnostic techniques, new generator systems and new radiolabelling techniques will enhance the importance of the radiopharmacy information centre as part of the nuclear medicine unit. For the centre to work efficiently, rigorous reporting of unusual occurences is essential.

REFERENCES
1.   Morrow, N C The community pnarmacist's role in drug information. Pharm J 1982; 229:719.

2.   Smith J. Drug information comes of age. Br J Pharm Pract 1985; 7: 193.
3.   Spencer M G. Community pharmacy usage of the drug information centre. Br J Pharm Pract 1986; 8: 186.
4.   Williams E S. Adverse reactions to radiopharmaceuticals; a preliminary survey in the United Kingdom. Br J Radiol 1974; 47: 54.
5.   Keeling D H, Sampson C B. Adverse reactions to radiopharmaceuticals: incidence, reporting, symptoms, treatment. Proceedings of European Nuclear Medicine Congress 1986, Goslar.
6.   Sampson C B, Keeling D H. Adverse reactions to radiopharmaceuticals: a follow-up survey in the United Kingdom. Annual Scientific Meeting, British Nuclear Medicine Society, London, 1982.
7.   Cordova M A, Rhodes B A et al. Adverse reactions to radiopharmaceuticals: J Nucl Med 1982; 23: 550.
8.   Abra R M., Bell N D S. et al. A survey of radiopharmaceuticals in the United Kingdom Hospitals. J of Clin Hosp Pharm 1980; 5: 11.
9.   Adams E N, Chandler M P et al. Sulfur colloid flocculation due to acid leached aluminium. J Nucl Med 1972; 13: 707.
10.   Slater D. & Anderson M. Syringe extractibles: effects of radiopharmaceuticals. Lancet 1983; ii: 1431.
11.   Millar A M, Wathen C G et al. Failure in labelling of red blood cells with Tc-99m: interactions between intravenous cannulae and stannous pyrophosphate. Eur J Nucl Med 1983; 8: 502.
12.   Hladik W B, Nigg K K et al. Drug induced changes in the biologic distribution of radiopharmaceuticals. Semin Nucl Med 1982; 2: 184.
13.   Sampson C B. Altered biodistribution of radiopharmaceuticals as a result of pharmocological or chemical interaction. In "Radiopharmacy and Radiopharmaceuticals", ed. A.E. Theobald; Taylor & Francis, London and Philadelphia 1985.
14.   Ohta H, Yamamoto K et al. A new imaging agent for medullary carcinoma of the thyroid. J Nucl Med 1983; 25: 323.
15.   Sampson C B. Preparation of Tc-99m(V)DMSA. Nucl Med Commun 1987; 8: 184.
16.   Bharij A K & Theobald A E. Preparation and analysis of complexes of Tc-99m DMSA and Tc-99m DMSA(V) Nucl Med Commun 1987; 8: 281 (abstract).
17.   Sampson C B. A survey of paediatric radiopharmaceuticals in America. Br J Pharm Pract 1980; 1: 17.
18.   Short M D. Radiopharmaceuticals for lung ventilatation studies. In "Radiopharmacy and Radiopharmaceuticals", ed. A.E. Theobald; Taylor & Francis, London and Philadelphia, 1985.
19.   Danpure H J. Cell labelling with In-111 complexes. In "Radiopharmacy and Radiopharmaceuticals", ed. A.E. Theobald; Taylor & Francis, London and Philadelphia, 1985.
20.   Danpure H J, Osman et al. In-vitro studies to develop a clinical protocol for radiolabelling mixed leucocytes with Tc-99m HMPAO Nucl Med Commun 1987; 8: 280, (abstract).

362

21. Sampson C B. & Solanki C. Tc-99m labelled leucocytes using diethyldithiocarbamate (DDC) and DDC/DTPA: a preliminary study. Nucl Med Commun 1987; 8: 280.
22. Mather S J. Immunoscintigraphy. In "Radiopharmacy and Radiopharmaceuticals", ed. A.E. Theobald; Taylor & Francis, London and Philadelphia, 1985.
23. Sampson C B. & Hesslewood S R. Radiopharmacy information and reporting systems: an overview. In "Progress in Radiopharmacy", eds. P H. Cox, S. J. Mather, C B. Sampson, C R. Lazarus: Martinus Nijhoff, Netherlands 1986.
24. Keeling D H. Sampson C B. Adverse reactions to radiopharmaceuticals. United Kingdom 1977-1983. Br J radiol 1984; 57: 1091.
25. Hladik W B, Gregorio N et al. Radiopharmaceutical Information and Consultation Services. In "Essentials of Nuclear Medicine Science" eds. W.B. Hladik, G. B. Saha, and others. Williams and Wilkins, Baltimore, London, 1987.

27. CURRENT TRENDS IN THE TRAINING AND EDUCATION OF PHARMACISTS IN RADIOPHARMACY

P.H. COX and F.A. GARRITSEN

1. INTRODUCTION

At the previous European Symposium on Radiopharmaceuticals, held in Cambridge in 1985, Lazarus reviewed the findings of an independent survey on the subject of the training of radiopharmacists (1). Despite the limited response to the survey it was abundantly evident that the degree of attention paid to radiopharmacy was extremely variable from country to country. At the time the only country offering a structured university education leading to a recognised degree in nuclear pharmacy was the United States.

Several countries had Master of Science in which the radiopharmaceutical sciences can be offered as one of the subjects for combined study. Variable amounts of time were expended on undergraduate and postgraduate education and in the Netherlands provision was made for registration by the Netherlands Society of Nuclear Medicine after four years of practical experience and aquisition of a recognised diploma in radiation protection.

The prime source of expertise in Europe was, and still is, practical experience supplemented by short postgraduate courses on a base, in many cases, of undergraduate education in radiochemistry and the nuclear sciences.

The status quo has not changed significantly in the intervening two years since the survey.

The international organisations such as IAEA and WHO are expressing a continued interest in the establishment of radiopharmacy in developing countries. In the case of the former this has led to the further development of undergraduate and postgraduate education in South America and the establishment of a regional postgraduate training course which will soon be held at the University of Montevideo for the second time.

In Western Europe there have been a number of developments which could affect the practice of radiopharmacy whilst techno- logical advances have also served to compound the problems. It is the authors opinion that the time is now opportune for the Pharmaceutical Profession to take steps to provide standards for a co-ordinated and uniform level of training for Radiophar- macists in Europe and we propose to examine the possibilities within a Western European context.

2. NEW LEGISLATIVE ASPECTS.

There have been several developments within the European Economic Community which are relevant to the practice of radio- pharmacy in member countries. The foremost, which is of funda- mental importance, is the EEC directive regulating the mutual recognition of pharmaceutical training (2). This directive is now effective and has to be implemented in member states by october 1987. The same regulation also establishes the right of free movement of Pharmacists within the community to practise their profession. Clearly once this is fully established it will be desirable to have recognised standards for specialist professional functions such as radiopharmacy which are appli- cable to the circumstances extant in each member country.

The second is the EEC directive with respect to Product lia- bility (3) which also applies to pharmaceuticals. Within the context of this directive a hospital pharmacist who prepares a medicinal preparation to prescription order and in particular in multidose form may be classified as a producer and as such is liable for the quality and efficacy of the product. This would be particularly relevant to radiopharmacies supplying other centres or who manufacture their own labelling kits.

The implications of this directive for radiopharmacy need to be clarified but it remains doubtful as to whether the radiopharmacist is able to exercise adequate control over the quality and performance of many radiopharmaceuticals such as labelled immunological or blood products.

3. TECHNOLOGICAL DEVELOPMENTS INFLUENCING TRAINING REQUIREMENTS.

The ideal radiopharmaceutical will provide an optimal accumulation in the target organ with a rapid clearance from the body to yield maximum diagnostic information with a minimal radiation dose to the patient. The carrier molecule should preferably be a compound with a known metabolism in order to provide information about organ function.

In the past the main groups of radionuclides available were metallic elements which could only be bound to a limited number of carrier molecules relatively few of which were actively metabolised or organ specific. The development of positron emmission tomography has opened the way to the use of ultra short lived radionuclides such as C-11 and N-13 to label true metabolites such as glucose and amino acids.

The preparation and evaluation of these compounds requires a good knowledge of organic chemistry and biochemistry. The short life of the label requires the use of automated preparation methods and direct administration to the patient which may preclude quality control after manufacture and prior to administration. (4). This is also true of the generator systems producing ultra short lived nuclides for organ blood flow studies. To guarantee quality an intimate knowledge of generator technology is required.

In the single photon field the use of antibodies and labelled blood cells require special knowledge not normally included in the pharmaceutical curriculum. (5).

The steadily increasing emphasis on organ function evaluation makes it imperative that extraneous factors which may influence the biodistribution of a radiopharmaceutical should be well documented, particularly with respect to the effects of drugs and other forms of therapies whereby there would appear to be an important contribution to be made by the pharmacist. (6).

4. THE BASIC REQUIREMENTS FOR A EUROPEAN RADIOPHARMACY TRAINING PROGRAMME

The concept of a standardised training and registration programme for radiopharmacy is attractive but would be difficult to achieve in practice because of the differences in organisation and legislation at the national level. Within the EEC, bearing in mind the Pharmacy directive, a basic standard level of technical and professional knowledge would be of direct practical value.

When considering the depth of knowledge required on individual topics it should be acknowledged that many of the procedures utilised to evaluate radiopharmaceuticals, which the pharmacist will require to evaluate the quality and efficacy of a radiopharmaceutical, will be carried out by graduates from other disciplines. An example of this are tests of cell viability or of immunobinding capacity. With respect to such procedures the pharmacist should have and adequate level of knowledge to evaluate the data with respect to determining the implications for the quality and performance of the labelled compound.

It is a universal requirement that the preparation of radiopharmaceuticals should be carried out by a suitably qualified pharmacist.
It is also the case that the preparation must be carried out under the direct supervision of a licensed radiation protection officer. In the optimal situation the pharmacist should also be the radiation safety expert.

The first requirement for entry to a European training scheme would therefore be that the candidate should be a registered pharmacist with a recognised diploma in radioprotection from the country of origin.

The majority of radiopharmacists are only part time and combine their work with more traditional pharmaceutical pursuits.

In order to benefit from a postgraduate training scheme the candidate should be required to demonstrate an adequate level of practical experience.

This could be achived by requiring the candidate to produce a signed statement from their employer countersigned by the national nuclear medical or pharmaceutical society confirming that they have, for instance, two years of practical experience.

On this basis a course on the theory and practice of radiopharmacy would be undertaken, at an approved centre, which would last +/- 30 days at the end of which practical and theoretical evaluation of the candidates knowledge would be made and certificate of competence in radiopharmacy would be issued to succesful candidates.

The training course would consist of theoretical and practical instruction in all aspects of radiopharmacy including:
- Radiation safety and materials handling
- Planning and layout of a radiopharmacy
- Administration
- Principles of tracer techniques
- Clinical nuclear medicine
- Radiochemistry
- Analytical quality control
- Design of animal experiments and alternative techniques
- Biodistribution
- Effects of drugs and therapy on biodistribution
- Adverse reactions
- Dispensing methods

In addition to the laboratory studies part of the course would be spent in a clinical nuclear medical department.

In view of the probable limited numbers of candidates from individual European countries it would probably be of practical value to hold the course at one central point. With this in mind the authors are preparing a proposal to hold a pilot course at the Reactor Centre of the University of Delft and The Rotterdam Radiotherapeutic Institute in the Netherlands. The

University Reactor Centre Delft has a wide experience in organising courses of this nature and has previously collaborated with the Radiotherapeutic Institute to organise short Radiopharmacy Courses and to carry out collaborative scientific projects.

A proposal will be submitted for discussion and approval by the European Joint Committee on Radiopharmaceuticals at their next meeting in Budapest after which, hopefully a definitive proposal can be made to the European Association of Nuclear Medicine.

References
1. Lazarus C. Training and education of radiopharmacists for radiopharmacy. In: Progress in Radiopharmacy. Editors P.H. Cox, S.J. Mather, C.B. Sampson and C.R. Lazarus. Marinus Nijhoff Dordrecht. 1986: 300-311.
2 EEC Training Directive 85/432/EEC
3. Product Liability and the Pharmacist. Pharm J 1986; 237: 744-745.
4. Kilbourne M.R. et al. Quality assurance of short life radiopharmaceuticals. In: Quality assurance of pharmaceuticals manufactured in the hospital. Editors: A. Warbick Cerone and L.G. Johnston. Pergamon Oxford 1984; 243-250.
5. Immunoscintigraphy Editors: K. Britton and L. Donato. Gordon and Breach London. 1985.
6. The Effects of Drugs and Therapy on the Biodistribution of Radiopharmaceuticals. In: Radiopharmacy and Radiopharmacology Yearbook 3 Editor: P.H. Cox Gordon and Breach London. In Preparation.

SUBJECT INDEX